Living Beauty

Feel Great, Look Fabulous & Live Well

Living Beauty

Feel Great, Look Fabulous & Live Well

LISA PETTY

Fitzhenry & Whiteside

Fitzhenry and Whiteside Limited
195 Allstate Parkway
Markham, Ontario L3R 4T8

In the United States:
311 Washington Street,
Brighton, Massachusetts 02135

www.fitzhenry.ca   godwit@fitzhenry.ca

Fitzhenry & Whiteside acknowledges with thanks the Canada Council for the Arts, and the Ontario Arts Council for their support of our publishing program. We acknowledge the financial support of the Government of Canada through the Book Publishing Industry Development Program (BPIDP) for our publishing activities.

Library and Archives Canada Cataloguing in Publication
Petty, Lisa
    Living beauty: feel great, look fabulous & live well / Lisa Petty.
ISBN 1-55041-870-X
    1. Health. I. Title.
RA776.P427 2005   613   C2005-900814-8

United States Cataloging-in-Publication Data
Petty, Lisa.
    Living beauty: feel great, look fabulous & live well / Lisa Petty.
[200] p. : ill. ; cm.
Summary: An informative look at how our appearance is key to monitoring our health and well-being, along with advice on how to achieve a healthy appearance and body through the foods we eat.
ISBN 1-55041-870-X (pbk.)
1. Beauty, Personal. 2. Health behavior. 3. Women – Health and hygiene. 4. Nutrition. I. Title.
646.7/042 22   RA778.P488 2005

The two lines that appear as an epigraph on page 251, are from *You Own the Power*, by Rosemary Altea. Copyright © 2000 by Rosemary Altea. Reprinted by permission of HarperCollins Publishers.
Interior design: Darrell McCalla
Cover design: Karen Petherick, Intuitive Design International Ltd.
Cover photograph: © FirstLight Images
Inset author photograph: Kenneth Schiff, New York, New York
Printed in Canada

1 3 5 7 9 10 8 6 4 2

Contents

CHAPTER FOUR

Living Beauty Essentials at a Glance   67

PART II   **Beauty Prescriptions**

CHAPTER FIVE

Facing *Candida* in the Mirror   71

CHAPTER SIX

Hormones and Your Healthy Glow   91

CHAPTER SEVEN

All About Skin

CHAPTER EIGHT

Your Skin Doesn't Stop at Your Neck

CHAPTER NINE

The Story of Hair

CHAPTER TEN

The Nail File

Foreword

Too often in life our choices are based on extremes: things are good or bad, right or wrong, fashionable or out of style. Following the same line of thinking, many people think that taking a healthy approach to life ultimately means that they have to give up everything that is fun, glamorous, or fashionable. But the truth is you don't have to give up looking fabulous or enjoying life to do some good for yourself.

For many of us, the problem is that we lack information. And when we can find the information, we aren't shown how to use it. Until now. In *Living Beauty*, Lisa Petty tells us in plain English how to regain control over many of our beauty concerns, from clear skin to beautiful hair to long and lovely fingernails. And all it will take is a few small changes in the way you go about your day.

Lisa doesn't talk about beauty potions, lotions, or magic ingredients that you will apply topically for a quick fix. Instead, she describes the cause of many of your beauty issues, and often the cause may surprise you. But once you've taken care of the source of the problem, you'll be happy to watch your natural beauty emerge.

You'll also learn how some of the beauty decisions you make on a daily basis might actually be doing you more harm than good. In *Living Beauty*, Lisa talks about how some ingredients in our cosmetics and beauty products are not only linked to conditions that age us, but also to serious health problems. As my mother taught me, we shouldn't put anything on our skin that we wouldn't eat.

I've been interested in the impact of chemicals on the environment since I was a teenager. That might seem out of synch to some of you who know my work as a model. It goes back to our tendency to live in extremes: many people picture an environmentalist as a hermit who lives without modern conveniences, rather than someone who also wears high heels.

But I believe that it's possible for everyone to live well while at the same time respecting our bodies and our planet. We can wear lipstick and still find ways to divert garbage from the landfill. We can have great skin now without paying for it with our health later. There is a lot of room between the extremes. Find your own balance.

Use this book as a first step in improving your beauty, naturally. You might be surprised where that step will take you!

Angela Lindvall
New York, New York 2005

Acknowledgments

I have to admit that, like millions of others, I do enjoy a televised award show like the Oscars® on occasion. Apart from watching for what everyone is wearing, I am quite interested in listening to the winners as they give their acceptance speeches. It's one time that we get a glimpse into the hearts of some of the celebrities of the day. I also have to confess to having been quite envious of those who have the opportunity to stand in such a great forum to thank the people who have helped shape their lives. Now, of course, I have the privilege of doing that too. So imagine me in a fabulous designer dress, standing at the podium, without any fear of the orchestra playing me off for acknowledging too many people.

First of all, thank you so much, Deane Parkes, for guiding me through the process of turning an idea into a book. Your generosity is an inspiration. Nancy Cheeseman, you are a mentor and a friend, and I am grateful for having you in my life. I also thank David and Elyse Chapman for helping me start this journey. To James Rouse, N.D., Dr. Bob Martin, and Lorna Vanderhaeghe, whose lead I have followed, I thank you for your example and encouragement.

I would like to thank Stewart Brown for your advice in the early stages of writing and Dr. James Meschino for your generous input. For your help in making sure I got the details right, thank you, Shelagh Jamieson and Janice Brenner of Bioriginal Food & Science Corporation. Kathryn Dean, editor extraordinaire, I am grateful for your attention to detail and for sharing my vision.

To Sonya Clarke, my sister and friend, I thank you for always being in my corner even when that might not have been a popular place to be! You remind me of my strength when I start to question it, and you are an example of unshakeable commitment to family. Bless you. To Jane Irwin, I thank you for many years of friendship, love, and support—and for a common interest in keeping our kids healthy despite their frequent protests. I'm sure they'll appreciate it one day!

I would be remiss if I did not acknowledge Susan Dean, for reading trial chapters of the book and for sharing your son with mine so I could write while they played. Thanks for the gift of time. Thank you, as well, to Laurie Lamothe, for reading, re-reading, critiquing, and debating my direction throughout the writing of this book, and as I navigate life's course. You are a good friend. Michael Jorgensen, for your constant encouragement, insight, and friendship, I am truly grateful. To Rose-Marie Swift, a fabulous make-up artist and passionate advocate for products that won't cause harm to our bodies or the planet, I am so thrilled to have you as my dear friend. Thank you so much for sharing your talents in this book. I look forward to having a front-row seat as you change the world.

I would also like to thank my grandmother Dorothy Waller, who is an amazing role model of love, patience, and living without judgment of others. Many times, Gramma, I have retraced the steps you walked in your life, and I thank you for being my guide. I love you. My love and appreciation also goes to my parents, Charles and Georgena Petty, for, in the most real sense, this book would not have been written without you! Thank you, Mom and Dad, for your strength and generosity.

And, finally, I would like to thank my children, Cassie and Cameron, for coming into my life, for being such great teachers, and for allowing me to give and receive unconditional love. It is because of you that I so value the gift of health. It is because of you that I want others to value their own health, their own lives, and the life of our planet.

I dedicate this book to mothers and fathers, who, by their example, teach their children to value their own bodies—and the world around them. *Namaste.*

Lisa Petty

For attractive lips, speak words of kindness.
For lovely eyes, seek out the good in people.
For a slim figure, share your food with the hungry.
For beautiful hair, let a child run his/her fingers through it once a day.
For poise, walk with the knowledge that you never walk alone.
People, even more than things, have to be restored, renewed, revived,
reclaimed, and redeemed; never throw out anyone.
Remember, if you ever need a helping hand, you will find one
at the end of each of your arms.
As you grow older, you will discover that you have two hands;
one for helping yourself, and the other for helping others.

Sam Levenson

In the Beginning

To get back my youth I would do anything in the world,
except take exercise, get up early, or be respectable.

—Oscar Wilde

I t was more years ago than I care to admit, but there I was, sitting in my friend's kitchen, watching her prepare a wheat-free, dairy-free lunch for her family while we sipped on caffeine-free herbal tea. I'd always considered myself a healthy eater—I tried to eat some fruit and a few vegetables every day and was never one for dessert or creamy sauces—but this woman was a fanatic! I knew that Jane was helping her husband with some of his health goals, but I had no idea what was involved. She explained food sensitivities to me, and described how much better she and her husband felt by avoiding certain foods, but this wasn't enough to convince me that her new way of living was worthwhile. I remember telling her that her new road to health looked like a one-way street that didn't allow U-turns. I didn't think I was up to the challenge. But Jane's venture was a great spectator sport, and I picked up a few tricks as I watched her from the sidelines.

Fast forward a few years to the day I learned that my infant son had been born with a heart defect. Having a bicuspid aortic valve means that Cameron has only two leaflets in his aortic heart valve, while the rest of us have three. As a result, he has a heart murmur that may or may not get worse as he ages; he might live a long and healthy life with no sign of heart trouble or he might require surgery as an adult if his valves harden. Think about how a mother bear protects her cub from a threat, and you'll have a picture of how I responded to the news about my baby's heart.

I immediately turned onto that one-way street. I started to educate myself, and the more I learned and the more I tried, the better I

3

felt. I cured myself of a decades-long battle with eczema, and I learned how to help my adolescent daughter when growing pains wake her up at night. I watched my skin clear, my nails harden, and the shine reappear in my hair. I finally even lost the ten pounds of "baby fat" that I'd held onto after my children were born. Wow, I thought, forget what health feels like—health *looks* fabulous! I realized that if other people knew that making healthy choices would make them look good, they'd be more willing to give it a try.

Think about the times you've been motivated to drop a few pounds because of an upcoming wedding or high school reunion. Was health your motivation? Don't kid yourself—it's vanity all the way. A nurse once told me about a woman she was treating who was anxious to leave the waiting room to have a cigarette. As this stylishly dressed and apparently intelligent woman was sitting with the nurse filling out forms, she made an off-hand comment about some new wrinkles she'd noticed around her mouth. When the nurse pointed out that the cigarettes were likely causing the wrinkles, the young patient decided to quit smoking—on the spot. Her blackened lungs weren't the motivator—no one could see those—but the wrinkles around her mouth made her rethink her habits. After all, they were there for the world to see.

As a nutritional consultant and health coach, my first job is to find my client's motivation. While some people come to me because they're concerned about a health issue, many clients are interested in learning a few anti-aging tricks. In fact, I haven't met anyone yet who's told me that what they really want is to look older, sicker, and more tired! Surprisingly, however, many of our habits and the choices we make each day do contribute to our aging. The condition of our skin, hair, nails, and smile broadcasts the state of our internal health and provides valuable clues as to what foods and nutrients are missing—or are excessive—in our diets. Often simple dietary changes not only improve health, but also banish pimples, strengthen nails, and put shine back into damaged tresses without anyone having to spend a dime at the cosmetics counter.

In fact, the way you look is such an important indicator of health that before the advent of our many modern diagnostic tools, doctors would look very closely at external clues to determine treatments for their patients. The exciting truth is that beauty really does come from the inside and is a direct result of how well our bodies are working. And who controls that? You do!

But you have more concerns in your quest for healthy good looks than simply learning what to do for the inside: products used on the outside of your body also have an impact on your reflection in the mirror. Unfortunately for consumers, many cosmetics companies have also figured out that you want to look your best. They ply you with products that may give you what you want in the short term, but in the long term, these items contribute to the aging process. Many skin-care products and cosmetics contain harmful chemicals that have proven links to illness and disease, including cancer.

So why, you may ask, are companies allowed to use these chemicals? Well, for one thing, most consumers don't know that their hair dye could kill them. Secondly, many people may be lulled into a false sense of security, trusting that governments will watch out for their health and safety. Unfortunately, this may not be the case. Finally, and perhaps most significantly, most of us are creatures of habit and like to use the products we know and love. Or maybe we think, "Man, I gave up booze and cigarettes for my health—leave my mascara alone!"

Trust me, I hear you. I'm not asking you to give up all the things you enjoy using. (I know I won't forsake my lipstick until I'm called to meet my Maker—and even then I might want to do a little touch-up!) What I'd like you to do is open your mind to the possibility of finding safe and effective alternatives to the dangerous products you may have been using for years. If you can achieve similar results without putting your health at risk, it's worth considering, right? As in all things, the consumer drives what manufacturers produce. If we won't buy toxic products, companies won't make toxic products. It's that simple.

I'm sure you're now feeling a bit the way I did, that day in Jane's kitchen. But the road to health doesn't have to be as scary as I thought it would be as I watched my friend prepare her lunch. For starters, the road to health is not one-way. You're allowed to take detours and enjoy the scenery. You can have that glass of wine with your dinner in a fancy restaurant and a nice slice of cake on your birthday. The key is to make small changes every day. Smoke one less cigarette. Have a glass of water instead of a fourth cup of coffee. And U-turns are definitely allowed. In fact, I encourage them. If you find that your detour took you too far off the path, and for too long, you can get back on the road anytime you want to. There is no such thing as "too late" on this highway.

This book is not about vanity; it's a book about beauty. It's about not risking your health in pursuit of it, yet it's also about improving your health to achieve it. It's a book that will help redefine beauty so the word becomes synonymous with health.

PART ONE

Living Beauty Essentials

CHAPTER ONE

A Healthy Dose of Vanity

Beauty is truth—truth, beauty—that is all Ye know on earth,
and all ye need to know.
—John Keats

As we look around at people in television, movies, fashion—and even in the grocery store—we see that society's definition of beauty seems to have changed. Individuality appears to have lost some of its appeal, and for many, the new ideal of beauty conformity comes at the hands of a plastic surgeon. That is certainly one definition of beauty, but it's not the one we'll be focusing on in this book. If, on the other hand, your goal is to become a more vibrant, youthful, and sparkling version of yourself, welcome to an exciting new approach to creating beauty.

Some people might argue that having beauty goals is superficial, but in reality, modern society has lost sight of one important truth about the way we look: our appearance speaks volumes about our health. Ignoring some of the issues that confront us daily in the mirror is, in essence, turning a blind eye to possible health concerns. You'll learn more about that in the coming pages. And knowing that our physical magnificence is a natural extension of good health frees us to pursue our beauty goals without concerns about shallow vanity. You could say that you are interested in beauty for sake of your health. On the flipside, if your wish is simply to improve the way you look, I'm all for that too.

The Whole Beauty Truth

While our pursuit of beauty through health is far from superficial, our approach to the quest for health is sometimes shallow. Consider for a moment the methods we use to treat health issues. In the West, we constantly focus on making our symptoms go away. Got a headache? Take a pill. Got a skin problem? Put cortisone cream on it. We barely scratch the surface of the problem and put little effort into investigating what caused it.

Many of us have grown up thinking that we don't have to worry about our diet and lifestyle choices because modern medicine will fix us if we break. As our waiting lists grow for diagnostic procedures and treatments for disease, however, it has become obvious that we need a new health philosophy. Our focus should change from "cure" to "prevention." Taking a painkiller for a headache is like responding to the alarm from your home's smoke detector by removing the batteries: you get rid of the immediate discomfort but you haven't addressed the source of the problem. To protect your home and family, you should also make sure that the loud, obnoxious ring of the alarm isn't warning of a hidden fire that you haven't yet noticed. To protect your body, you should investigate whether the "symptom" alarm is a warning that your health is in danger.

If you suffer from chronic headaches, instead of being on the constant lookout for the next great pain reliever, you should focus your energy on discovering what triggers the throbbing. Head pain is often a symptom of dehydration, and many of us simply don't drink enough water. Headaches are also frequently a symptom of food sensitivities— sensitivities that may not be detected through standard laboratory allergy tests. It's worth your while to find a professional who can help you isolate your headache triggers and remove the pain at its source.

The same philosophy holds true for skin conditions. Most of the time, a skin condition is not simply a skin condition. As you will discover in the pages of this book, acne, eczema, and other concerns are often symptoms of a larger issue. Problems with skin frequently indicate a dietary deficiency or nutrient absorption problem. Skin eruptions may simply be the silent alarm, letting you know that all is not right in the inner workings of your body. While medicated creams might work to make the most recent outbreak of a problem vanish, they do not address the cause of the trouble. The rash, spot, or eruption might disappear when you use your fancy creams, but make no mistake, it will be back. Just as in the case of the recurrent headache, you must also shift your focus away from treating your skin symptoms to treating the cause of the problem.

Beauty Equals Health

In addition, we must certainly not forget that our skin is attached to the rest of our bodies. The same blood that feeds the heart and brain nourishes the skin. The same systems and cells that protect our bodies from bacteria, viruses, and disease are found in our liver, lungs, and, yes, skin. The same chocolate or asparagus or wheat that triggers a headache or tummy trouble travels through the digestive system to the bloodstream and eventually to our skin cells. Our skin cells are also washed with a special cleaning solution called lymph. If an infection causes a problem in the glands that produce lymph or if the system designed to move the lymph around our bodies is sluggish, the evidence shows up in the mirror.

The reason is simple. Just as nature operates according to the harsh reality of "survival of the fittest," there is a similar pecking order in our bodies. I'm sure you will agree with me that you will survive a pimple or a wrinkle, but addressing problems with organs like your heart and brain is quite important if you wish to see another day. Your body thinks so too, and it makes sure your essential organs are first in line at mealtime. The skin, while still very important to your survival, gets the leftovers. If there aren't enough nutrients left for the skin, it will weaken. Weakened skin starts to sag, loses its healthy glow, and heals more slowly from injury. If those beauty issues seem familiar, your body may be prompting you to adjust your diet.

Your outer appearance is also ignored in the case of an emergency in one of your vital organs, because all energy is diverted to managing the crisis. That's why doctors want to know when your cuts or wounds take a long time to heal. Slow wound healing is a strong indication that your body is fighting an internal condition that is potentially life threatening, such as cancer or diabetes. Remember that the body parts you can see are not the only body parts you have.

Pay attention to the signals: in order to have healthy hair, you need to have healthy hormone function. Hormones are chemical messengers that help coordinate and control cells in the body. They play a role in everything from development and reproduction to adjusting the chemistry of the blood. When hormones are out of balance due to poor diet, excessive stress, or a body that is overburdened with toxins, visible symptoms start to appear.

For great skin, your immune system has to be humming and your digestive system firing on all burners. Your immune system is in charge of preventing you from becoming sick, and it heals you when you do fall ill. A tired immune system is associated with aging and disease. Strong and lovely fingernails tell you that you are eating the right diet. Problems with your nails might indicate that you are deficient in certain nutrients or are having difficulties with digestion. Most people don't give their digestive processes a second thought. But consider this: if your body's fuel-burning system is out of whack, how are you going to benefit fully from the foods you eat? The answer is that you won't, and deficiencies will make themselves known in noticeable ways. If you have any of these beauty issues, it's time to do a little inner-body investigation.

The challenge for most people is that they don't know what they're looking for, because they don't know how body systems are supposed to work. I'll compare this dilemma with the relationship I have with my computer. Because I am a writer, I depend on have a working machine. It's not a good day for me when my computer crashes or stalls or won't cooperate in some other way. A wise self-employed person who works without the luxury of a "technical department" to fix computer woes would have a reasonable understanding of how computers operate in order to prevent many of the little problems that could potentially put a kink in his or her day. I am not that wise person.

Although I am very familiar with my computer's power switch, that is where my knowledge of computer technology ends. As a result, every minor computer glitch sends me into a tailspin. I call in favors, pester the technical people at the company that sold me my machine, and usually start checking my bank account to see how much money I have to fix the problem. It doesn't have to be that way, of course. I could read a book or take a course to learn about the inner workings of my computer. I don't need to know how to build a machine, but if I understood what all the parts did and what they needed from me as preventive maintenance, I wouldn't have as many catastrophes.

As with me and my computer, you might want a few instructions to maintain and enhance your health and beauty. And you don't have to wade through a bunch of biology and anatomy lessons. In the chapters that follow, I will explain how some of your important body systems work in words that are as easy to understand as the ones you're reading now. Then, after you've acquired a basic understanding of your inner workings, your mirror will become your partner in health prevention. Many clues about potential health problems are as plain as the skin on the nose of your face or the quality of your hair or the puffiness around your eyes. Always remember that the parts of the body we can see are attached to the parts of the body we can't see. Our outward appearance provides our only glimpse into the inside of our bodies. Relegating appearance to the realm of the superficial or vain might actually do your health a disservice. From a whole beauty perspective, looks matter.

Enduring Gratification

No doubt about it, people are in a rush. As kids, we're in a rush to grow up. As adults, we rush to work, to meet deadlines, or to take the kids to their activities. We gulp down drive-through dinners in the comfort of our cars, and at home, we zap our meals in the microwave. We eat instant rice, instant noodles, instant oatmeal. If it takes longer than an instant, it's too long.

When it comes to our looks, we also want instant results. And we want those instant results with minimal effort: we'll take a magic bullet to melt away fat instead of adopting a sensible plan of diet and exercise, and we'll endure an injection to banish wrinkles caused by a lifetime of sun worship. But let's be honest. How effective have these approaches been in the past? I don't think you got the results you were looking for or you wouldn't be reading this page.

Using the whole beauty approach, you can improve the quality of your skin and restore a glimmer of that youthful glow you didn't notice or didn't appreciate when you were young. You can have strong and healthy hair, and you can help to prevent or stall the appearance of gray hairs that seem premature at any age. You can have beautiful finger-nails that don't split, crack, or peel. You can have sandal-worthy feet. You can shed a few unwanted pounds, find your waistline, and be able to climb a set of stairs without panting for breath. You can polish the twinkle in your eyes, oil the spring in your step, and hold back the hands of time just a little bit—if you take a novel approach to your life.

The first thing you have to do is stop watching the clock. There is no magic beauty bullet. Let's trade in our quest for instant gratification for the option to have an energetic, healthy, and beautiful life. The second thing you have to do is accept the fact that you may have to make a few changes in the way you do things. And I know, change is hard. We all tend to follow the path we've always followed, making the same choices we've always made. If we do that, the results, of course, will continue to be the same as well.

But in your defense, how can you possibly be expected to make different choices in your life when you don't know and understand all your options? Consider this book the introduction to your options. Armed with information, your only challenge will be to find that elusive "willpower." All the same, willpower has little to do with your chances of success in your whole beauty endeavor. In fact, it has very little to do with your success at anything. Rather than bemoaning a lack of willpower, you should focus instead on learning information that will give you the power to make different choices. When you understand that your need for sugary snacks might be triggered by a digestive tract problem, for example, you will have the power to fix the problem and put an end to the physical craving. You don't need to rely on willpower when you have knowledge.

Commit to learning about the multitude of options that surround you. If you don't like jogging for exercise, don't jog. Try martial arts or dance or swimming instead. If you always eat when you are stressed, find out what else is available to help you cope with your troubles. Meditation, yoga, and volunteering, for instance, are some of the activities that have worked for others. If you've had dry skin your whole life and none of the creams on the market seem to help, maybe you should consider some dietary changes. Rather than focusing on the problem area, focus on finding a solution that you will enjoy and that can be incorporated into your life.

Make sure that your whole beauty ambitions receive the same attention as other projects that fill your day, and set reasonable goals.

How many times have you heard from your human resources department that your goals should be specific, manageable, and measurable? Why should your personal goals be any different? Let's assume that you are overweight and you have 50 pounds between you and your favorite pair of jeans. Well, your goal is specific and it is also measurable. Now all you have to do is make it manageable.

Since you didn't gain the weight overnight, it's highly unlikely that you're going to rid yourself of it overnight, so find a manageable goal. Why don't you aim for a pound per week? Now I can hear the calculator in your head quickly computing that it will take you nearly a year to get there. That might not give you the instant gratification you're looking for, but I'm betting that you're more likely to make it if you tread slowly and reward yourself with a weekly loss of one pound.

Ease into change. Drink one less glass of wine today or choose fruit over a chocolate bar. You'll slowly start to feel better as you gradually alter your habits, and the way you feel will motivate you to continue on your new path. Most importantly, remember that mistakes are part of the journey and not the end of it. Forgive yourself for minor indulgences and get right back on the path where you left off. Value yourself, and change will be easy. Finding a long-term solution to beauty concerns will take a little time. But remember that you're renovating your beauty from the inside out. If you were building a new home from the ground up, you wouldn't want the contractor to skimp on the foundation. If he did, in time you'd start to notice creaking and cracks, and you'd likely begin to question the stability of your house. Apply the same principle to your personal reconstruction, and you'll reap the benefits of improved energy, increased confidence, and youthful vitality. *Beautiful!*

How to Use This Book

This book is divided into two parts. The first one, which we've already begun, is entitled *Living Beauty Essentials*, and it will provide important information that applies to absolutely everyone. In order to improve your health and energetic glow, gradually adopt the suggestions in this section into your life. In no time at all, you'll notice improvements in your life—and others will notice them too!

The second part of the book, *Beauty Prescriptions,* addresses individual concerns and what your beauty symptoms might be trying to tell you. Each chapter of that part ends with a *Beauty Prescription*, including the *Living Beauty Essentials*. I encourage you to read through every section carefully, because you might learn that certain symptoms you'd accepted as an unavoidable part of the aging process might be avoidable after all.

As you start any health regimen, you should proceed slowly. Doing too much too soon can cause your system to overload, and instead of helping yourself feel better, you could actually trigger complications. Research shows, for example, that when some people start taking a multivitamin, they can temporarily raise their blood pressure, simply because the added nutrients start to move cholesterol through the body toward elimination. Talk to your doctor, chiropractor, naturopath, or other health-care provider for advice about your own particular situation. Along with that medical advice, recommendations from a nutritionist can also help you improve your health by addressing nutrient deficiencies that may not be covered in this book.

Now let's get started.

Do note: If you are pregnant, or if you are breast feeding, remember the only safe levels of nutrients are those found in standard prenatal vitamins unless advised otherwise by your doctor for certain health conditions. Follow the Beauty Prescriptions only when you are not pregnant or when you are not breast feeding. Besides, with the maternal glow of pregnancy and new motherhood, you are already simply beautiful!

CHAPTER TWO

Protecting the Body Beautiful: The Immune System

Whatever is in any way beautiful hath its source of beauty in itself, and is complete in itself; praise forms no part of it.

—Marcus Aurelius

Keeping yourself looking gorgeous means that you're staying at least one step ahead of all the things in the world that are trying to take your health away from you. Every day of our lives, our bodies work against time; genetics; pesticides and fertilizers in our food supply; pollution; dietary choices; and every single germ, virus, or parasite that crosses our paths. And our bodies fight this fight every second of every hour while we are asleep and when we are awake. It's no wonder that sometimes the great defender of our health, the immune system, becomes so overworked that a cold virus sneaks in or an allergy develops or serious disease takes hold. As I mentioned earlier, although many serious health conditions can take years to make themselves known through standard medical tests, our bodies often send us signals that there is trouble in paradise. These signals come in the form of what we know as "symptoms" and can include everything from aches, pains, and fatigue to gray hair, undereye bags, cracked fingernails, and skin conditions. If we respond to the symptom in the appropriate way—by addressing it with lifestyle and nutrient changes rather than covering it up—we might be able to prevent a future health crisis. And of course, the only way we can decipher these symptom signals is to understand the language of our bodies.

The Immune System Translation

If you've ever been to a rock concert—or seen a movie about a rock concert—you know that the stars are always surrounded by Big Burly Men. With biceps the size of small children and thighs like tree trunks, these bodyguards are charged with the responsibility of making sure the stars aren't bothered by annoying fans or by people who are distinctly non-fans. Let's pretend that you've secretly fantasized about being a rock star and for the rest of this chapter (poof!) you are a rock star. The Big Burly Men have been hired by The Immune System, an organization that specializes in body protection. They are your security team, and their job is to make sure that no harm comes to you. They are very accomplished at their task: every entry point to the auditorium where you are performing has been thoroughly covered. The Men know how unseemly characters like germs operate, and they know how those villains and other nefarious elements will try to get in. The security men have heard every con in the book, so it's not easy for intruders to talk their way past these formidable guards. And woe to the unfortunate one who tries to bully his way in. The Men stay connected to each other through a high-tech communication system, and they all wear headsets with small microphones that allow them to call for backup if necessary.

Anyone who tries to enter has to show identification or somehow prove that they have the right to be there. Invited guests are allowed to enter through one door only, and they have to show a ticket to gain admission. For a delicate security detail such as this, there can be no deviation in the system, or chaos may ensue. Unfortunately, deviations sometimes do take place. Let's assume that on opening night, one of the Big Burly Men is a bit distracted. We'll call him Mike. To make some extra money, Mike stayed up most of the night helping the crew set up the stage. Early morning rehearsal found him exhausted from the night's work, and his intravenous coffee supply wasn't cutting it anymore. With his spidey senses slightly askew, Burly Mike listens to a cute little brunette called Germella as she begs to be let in backstage. She's the sister of a friend of a guy in your band, and she has something to deliver. She can't just hand "it" over to Mike, because "it" is private. Normally, being the professional that he is, Burly Mike would have quickly given this woman her walking papers, but tonight—he's not sure why, but there's just something about her that he trusts. She looks familiar somehow, like maybe he's seen her with the band. He lets her in.

It doesn't take long for Burly Mike to remember why she seemed so familiar. She's the sister of a woman your drummer dated last summer, and the relationship didn't end well. In fact, tonight, Big Sister is in the mood to serve up a little retribution. Suddenly, there's a great commotion onstage. Big Sister has run out to "talk" to your drummer during the opening number. Pandemonium breaks out as drumsticks fly through the air and the drummer heads for cover. Big Burly Men leave their posts at the front of the stage to try to grab the sister-on-a-mission, and excited fans rush the stage. In a frenzy, your bodyguards now swoop in from all directions, trying to restore order. Of course, this leaves the auditorium doors open and unprotected, and disgruntled fans who've been unable to buy tickets to the show steal the opportunity to finally get in. Bruised and broken bodies surround you on the stage, and you realize you have to escape. You finally push your way offstage and lock yourself in your dressing room. The action outside your door is busy and frightening and seems to go on forever. Finally, you hear the wail of police sirens (thank goodness for those high-tech communication devices!) and ever so gradually calm is restored. Exhausted from your trauma, you fall asleep, still safely locked in your dressing room.

Do you still want to be a rock star?

Actually, you already are the star of your own show, but the players are a little different than the ones in this little drama. You are still you, but your bodyguard team is actually your immune system, and the role of the sister-with-a-mission goes to every germ, virus, or parasite that needs a place to live and thinks your body is a nice neighborhood. You have many points of entry: your eyes, nose, and mouth are obvious examples, but every opening in your body is a potential access point for undesirables. Most people don't think about it, but your skin also provides a large entryway, particularly if it is impaired by open sores, acne, cuts, eczema, itchy psoriasis, or other skin conditions. Fortunately for you, your bodyguards are usually very efficient at their work, keeping bugs out and ganging up on the sneaky ones that find a way in.

Problems occur, however, when your bodyguards become distracted, and there are plenty of distractions. Stress, recovery from a previous illness, bad food, lack of proper nutrients, drugs, synthetic chemicals, and electromagnetic radiation from your television or computer screen are a few of the factors that have an impact on your immune system's ability to function.

Like poor Big Burly Mike, your immune system also gets fooled sometimes. Burly Mike thought that Angry Sister looked familiar, so he let her in. Similarly, bugs often rely on their resemblance to something harmless in our own bodies to gain entry. Unfortunately, research is revealing that some poisonous chemicals have the ability to do that as well. Certain chemicals used to make fragrances, cosmetics, body-care products, toys, and items in our homes are so like our own hormones that our immune systems let them stay because they do not recognize them as foreign. These xenoestrogens (pronounced "zeeno"-estrogens) are also known as estrogen-mimics and include the dioxins often used to treat paper for our toilet tissue, feminine pads, and tampons. Some chemical fertilizers and pesticides used on our foods have estrogen-mimicking properties, as well. These body-fooling chemicals have been linked to various forms of reproductive changes and cancers. In the coming pages, I'll be discussing these chemicals and their effects on our bodies in more detail. Sometimes flaws in our immune systems work in the opposite way—by not recognizing certain cells that are actually parts of our own bodies and launching attacks on them. This occurs with autoimmune conditions like rheumatoid arthritis, in which the immune system thinks that part of the body is foreign and tries to eliminate the perceived threat. Similarly, allergies result when our bodyguards overreact to a harmless substance, launching a full-blown attack on pollen or dust, which leads to runny eyes and nose and various other problems. The key to reducing the impact of allergies and autoimmune conditions is to improve the functioning of your immune system.

How It Looks

Do you remember how you looked the last time you were sick or your allergies were acting up? Dry skin, puffy eyes, and pallor result from the measures your immune system uses to evict the bugs and other intruders and set the stage for healing. Runny nose, diarrhea, fever, and vomiting quickly lead to dehydration as your body pulls water from all of your cells. As much as your body wants you to look good, its first priority is to survive. So it only seems logical that repeating the process of getting sick too frequently will have a long-term impact on your appearance. Think about this: if you have a sore somewhere on your skin that will not heal, it's a major clue for doctors that you have a serious internal problem like diabetes or cancer. When your bodyguards are all engaged in the melee on the stage, no one is available to watch the door. Similarly, your healthy good looks are going to suffer if your immune system is constantly working on allergies, food sensitivities, arthritis, or the flu—or if it's working overtime because of inflammation caused by your stress levels, lack of sleep, or lack of good nutrition. So keeping your immune system healthy is important not only because no one likes to get sick, but also because no one likes to look sick when they are not.

Payback

Another problem with being a star is that your success is never completely your own. Because you are such a big hit, you can't keep track of everything that's going on in your life and you've had to hire help. This management team takes a little piece of your earnings and so do your assistant, your publicist, your agent, and the government. Sometimes you feel as if you have to keep working just to make sure that no one goes hungry. A similar process is going on in your body right now, and it's responsible for much of what we consider to be aging.

Free Radical Theory of Aging

Think of free radicals as all the people who want a little piece of you—who pick and pick until, at the end of the day, you hardly recognize yourself. (You don't have to be a rock star to go through that!) Free radicals are naturally occurring atoms in our bodies, and they're the byproducts of eating, exposure to sunlight, and breathing. These atoms cause problems because they are missing an electron, and atoms are only stable with an even number of electrons in their outer shell. Because atoms want to be stable, the free radical bounces around from cell to cell until it can find and rob an electron. In the process, it causes damage to every cell it touches and turns the donor atom into another free radical when it steals the electron.

Our use of oxygen is a major contributor to the formation of free radicals, so free radicals are also known as radical oxygen species (ROS). And since we need oxygen to survive, free radicals are an inevitable byproduct of living. The damage that they do to your body is known as oxidation. You've likely heard that word before, but most often in terms of what happens when you leave a metal object in the rain. In the case of a tin can, oxygen and water react with the metal to cause it to rust. Free radicals cause similar destruction in your body by constantly picking away at our cells and causing them to weaken. And as the ROS bounce around trying to complete themselves, they leave a slew of damaged cells in their wake. The immune system becomes involved at this point, because it no longer recognizes the ravaged cells as part of the body and launches an attack. The first step that your bodyguards take in fighting any assault is to induce inflammation. Inflammation refers to the swelling, heat, redness, and pain that occur as a result of any injury. Think of the swollen and deformed joints associated with arthritis as an obvious example. In a vicious cycle, inflammation starts a chain of events that leads to the production of more ROS, and the cell damage continues. The Free Radical Theory of Aging holds that this continual injury to the cells leads to organ and system damage—and results in conditions and diseases that we often associate with aging, ranging from Alzheimer's disease to heart disease to wrinkles. Fortunately for us, there is an antidote to free radicals. Free radical scavengers, or antioxidants, thwart the damage caused by ROS by sacrificing an electron (giving the free radical what it wants). Antioxidants are found in plant nutrients such as vitamins A, C, E, and B complex, and in minerals like selenium and zinc, which occur in various fruits, vegetables, and herbs—in short, in our food. These nutrients are essential for your Big Burly Men to perform at the peak of their game.

When we are young, antioxidants balance out the free radicals quite beautifully. As we approach our 30s, however, the balance of power shifts decidedly in favor of the free radicals, and we noticeably begin to age. It doesn't help that damage occurs from the unavoidable activities of eating, breathing, and being exposed to sunlight, but free radicals are also generated by cigarette smoking, alcohol consumption, toxic chemicals in our environment and in our food, and electromagnetic radiation from our computer and television screens. Compounding the problem, most people in contemporary Western cultures don't eat a wide enough variety of fruits and vegetables to take in an adequate supply of antioxidants. And free radicals gain even more power because many of our foods don't pack the same nutritional punch as they did in the past. Soil quality has diminished because many farmers rely on chemicals to protect their crops instead of using more earth-and-food-friendly practices like crop rotation and natural fertilizers. As a result, the quality of the antioxidants in our food has declined.

At the same time, these modern farming methods mix chemical fertilizers and pesticides with our foods, so we are ingesting free radicals with every bite.

Whenever possible, boost the antioxidant status of your food by choosing organic products. Very simply, organic foods are grown without chemical fertilizers, pesticides, or herbicides. In addition, organically raised livestock are not injected with hormones or antibiotics and they're fed organically grown grains. Organic foods are more similar to the foods our ancestor George the Caveman would have eaten than to modern foods.

Busy, Busy, Busy

Although you may have a crazy schedule, find a way to add some more fresh organic produce to your day. The great thing about eating an orange is not sim-

> ### Tasty Berries for Gorgeous Skin
>
> Looking for antioxidants to go? Grab a handful of berries. Vitamin A, found in blueberries and bilberries, is necessary for producing mucus and secretions from the cells that line the mouth, throat, and stomach. Due to their vitamin C content, berries also boost collagen. (Collagen is the most abundant protein in the body, used to provide support for the skin and to promote the healing of skin and bones.) Look to blueberries and blackberries for healing vitamin E.
>
> A component in berries called proanthocyanidins may also help prevent the breakdown of elastin, the component responsible for giving our skin a youthful "snap." And quercetin, the flavonoid that colors raspberries and strawberries, provides excellent protection against ultraviolet light.

ply the amazing influx of vitamin C that you will get. The bonus is that the vitamin C exists in exactly the right proportion with the other vitamins in the fruit for your body to best benefit from it. Vitamins and minerals have a way of canceling each other out if you take in an oversupply of one. The B vitamins, for example, must always be taken together in what is known as a "complex" because excesses of one B will cause or hide deficiencies in another and potentially lead to serious consequences. You also don't want to pass up the delicious experience of the tangy liquid squirting in your mouth as you eat your orange on a hot summer day or the benefit of the fiber as it passes through your system. You'll learn more about the value of fiber in Chapter 3.

Although I've just pointed out that a whole foods approach to taking in your antioxidants is best, I also live in the real world. Actually, like many of you, I live in a place where winter seems, to me at least, to linger a very long time. Finding fresh produce is difficult when the roadside stands are buried under snow, so we often rely on our local grocers to ship fruits and vegetables in from the sunny south. I can only speak of my own experience, but such long-distance traveling is exhausting. I know that by the time I come home from a long trip, I'm ready for a shower and a nap. By the time long-distance produce arrives on the store shelves, it sometimes looks a bit tired too—and it's not in the same nutrient-packed, energy-filled condition it was when it left its sunny home.

Because of the low levels of nutrients in many of our foods, I recommend that you start taking a quality multivitamin/mineral supplement every day just to have a fighting chance against the aging caused by free radicals. A supplement—whether a capsule, tablet, powder, or drink—is designed to offer you nutrients that you might not be acquiring through your diet. But not all supplements are created equal: when choosing your vitamin supplement, look for "whole food" products, rather than synthetic versions. Unlike those designed in a lab, whole food supplements are derived from food. In a whole food supplement, vitamin C would come from oranges, for example, rather than a test tube. The benefit is that your body knows how to process the natural nutrients from foods much better than from manufactured varieties. Product labels will state when nutrients have been derived from whole food.

And remember that the key here is the word "supplement." You can't eat greasy hamburgers, fries, and a shake containing free-radical-producing hydrogenated and saturated fats and sugar, then pop a vitamin and think you've had a good anti-aging, antioxidant day. Instead, eat as well as you can and supplement your efforts with a multivitamin. Make sure that your family does the same.

How Much Is Enough?

You might be familiar with the Recommended Dietary Allowance (RDA) of nutrients, which refers to the minimum amount of a nutrient that healthy humans need to survive. Unfortunately, the RDA might not necessarily be the amount an individual requires to thrive. Often, people need more of a particular nutrient than suggested by the RDA in order to achieve optimum health. Some people have more difficulty assimilating different nutrients, for example, so they might have to supplement at greater levels or in different ways. Think, for example, of people who have vitamin B12 injections. Typically older people, these individuals must have B12 injected directly into the bloodstream because B vitamins are difficult to absorb and digestion often slows as we age. Deficiencies call attention to themselves through different symptoms, some of which we will address throughout this book. In the meantime, however, the following descriptions will provide information about important nutrients, as well as providing general guidelines for daily requirements.

What Do All These Antioxidants Do?

Vitamin A

Vitamin A is required for the production of mucus and secretions from the cells that line the mouth, throat, and stomach. It also helps to reduce the production of pore-clogging oil, so it is valuable in the treatment of acne. Vitamin A is necessary for new cell growth, and it's essential for protecting the skin from sun damage. If you have ever experienced rough, sandpaper skin on the backs of your arms, that's the result of a vitamin A deficiency. Acne, dry skin, dry hair, and dandruff are also common signs of a vitamin A shortage. Many people are deficient in this oil-soluble vitamin, and would benefit from using a vitamin A supplement.

Although some medical professionals prescribe treatments that involve up to 25,000–50,000 IU of supplemental vitamin A per day to combat skin conditions such as acne, for most people this amount is excessive. In fact, because vitamin A is stored in the liver, it is possible to take too much, leading to liver toxicity. Signs of excess A include abdominal pain, loss of menstrual periods, and hair loss. Most people should be sure to get 2,500–5,000 IU of vitamin A daily, but pregnant women should not exceed 2,500 IU per day. Talk to your health-care provider about appropriate supplementation of vitamin A if you have concerns about your liver. Food sources of vitamin A include animal livers and fish oils, as well as a variety of fruits, vegetables, and herbs such as paprika, alfalfa, and carrots. If you are one of those people

> **Measuring your Nutrients**
>
> Fat-soluble nutrients are typically measured and recorded on labels in International Units (IU), while water-soluble nutrients are measured in milligrams (mg) or in smaller units, called micrograms (mcg).

who need more than the average amount of vitamin A, consider supplementing with beta carotene, the flavonoid that makes carrots orange. Beta carotene is actually stored in the liver, where it is transformed into vitamin A as you need it. The only known side effect of taking too much beta carotene is that, like the carrot, you may develop an orange hue! Most people will benefit from supplementing 10,000 IU beta carotene daily.

Unfortunately, however, some people can't make the switch from beta carotene to vitamin A. If you've been diagnosed with diabetes or hypothyroidism, for instance (see Chapter 6), you may not be able to convert adequate amounts. You may need to take a minimum of 10,000 IU of supplemental vitamin A daily. Talk to your health-care provider if you are concerned.

The B Vitamins

You probably know by now that there are a whole bunch of B vitamins. Anyone who has ever bought a box of cereal is also familiar with some of their technical names: niacin, riboflavin, and thiamine are some of the more well-known ones. B vitamins are vital in the production and maintenance of healthy blood; the metabolism of carbohydrates, fatty acids, and proteins; cellular integrity; a healthy nervous system; support of the immune function; and prevention of some cancers—and they are also required for the maintenance of healthy skin, hair, and nails. Deficiency in the B vitamins can lead to fatigue, depression, sleep disturbance, poor appetite, anemia, loss of coordination, and in the worst cases, paralysis and death. Studies indicate that low to normal levels of the B vitamins are found in two out of five North Americans, including meat eaters. Low levels in meat eaters may exist because vitamin B is tightly bound to the proteins in meat and dairy products, and high acidity is required to cut it loose. As we age, we lose some of the acid-secreting cells in the stomach. Consumption of alcohol, and coffee also plays a role in the stomach's inability to absorb vitamins.

In addition, many people have B vitamin deficiencies simply because stress depletes the body of these vital nutrients—and who doesn't have stress? All vitamins play roles in maintaining our health, but the B vitamins work best in concert with one another, and a deficiency in one often indicates a deficiency in another. In fact, randomly supplementing a single B vitamin can actually mask a shortage in another. For example, too much folic acid can hide a B12 deficiency, leading to depression, fatigue, and eventually, pernicious anemia.

Having said that, there are times when a health-care professional might recommend supplementation of a single B vitamin. Niacin, for example, is often used to treat high cholesterol. Because of the intricate interaction between the many B vitamins, however, it is best to take them in a B complex formulation unless you are under a physician's care. A client once phoned me, a little unnerved, because whenever she took the nutrients I recommended to help with her digestion, she would get a tingle that started at her scalp and worked its way downward. She thought the reaction was simply the nutrients at work, but after a few days of her new regimen, she broke out in red blotches in her face and neck area. Finally, she called me.

As she had purchased her own supplements, I asked her to bring them to the phone and read me the labels of everything she'd been taking. Lo and behold, along with the nutrients I'd recommended, she'd also started taking supplemental niacin. In doses greater than 50 mg per day, niacin is known to cause a "flush" in the skin, and she'd been taking 100 mg! After confirming that her doctor hadn't recommended niacin for a cholesterol problem, I told her to stop taking it and to use B complex vitamins instead. The flushing stopped immediately. Unless otherwise advised by a physician, most people would benefit from a B complex supplement (minimum 50 mg) every day. Folic acid, an important B vitamin, is required in smaller amounts. Most healthy people should aim for 400 mcg of supplemental folic acid daily.

What Do All Those B Vitamins Do?

Vitamin	Effect	Food Sources
B1 Thiamine	Adrenal gland function, immune performance, metabolism of foods and alcohol	Brown rice, wheat germ, whole grains, brewer's yeast, broccoli, Brussels sprouts, dried prunes
B2 Riboflavin	Prevents migraine headaches, alleviate arthritic pain	Egg yolks, fish, legumes, leafy green vegetables, whole grains, almonds
B3 Niacin	Treatment of high cholesterol, neurological diseases	Beef liver, brewer's yeast, peanuts, potatoes, whole wheat, tomatoes, dates
B5 Pantothenic acid	Works with all other B vitamins to help cope with stress, required for proper immune function and adrenal hormone function	Organ meats, brewer's yeast, eggs, milk, fish, tomatoes, wheat germ, mushrooms, nuts, strawberries, bananas, cantaloupe
B6 Pyridoxine	Supports immune function, reduces homocysteine, supports cardiovascular health	Brewer's yeast, meat, fish, eggs, spinach, sunflower seeds, brown rice and whole grains
B12 Cobalamin	DNA synthesis, blood cell development, cleans up byproducts of protein metabolism	Clams, herring, milk and dairy products, organ meats, sea vegetables (e.g., arame, kombu, wakame)
Biotin	Fatty acid production, utilization of all other B vitamins, required for healthy hair and skin	Milk, poultry, meat, whole grains, brewer's yeast, mushrooms, cauliflower, salmon

Vitamin	Effect	Food Sources
Choline	Brain and nerve function, gallbladder regulation, liver function	Egg yolk, lecithin, whole grains, legumes, meat, milk
Folic acid	Repairing DNA, reduces birth defects, required for cellular repair	Citrus fruit, asparagus, lentils, beef, barley, brown rice, salmon, tuna

Vitamin C

You probably already know plenty about vitamin C, as it is definitely the media darling in the vitamin family. This water-soluble vitamin plays a key role in everything from immune-system health to adrenal-gland function, to protecting us from pollution. It helps keep our blood from abnormal clotting and protects against bruising. Vitamin C is a crucial component in the formation of collagen, so it is essential for our bones and skin. Collagen is the most abundant protein in the body, used to provide structural support for the skin and to promote the healing of skin and bones. Vitamin C also preserves the integrity of blood vessels, muscle, and tissue and increases the absorption of iron. As an antioxidant, vitamin C scavenges free radicals in our body fluids. It also promotes wound healing and protects against DNA damage from the sun.

This nutrient is plentiful in green peppers, citrus fruit, and berries, but even healthy people with good eating habits should take a minimum supplement of 500–1,000 mg of vitamin C daily. A common indication of vitamin C deficiency is pinpoint red spots around hair follicles, particularly on the arms, thighs, and buttocks. Known as petechiae, these spots are the result of leaking blood vessels. Other signs of deficiency include bleeding gums, slow wound healing, and easy bruising. Excessive hair loss may also be an indication of a vitamin C shortfall.

> ### C is for Colds
> If you are anticipating or suffering through a cold, or if you have a cut or burn that you would like to heal, take 500 mg vitamin C in increments throughout the day up to at least 3,000 mg. You'll know when you've gone far enough because too much vitamin C can lead to diarrhea. If you reach that level, cut back 500 mg and continue supplementing at the reduced level until you've healed or recovered from the cold.

Vitamin D

When most people think vitamin D, they think bones. While it's true that this vitamin is necessary for calcium absorption, it is also important for your skin because it promotes the healthy development of immature skin cells as they journey from the lower epidermis to the outer layers. Vitamin D is considered, as well, to be both an antioxidant and an anticarcinogen, and because it helps to slow cell division, it is valuable in the treatment of psoriasis, a skin condition involving rapid cell turnover. Ironically, as much as we have been told to protect our skin from the sun to prevent skin cancer, liver spots, dry skin, and wrinkles, we also need exposure to sunny rays in order for our bodies to manufacture vitamin D. Twenty minutes of sunlight each day should do the trick for most people.

Unfortunately, anyone who lives in the more northern climates will have a difficult time reaching that level in the winter months. (You can try it, but watch out for frostbite!) And even in the summer, we have to worry about our sunscreens possibly blocking our ability to synthesize vitamin D. Another concern with this fat-soluble vitamin is that problems with digestion, liver, or gallbladder can impede its absorption into our bodies. This is because the form of vitamin D that we get from our food must be converted to a usable form in the liver, so any liver weakness will slow the conversion. Our gallbladder helps to emulsify fat, making it easier for the body to digest. You can see how problems in the gallbladder will also affect absorption of vitamin D. Food sources of vitamin D include fish liver oils, eggs, dandelion greens, and herbs such as alfalfa and parsley. Most people should supplement with at least 400 IU of vitamin D daily.

Vitamin E

I mentioned earlier that vitamin C is a powerful antioxidant in our body fluids. Vitamin E is a fat-soluble vitamin that performs a similar function within the fats that make up cell membranes. It also protects other fat-soluble vitamins and Essential Fatty Acids from the ravages of free radicals and promotes the use of vitamin A. It helps with circulation and heart health and is also vital for tissue repair, wound healing, and scar reduction. Vitamin E is also partly responsible for giving us healthy hair and skin. You will find vitamin E in dark green leafy vegetables, nuts and seeds, and kelp, as well as in flaxseed and wheat germ. Although everyone has different requirements, most people should supplement with at least 400 IU of vitamin E daily. Go for vitamin E supplements in the form of natural d-alpha-tocopherol, as it is used best by our bodies. The synthetic form of E (dl-alpha-tocopherol) costs much less, but it is also a much less effective form of the vitamin.

Calcium

As in the case of vitamin D, when we think of calcium, we usually think of bones. This is a good first step, but we shouldn't underestimate the power of this mineral. As the most abundant mineral in the body, calcium not only helps to build strong bones, teeth, and gums, but also helps to maintain a regular heartbeat. It may also lower blood pressure. New studies suggest that calcium plays a role in weight loss and weight maintenance and that a deficiency in calcium actually leads to fat accumulation. By helping to maintain the integrity of cell membranes, calcium also promotes healthy skin, and working in concert with zinc and iron, it helps you grow strong, beautiful nails. Nails that chip and break easily may be a sign of a calcium deficiency.

Sesame seeds and dark green leafy vegetables are often overlooked food sources of calcium, along with asparagus, almonds, and chamomile. To improve your calcium status, take at least 500–1,000 mg of supplemental calcium daily, along with your 400 IU of supplemental vitamin D. Women who are starting to experience premenopausal symptoms may choose to supplement more calcium, depending on dietary intake. Calcium can be difficult to absorb, so you will also need to correct any digestive problems you may have to be sure that you are acquiring all the benefits of your food and supplements. It's also important to avoid coffee, as caffeine leaches calcium from the bones and sends it straight to the urine stream.

Magnesium

Magnesium is needed for us to use calcium, and it also helps prevent the calcification of soft tissue. Along with its many other duties, this mineral supports muscle function, helps to prevent stress to the lining of arteries caused by rapid changes in blood pressure, and is important for healthy heart function. Deficiencies show as irritability, muscle twitches, pre-menstrual syndrome (PMS), and for young people, growing pains. Eat your magnesium in grapefruit, bananas, whole grains, and paprika. Supplement with 200 mg daily.

Selenium

Selenium is a very powerful antioxidant on its own, as well as being required for the activation of an extremely potent antioxidant enzyme called glutathione peroxidase. It's also essential for skin integrity, and people with eczema, psoriasis, or dry or thin hair may have a deficiency of this nutrient. Look for selenium in garlic, onions, Brazil nuts, and whole grains. Be sure to get at least 100–200 mcg of supplemental selenium in your multivitamin each day.

Zinc

When it comes to the health of your skin, zinc is definitely one of the good guys. It's vital to the formation of cells, tissue, and collagen, and it promotes wound healing. By controlling oil production, it also helps to prevent and treat acne. Zinc works as an antioxidant, increasing the absorption of vitamin A and enhancing immune system function. White spots on fingernails and hair loss may indicate that you aren't meeting your requirements for zinc, and if you find that your taste buds aren't as efficient as they once were, boosting your zinc might give you more flavor with every bite. For most people, a supplement containing at least 15–25 mg of zinc should make up for nutritional deficiencies.

Storing Your Vitamins

Vitamins and nutritional supplements aren't cheap, so be sure to protect your investment by storing them properly. The Rules:

1. *Never assume.* Always read the product label for storage and handling instructions—and be sure to follow them.

2. *Keep a lid on it.* Air is extremely damaging to vitamins. Don't buy a product in bulk to save money if you know it will take you years to use it all.

3. *Made in the shade.* Keep vitamins out of direct sunlight, as the sun's rays can speed chemical breakdown and diminish the effectiveness of the product.

4. *High and Dry.* Store supplements away from humidity (the bathroom is off-limits!) and avoid areas that experience temperature extremes. Room temperature is usually best. See Rule 1!

5. *If in doubt, throw it out.* If you are concerned about the freshness of a product that you've had for a while, look for changes in color, taste, or odor, as well as flaking or cracking. If any of these have appeared, throw the supplements out and start again.

Protein

Proteins are essential to every living cell in our bodies and rank second only to water in providing the majority of our body weight. As well as being extremely important to our immune systems, proteins are a factor in maintaining healthy bones, ligaments, muscles, organs, body fluids, skin, hair, and nails. Because this nutrient helps keep blood-sugar levels stable, it can stop food cravings caused by wild fluctuations in blood sugar. Various proteins are also crucial for the absorption and effective use of vitamins and minerals.

It may be surprising to learn that our bodies don't use the proteins we eat in the form that we eat them. Instead, dietary protein is broken down into chemical units called amino acids. These various amino acids are then reorganized to build the specific proteins our bodies need. Think of amino acids as a box of building blocks that can be used to create many different kinds of constructions.

The liver provides 80% of the amino acids that we require, but the remainder must be supplied by the diet. Any nutrient that our bodies need for optimum functioning that cannot be manufactured from other chemicals (and must therefore be obtained through our diet) is considered to be "essential." The following chart shows the nine essential amino acids and some of their effects on the body, as well as examples of food sources. You may be surprised to see how many of these essential amino acids are not found in meat!

Nine Essential Amino Acids

In the following table, I've included important indications that you might be experiencing a deficiency of a particular amino acid, or in some cases, that you might have an excess in your diet.

Amino Acid	Effects	Sources	Indication of Deficiency or Excess
Histadine	Growth and repair of tissue	Rice, rye, and wheat	Deficiency: poor hearing CAUTION: Do not supplement if you experience bipolar disorder or depression

Amino Acid	Effects	Sources	Indication of Deficiency or Excess
Isoleucine	Metabolizes muscle tissue	Most seeds, almonds, cashews, chick peas	Deficiency: hypoglycemia
Leucine	Healing of bones, skin, muscle tissue	Brown rice, beans, nuts, whole wheat	Excess: can lead to pelagra, hypoglycemica Deficiency: poor wound healing
Lysine	Necessary for Calcium absorption, collagen formation, and formation of all proteins	Eggs, fish, red meat, milk	Deficiency: hair loss, enzyme disorders, bloodshot eyes, reproductive problems
Methionine	Supplies sulfur, aids digestion, breaks down fat, essential for detoxification	Garlic, beans, fish, eggs, onions	Deficiency: disorders of the skin, hair, and nails
Phenylalanine	Elevates mood, improves mental alertness; helps memory, decreases pain	Eggs, milk, bananas, meat	Excess: anxiety, insomnia, headaches, kidney damage Memory loss could be a sign of deficiency CAUTION: The artificial sweetener aspartame contains phenylalanine. Do not use aspartamine or supplement with phenylalanine if you are pregnant or if you have diabetes, high blood pressure, or phenylketonuria
Threonine	Tooth enamel, collagen, elastin, wound healing	Animal proteins	Deficiency: poor wound healing CAUTION: Content in grains is low, so vegetarians may have deficiency
Tryptophan migraine	Necessary to produce serotonin, combat insomnia, and depression; enhances release of growth hormone	Brown rice, meats, peanuts	Deficiency: insomnia
Valine	Tissue repair, muscle metabolism	Dairy products, meat, grains, mushrooms	Excess: sensation of crawly skin Deficiency: poor wound healing.

For maximum absorption, combine your protein with small amounts of vitamins C and B6. Protein deficiencies can cause depression, indigestion, and impaired growth, and they are also linked to skin conditions. In addition, a shortfall of protein can lead to edema (also known as fluid retention or swelling). Deficiencies may be the result of impaired protein digestion or insufficient intake of vitamin C.

It's important to have enough protein in our diets, but if we consume too much, we will stress the kidneys and the liver. Our kidneys break proteins down into toxic ammonia, which our bodies then transform into harmless urea, excreted via the urine. Excess protein overloads the kidneys and causes ammonia to flood the system, leading to serious damage.

If you choose to supplement with amino acids, it's best to take them in a complex formulation unless you really know what you're doing. Some amino acids (such as cysteine) become toxic at over 1,000 mg daily, while others become toxic at doses of over 6,000 mg a day. Talk to your health-care provider to learn whether supplementing amino acids is a good idea for you.

Age-Defying Essential Fatty Acids

As with the essential amino acids, Essential Fatty Acids are those that we must consume in our diets. Yes, you read that correctly: your body does require some fats. You can assume that you are not taking in enough Essential Fatty Acids (EFAs) in your diet if you have dry, fragile hair or skin that is rough, dehydrated, or flaky. If you are troubled by eczema or psoriasis, you should also up your EFA intake. (For treatment information, see the sections dealing with individual skin conditions in Chapter 7.) EFAs are involved in enzyme regulation, nutrient absorption into the cell, cell communication, and the creation of a healthy, fluid cell structure (the cell membrane). EFAs also nourish and help to retain moisture in your hair, nails, and skin. And they're used to create various hormone-like compounds that are involved in blood clotting, blood-vessel dilation, and inflammation. Inflammation is not only a factor in skin conditions such as acne and eczema; it is also associated with clogged arteries, high blood pressure, heart disease, and many other chronic conditions. Any one of these conditions can have an impact on skin quality.

Clogged arteries reduce the flow of oxygenated blood, causing skin cells to suffocate and die. High blood pressure may cause artery damage, brain damage, eye damage, heart damage, and/or kidney damage. Damaged kidneys can't filter blood efficiently, so your body will try to eliminate waste through your skin. Soon overworked, the skin cells inflame, infect, and die. A diseased heart can't pump optimal levels of nutrients into cells, so they starve. And because dead skin cells are dull, gray, and dehydrated, they don't look good on you. Inflammation is serious business. You want to minimize inflammation in your body as much as possible, and your choice of fats can help you do that. Researchers have learned that all of our cells take up EFAs from the bloodstream and convert them into several different products, but the main ones we will focus on here are the prostaglandins. There are three types of prostaglandins (PG), conveniently numbered PG-1, PG-2, and PG-3. PG-1 and PG-3 are what we will call the good prostaglandins; they are known to make the skin moist, smooth, and supple. PG-2, on the other hand, causes inflammation and problems with constricted blood vessels and blood clotting. I'll simply refer to them as beneficial or harmful compounds as we discuss Essential Fatty Acids.

Fats Simplified

This section will be full of short forms and big words, but the material we are dealing with is scientific stuff, which I've tried to simplify as much as possible. The bottom line is that you should try to know your Omega-6's from your Omega-3's so you can be sure you're getting enough of each in your diet.

Omega-6

Linoleic acid (LA) is an Essential Fatty Acid more commonly known as Omega-6 fat. LA provides us with gamma linolenic acid (GLA) and one of the helpful compounds that promotes anti-inflammatory benefits, as well as proper blood-vessel constriction and clotting. We get lots of LA

Minding Your 3s and 6s

This chart simplifies the question of fats:

Healthy Omega-3 Fats
alpha-linolenic acid (ALA)
eicosapentaenoic acid (EPA)

Beneficial Omega-6 Fats
gamma linolenic acid (GLA)

Omega-6 Fats (Harmful in Excess)
linoleic acid (LA)
docosahexaenoic acid (DHA)

from foods like meat and eggs, but may not benefit from GLA due to inefficient or absent conversion. Those who smoke, consume excess alcohol, or have allergy-related eczema have poor conversion. Cancer, diabetes, and some viral infections can also play a role. Aging weakens the D6D enzyme responsible for the conversion of LA to GLA, and an excess intake of dietary saturated fat (from certain meats, high-fat dairy products, and some common cooking oils) or trans-fats can hamper the switch. It's also essential to have adequate zinc, magnesium, and vitamins B3, B6, and C in the diet, so that conversion does not become a problem.

Through another conversion pathway, LA leads to the production of arachidonic acid (AA) and other compounds. AA is associated with promoting rapid cell division, which is an aspect of psoriasis and often a factor in cancerous mutations. Arachadonic acid also causes inflammation. As we get plenty of LA and AA in our diets, there is no need for us to supplement it. In fact, many of us have excess LA and AA and should be limiting the amount we consume. Only infants need large amounts of AA for growth and development.

If you think your diet is not providing you with enough GLA, however, you should supplement this nutrient directly. Borage oil (also known as starflower oil) is the best source, providing up to 23% GLA. Black currant oil also contains GLA (15–17%), and evening primrose oil contains 8–10%. If you enjoy using evening primrose oil, however, you should know that it contains high levels of LA, as well as GLA. As a bonus, supplementing with GLA helps with inflammation of all kinds in your body and may reduce the symptoms of muscle contraction, clotting, painful breasts, and depression associated with premenstrual syndrome!

Omega-3

When discussing Omega-3 fats, we're talking about alpha-linolenic acid (ALA). ALA eventually becomes eicosapentaenoic acid (EPA) or docosahexaenoic acid (DHA), and it is one of the beneficial prostaglandins. (Of course, not all of the ALA makes the conversion to these beneficial acids.) EPA is useful in fighting infections, while DHA is necessary for brain development and function and for the health of the nervous system. It also contributes to healthy, smooth skin. The same enzyme that converts linoleic acid (LA) to gamma linolenic acid (GLA) is also at work with the Omega-3s, but D6D will convert alpha-linolenic acid (ALA) to its derivatives before it works on linoleic acid (LA). For the same reasons mentioned in the Omega-6 section above, problems with the D6D enzyme can cause a breakdown in conversion.

If you are experiencing skin problems and increasing your ALA hasn't created noticeable improvements, you should supplement with EPA and DHA to be sure you're obtaining enough of each. EPA and DHA are found in coldwater fatty fish such as salmon, mackerel, and sardines. If you aren't a fish lover, however, you absolutely must use supplemental fish oils. Choose a concentrated oil (available in capsule form, as well as liquid form) that yields at least 30% EPA and 20% DHA content. Flaxseed oil is also an excellent source of ALA. Choose high-quality, cold-pressed flaxseed oil from the refrigerated section of your health products store, and use it in place of other oils in your blended drinks, salad dressings, or yoghurt—or drink it directly from the spoon. When fresh, it has a pleasant, nutty flavor. If your flaxseed oil tastes at all bitter, throw it out, as this means it has become rancid. Flaxseed oil must remain refrigerated after opening, and should not be used in cooking, as heat can turn the fats into toxins. Excess amounts can be stored in the freezer to extend shelf life.

For an added punch, buy flaxseeds in bulk and grind them yourself with a nut or coffee grinder. They must be mechanically ground, because our bodies can't break through to release the health benefits, and whole seeds will pass untouched through the digestive tract. Add two tablespoons of ground flaxseed to your meals for an inexpensive source of ALA, fiber, vitamins, minerals, and lignans. (Lignans have been associated with protecting the breast from cancer.) Ground flaxseed blends especially well with cereals and salads. While you will definitely benefit from the fiber and other health benefits of ground flaxseed, the seeds do not offer enough oil to be considered a replacement for the flaxseed oil. For best results, add both to your diet.

Balancing Your Oils

We need both Omega-6 and Omega-3 fats, yet to benefit most, we have to consume them in the proper ratio. Because of typical diets, North Americans commonly take in too much of the unhealthy Omega-6s in the form of linoleic acid (LA) and arachidonic acid (AA), consuming in ratios upwards of 10:1. This can lead to the deficiencies in Omega-3 that show up in inflammatory, autoimmune, and cardiovascular diseases, as well as in mood disturbances and difficulties with concentration. On the other hand, taking in Omega-3 at the expense of good Omega-6s can cause tissue, cell, and organ damage.

Those without serious skin conditions should try to take in twice as much Omega- 3 as Omega-6. If you feel that you have too much Omega-6 in your diet, change to olive oil, walnut oil, or hazelnut oil for your meal preparation, cut back on saturated fats (high-fat dairy products, some meats, and certain cooking oils), and be sure to eat enough protein. Look ahead to the treatment sections in Chapter 7 if you experience acne, eczema, or psoriasis, as you might require supplementation.

Move It, Move It

Keeping your immune system strong is not just about the foods you eat.

> ### What Are the Aging Fats?
>
> If you want to stay youthful, avoid partially hydrogenated and hydrogenated fats—also known as transfats. Hydrogenation is a process that alters the chemical structure of a fat through the addition of more hydrogen, effectively turning a liquid into a solid. The goal is to prolong the shelf life of a product by delaying the rancidity that occurs with natural oils.
>
> Problems with trans-fats occur because our bodies do not recognize this artificial chemical structure, and it does not have the tools to digest and metabolize it. Having too many of these trans-fats in your system causes cellular malformations that can impair the functioning of cells and organs.
>
> Trans-fats have been linked with cardiovascular disease and diabetes, and because of the role of fats in the brain, they may also contribute to the free radical damage associated with diseases like Parkinson's and Alzheimer's. Stay young. Avoid trans-fats.

Multiple studies show that physical exercise increases activity in the immune system. As with all things, however, balance is key: intense exercise for a long period of time suppresses immune system activity and may cause you to be more susceptible to infections. You also need to be sure to get your beauty sleep: much body repair takes place when we are sleeping. Denying your body the opportunity to make these repairs is courting trouble. Give your body the right mix of activity and rest. Eat properly and make sure that you take the following supplements daily to boost your intake of health- and beauty-promoting antioxidants and immune-system boosters.

Beauty Essentials for Your Immune System

1. High-Potency Multivitamin and Multimineral Supplements, including:

	Daily Amount	Nutrient Action
Vitamin A	2,500–5,000 IU	Antioxidant; helps with wound healing, especially of the mucous membranes; helps to keep skin smooth and moist
Vitamin B Complex	50 mg	Improves skin texture; necessary in formation of anti-inflammatory chemicals; helps with wound healing
Vitamin C with bioflavonoids	500 mg — 1,000 mg	Powerful antioxidant; necessary for formation of collagen; offers sun protection
Vitamin D	400 IU	Necessary for absorption of calcium; helps promote healthy cells; slows cell division to reduce risk of carcinogenic mutations; benefits healing of psoriasis
Vitamin E	400 IU	Protects cell membranes from free radicals; helps in formation of anti-inflammatory chemicals; offers sun protection
Beta carotene	10,000 IU	Converted in body to vitamin A; to produce and maintain cells
Calcium	500–1,000 mg	Strong bones, teeth, and nails
Magnesium	200 mg	Energy metabolism; protein synthesis

	Daily Amount	*Nutrient Action*
Selenium	100–200 mcg	Antioxidant that strengthens the immune system; promotes anti-inflammatory chemicals
Zinc	15–25 mg	Helps with wound healing; helps control skin inflammation

You could likely also benefit from nutrients not included in this list, but these are essentials for your immune system's health, and by extension, your vitality. You will also learn in the coming chapters that, from time to time, you might need increased quantities of some of these nutrients for healing purposes.

2. Essential Fatty Acids

These are available in liquid and capsule forms.

Supplement containing:	*Daily Amount*	*Nutrient Action*
EPA (30%) and DHA (20%)	1,000 mg twice daily, (total 2,000 mg)	For cell membranes; to provide sun protection; to decrease inflammation; also useful for brain function
Flaxseed oil	1 tbsp daily	Source of ALA; helps to promote anti-inflammatory and healing PG-3
GLA (Borage oil)	1,000 mg	Helps to promote anti-inflammatory and healing

CHAPTER THREE

The Beauty of Digestion: Getting the Most from Your Food

We ascribe beauty to that which is simple;
which has no superfluous parts; which exactly answers its ends.
—Ralph Waldo Emerson

I mentioned earlier that you would likely encounter a few detours on the road to healthful good looks. A discussion of your digestion may seem like one of them, but it is actually the most direct route from Point A to Point B.

Nothing affects our health and vitality quite as much as the foods we put into our mouths. Some food choices, like pizza and diet soda, are lacking in the antioxidants that drive the immune system—and in the nutrients that drive all the rest of our cells, tissues, and organs. Unfortunately, however, even really good food choices like fruits, vegetables, and lean protein don't do us any good if the digestive tract isn't working properly. And you might be surprised to learn that, for many people, it isn't. Of course, since your digestive system is the only one you've ever known, you've become used to its little quirks as the way things are meant to be. And because digestion is frowned upon as a topic for polite dinner conversation in most circles, you've possibly reached this point in your life without really understanding the importance of some very—hmmm, what's a good word?—"natural" functions.

So after the dinner guests have gone home and you're curled up in the privacy of your favorite reading chair, you can indulge in an exploration of the digestive tract.

Getting Back Some Va-Voom

Think about Agent 007, careening along one of those spectacular cliff-side roads on some exotic European coastline in a sexy little custom Ferrari—a Bond Girl at his side. (You can be James or the Girl in this little example. It's your fantasy.) But the sexy Ferrari in this escapade is your body. After arguing about who should drive, the undeniably gorgeous couple are racing against time to save the world from some fiendish scoundrel, but as life would have it, that fabulous sports car is now running on fumes. You swerve into a gas station, and while Bond Girl runs to use the ladies' room, 007 walks to the cliff to admire the scenery. Neither of them notices the attendant as he fills the gas tank with regular, unleaded gasoline. Doesn't he know that Q-designed custom Ferraris need super-high-octane gasoline? Or maybe he does know, but he's on the payroll of the fiendish scoundrel!

Bond and companion jump back into the car, anxious to take those treacherous corners at toe-curling speed. But what's this? Something's gone wrong with the car! It's sluggish. Bond forces the gas pedal to the floor as his hitherto trusty vehicle sputters to a crawl. The dynamic duo abandons the flashy sports car, and they wave down a local farmer. The three crowd into the front seat of the pick-up and lumber along in the faded old vehicle. Agent 007 and his Girl might make it to the lair of the fiendish scoundrel, but will they get there in time? If only Bond had paid attention to the fuel going into his car! Then he wouldn't have had to ditch the sweet ride. But he didn't pay attention, so now he and his Bond Girl are making the journey in a beat-up, broken-down farm truck. Of course, in Hollywood, Bond could conceivably take a running jump from the cliff, pull the drawstring hidden in the breast pocket of his tuxedo, and parachute gently to the ground. But life isn't a Hollywood movie, so what gimmicks do you have to regain and retain your speed, style, and effortless agility as you journey to your destination? Is it possible to hold onto the sports model just a little bit longer?

It's time to think of your body as that custom-built Ferrari. I know very little about the inner workings of cars, but I do know this: every three months I get an oil change and top up the fluids in my vehicle's engine. I do this because my Dad told me my car would last longer with regular maintenance. The mechanic at the garage also suggested that I add a fuel cleaner at every other oil change, to get rid of the sludge that can build up in the car's system. I also know I have to put gas in the tank every week or so, depending on my driving schedule, or I'm going to get stuck somewhere—and that could be embarrassing and incredibly inconvenient.

The same basic concepts apply to the engine that runs your body. It needs regular maintenance and the right fuel for maximum performance, and every once in a while, it needs a good cleaning to clear out the build-up of "gunk." (I do believe that's the technical word.) No one is going to admire a sports car that's been abandoned on the side of the road because the engine was unreliable: eventually that sports car is going to start looking like an expensive bag of bolts, covered with mud and rust. Let's see what we can do to prevent that from happening to you.

The Ultimate Engine

The first step in fixing any problem is determining what is broken. But in order to do that, you have to know how it's supposed to work and how it got broken. Only then will there be any hope of correcting the problem and preventing it from happening again

Very simply, it's important to understand that our digestive systems evolved over thousands of years and are well equipped to handle the rigors of digesting natural food like the fruits, vegetables, nuts, and seeds that our ancestors ate. But the more our "food" deviates from its natural state, the harder it is for our bodies to recognize it as food and digest it properly. Do you think that two hundred thousand years ago family dinners consisted of boxed instant mashed potatoes, microwaved pot roast that was ready to eat in five minutes (gravy included), and salty canned beans followed by coffee and a glazed donut? Unfortunately, our digestive systems have not kept up with the times, and they work on the same primitive principles as always. Our bodies' ancient processes don't know what a 20th-century artificial "trans-fat" is, let alone what to do with it.

> The more our "food" deviates from its natural state, the harder it is for our bodies to recognize it as food and digest it properly.

In trying to carry out their jobs efficiently, our bodies attach food chemicals to cells where they appear to make the best fit—and in some cases, this blocks nutrients that belong in those cells from gaining access. Other unrecognized or decidedly toxic compounds like those found in coffee, alcohol, and cigarettes end up in the liver, where a backlog quickly builds because there are only so many hours in the day and oh-so-many toxins. Eventually, of course, as systems become clogged with stuff your body doesn't know what to do with, there has to be a malfunction. The result may be a chronic condition like diabetes or a disease like cancer. Along the way, however, your body gives you clues that things aren't going so well—if only you were paying attention. A short list includes things like heartburn, morning aches, creaky joints, PMS, and headaches. But those are problems you can keep to yourself because no one can see them. Visible clues such as skin conditions including acne, eczema, and psoriasis, premature fine lines and wrinkles, dandruff, and even gray hair may all be broadcasting problems with your digestion, and these can often be traced back to problems with your food.

A Really, Really Simplified Overview of Digestion

Let me briefly describe the scenic route enjoyed daily by the food you eat. After we swallow, our food makes its way to our stomachs and past the duodenum, which is the first part of the small intestine. Partially digested food particles then pass through to the large intestine before reaching the colon, where the final stages of breakdown occur. Waste products are stored in the rectum until the final exit from the body occurs via the anus. Along the way, different organs like our gallbladder, pancreas, liver, and kidney contribute to the breakdown and use of our food.

We digest our foods through both mechanical and chemical means. The grinding of our teeth and churning of our stomachs help break food particles into smaller, more nutrient-accessible pieces. Meanwhile, the digestive juices work on the smaller bits in our mouths and stomach. (Digestive juices include the hydrochloric acid in the stomach, as well as different enzymes secreted by various organs involved in digestion, such as the amylase in saliva.) Obviously, then, digestion begins in our mouths. But after we've swallowed and the stomach has processed our food as much as it can, a valve at the bottom of the stomach opens to allow the liquefied food, now called chyme, to pass through to the beginning of the intestinal system. Since chyme is mixed with highly acidic stomach juices that would cause serious problems if they passed through our entire body, they must be made more alkaline immediately—and that is done by digestive juices in the intestines.

After the chyme enters the first part of the small intestine (known as the duodenum), the pancreas supplies enzymes that continue the digestive process. The food then moves farther into the small intestine, a 20-foot-long passage, where more alkaline digestive enzymes are added to the mix. Most of the nutrient absorption from our food takes place in the small intestine through millions of tiny suction tubes that vacuum up small digested food particles to transport them via the bloodstream to the liver. The liver has many roles in our bodies, but its role in digestion is to produce bile, a watery solution that is necessary for breaking down dietary fat so it can be used by the body. The liver also acts as blood filter, isolating and trying to deactivate any toxins or harmful particles that have entered the bloodstream.

If the liver is tired and can't fully neutralize toxins before they continue on their journey out of the body, damage appears in many ways. The first problems appear in the gall bladder. (The gall bladder is a tiny sac adjacent to the liver that stores bile.) When we eat a meal containing fat, the gall bladder squirts bile into the duodenum. When we are not digesting food, bile is concentrated in the gall bladder through the removal of water. Because the gall bladder is a storage site, it can become irritated if the bile contains toxins that have not been fully neutralized by the liver. This irritation can lead to gall stones, migraine, chronic neck problems, and most skin problems.

Back to the intestines for a moment. Leftovers leave the small intestine through another valve that leads to the large intestine. Naturally present bacteria in the large intestine continue breaking down any food particles that have survived the journey thus far. Larger proteins not broken down because of an inefficiency in the system are fodder for the bacteria in the large intestine, and they begin to rot. This fermentation leads to painful bloating and often foul-smelling gas. (Sorry, but that's what it is!) Through a squeezing action, the large intestine shuttles its contents along as it begins to extract liquid from the digested food. So by the time the waste products reach your colon, they have become more solid.

Problems and Solutions

Along with the obvious signs of digestive trouble like constipation and diarrhea, symptoms ranging from PMS to skin problems can also suggest that your digestive tract needs a bit of maintenance. Keep reading to learn what you can do to improve your digestive performance.

Mouth

Don't rush through your meals. Chew properly. The more that food is broken down before it enters your stomach, the easier it is on the rest of your digestive system. In fact, when some carbohydrates are chewed sufficiently and combined with adequate amounts of the alkaline juices in your saliva, they can be completely digested before they leave your mouth.

Stomach

Enzyme Deficiency

The stomach is the site of many digestive complications, most often the result of food selection, including too many refined, deep-fried, fast foods and sugary desserts. Along with the very acidic hydrochloric acid in your stomach are various enzymes that aid in food digestion. Protease, for example, helps to break down protein. The problem with enzymes is that when they are used, they don't come back, so our bodies are forced to create more. Fortunately, many of the whole foods we eat come with their own ready-packed enzymes. Raw apples are full of apple-digesting enzymes, and raw carrots come with their own carrot-digesting enzymes. Unfortunately, however, these important enzymes are destroyed by processing, cooking above 118 degrees Fahrenheit, and freezing.

> **Important enzymes are destroyed by processing, cooking above 118°F, and freezing.**

This wouldn't be a huge problem if we ate only a few of these enzyme-less foods, because we have backup mechanisms that can digest the food. But we eat so much cooked, frozen, or processed food that our enzyme stores are used up more quickly, and our bodies have to continue manufacturing them. Overeating can cause the same problem: we may have enough enzymes available to help process a bowl of pasta and vegetables, but not enough for the second or third helping. Constant manufacturing of these enzymes exhausts our glands, leading to weakness and fatigue. The other important thing you need to know about enzymes is that we use them for every single process in our bodies, from blinking to thinking. Of course, that includes providing energy to cells and repairing tissues, so enzymes are essential if you want to look good. As we age, however, our bodies become less efficient at producing enzymes—and it shows in our "aged" appearance. That means we need to get them from other sources.

One of the best ways to help in this process is to be sure to add adequate fresh, raw, enzyme-filled fruits and vegetables to your diet. You also need to take supplemental digestive enzymes whenever you have a cooked, previously frozen, or processed meal. A "processed" or "refined" food is any food that is altered from its natural state. Consider anything white (white rice, white bread, white pasta) to be refined. Consider anything from a box to be processed, including cereals. When shopping for your enzymes, at the very least look for ones that contain protease to digest protein, lipase to digest fat, amylase to digest carbohydrates, and lactase if you eat dairy. If you no longer have your gall bladder, you should also take a pancreatic enzyme. Everyone, including you, would benefit from taking digestive enzymes with every cooked, processed, or previously frozen meal.

Underactive Stomach

Because of our food choices in the last several decades, our stomachs have become very weak from overwork. An overworked stomach responds the same way you do when you're exhausted: it becomes less productive. Some signs of an underactive stomach include excessive gas, bloating and burping after meals, bad breath, nausea after taking supplements, undigested food in the stool, and acne. Many people who believe that they have an overacidic stomach actually suffer from a lack of acid. When food sits in the stomach for too long a time due to weak stomach acid, it begins to ferment, causing the release of gas. Gas rises and takes a bit of stomach acid with it, causing the heartburn that most people associate with too much acid. Taking an antacid then contributes to the problem because it further reduces the acidity of the stomach, creating a vicious cycle. Low stomach acid is also a risk factor for osteoporosis, because it prevents you from gaining access to all of the bone-building nutrients in your food.

To find out whether you have an underactive stomach, go to a health products store and purchase some betaine or hydrochloric acid tablets. Take a tablet on an empty stomach. If you feel a burning sensation, you do not likely have an underactive stomach. (To extinguish the burning, have a meal.) If you don't sense any burning, you likely do have an underactive stomach. Take a hydrochloric acid digestive tablet with every meal, and take another tablet with heavier meals. Note that these betaine tablets are in addition to the digestive enzyme tablets that everyone should be taking. (If you need help with your stomach acidity, consider taking supplements that include both betaine and digestive enzymes.) This may not be a lifelong process, but it's necessary as a first step in improving your digestion. Improved digestion leads to better use of food, better performance, and of course, better looks. Make sure you eat smaller meals more frequently. Avoid cold drinks with meals, and take only small sips of water at mealtime. Keep your dinners relaxed and stress free.

Overactive Stomach

Some symptoms of an overactive stomach include a burning sensation in the stomach, stomach pain an hour after eating, blood in the stool, gastric ulcer, and hiatal hernia. The test to determine stomach acidity described in the "Underactive Stomach" section will work here too. If you know that you have an overactive stomach, avoid spicy foods, alcohol, tobacco, caffeine, sugars, and nitrates. (Nitrates are chemicals often added to meat products such as bacon, sausage, and sliced meats.) Also be sure to get adequate fiber in your diet. Raw cabbage juice is useful for healing your stomach, as is aloe vera juice. Try liquid vitamins, as capsules may irritate your condition. Vitamins A, C, E, and zinc are useful in healing.

Pancreas

In digestion, the role of the pancreas is to manufacture digestive enzymes such as amylase, lipase, pancreatin, and protease. Problems with your pancreas are often associated with an underactive stomach and protein malabsorption. Because the pancreas is also involved in the production of insulin and glucagon to regulate blood sugar, any problems with this gland should be reported immediately so your medical adviser can check for diabetes. Whether or not you are at risk for diabetes, you can help ease the burden on your pancreas with the use of digestive enzymes.

Liver

The liver is probably the least understood and yet the hardest-working organ in our bodies. I won't recite the entire list here, but know that without your liver, you would die within 24 hours. The liver's role in digestion is to filter two liters of blood per minute, neutralize toxins, regulate metabolism, and produce the bile needed for digestion of fats. Signs of an overworked liver include, but are not limited to, fatigue, immune weakness, and compromised thyroid function. If toxins build up in the blood, other eliminative organs such as the kidney and the skin try to get rid of them. Skin can erupt in acne, rashes, and eczema, or you can suffer from itching, peeling, dry skin. Puffy eyelids in the morning may also indicate a stressed liver.

One way to determine whether your liver is stressed is to watch your urine. If it is dark in the morning and becomes clear and more copious as the day wears on, your liver may be overworked. The best thing you can do for your liver is to decrease its toxic burden. Avoid alcohol, cigarettes, refined sugar, and chemical additives in your food. Stay away from fried foods and junk food, and switch from coffee to herbal tea. Instead, eat fresh, raw, organic fruits and vegetables; whole grains; and organic meats and fish. Organic foods are grown or raised without chemical fertilizers, hormones, or other additives that may stress your system.

> The best thing you can do for your liver is to decrease its toxic burden. Avoid alcohol, cigarettes, refined sugar, and chemical additives in your food. Stay away from fried foods and junk food, and switch from coffee to herbal tea.

Gall Bladder

After toxins are filtered by the liver, they are sent to the gall bladder with bile for storage. Bile is necessary for the breakdown of fats and the absorption of the fat-soluble vitamins A, D, E, and K, as well as for converting beta carotene to vitamin A. (The fat-soluble vitamins are essential for healthy skin.) Bile is secreted into the small intestine and eventually passes out of the body with your feces. Problems with your gall bladder include gallstones and inflammation. To keep your gall bladder healthy, avoid fried and fatty foods. If you have had your gall bladder removed, be sure that your digestive enzymes contain bile and pancreatin.

Kidneys

We didn't mention kidneys in our earlier discussion of digestion, because we were focusing on solid food. But every day the kidneys filter gallons of fluid from the bloodstream, allowing wastes and toxins to leave the body in urine, while returning necessary substances to the bloodstream. They also regulate blood volume and balance the chemical components in our blood. Problems occur in the kidneys as a result of drugs, toxins, poisons, and viruses. To help your kidneys do their job, make sure you are well hydrated at all times by consuming approximately eight 8-ounce glasses of pure, filtered water per day. Puffiness under your eyes might be linked to underperforming kidneys, as can kidney stones, lower back pain, and fatigue. It is even possible that an inability to lose weight might be due to a kidney problem: deficiencies in the kidney cause the liver to take up the slack, and one of the key functions of the liver is fat metabolism. But if the liver is on kidney-duty, it can't perform the fat metabolism role as efficiently.

Intestines

Your intestines are home to trillions of creatures that play a key role in your digestion. They help to break down food, create vitamins, and prevent yeast and other bacteria from taking over the system. Unfortunately, modern realities like antibiotics, chlorinated water, nutrient-empty food, alcohol, and stress can cause imbalances in intestinal harmony, and this can lead to all sorts of complications. One of the most common conditions is an overgrowth of *Candida albicans*, a normally harmless bacteria that proves to be very aggressive in certain circumstances. An overgrowth of *Candida albicans* is so common, in fact, that I have devoted an entire chapter to it (Chapter 5). You might be surprised to discover that many of the symptoms you've blamed on your age—including muscle aches, PMS, and itchy skin—might actually be the result of *Candida*. It is also a major factor in food sensitivities. Be sure to fill out the "*Candida* Questionnaire" in Chapter 5 to see if *Candida* might be an issue in your life.

The other intestinal complication that's often overlooked in our part of the world is intestinal parasites. It's important to remember, however, that thanks to airplanes, our world is shrinking, and many of us have traveled outside of North America to places where it may be easier to pick up a parasite. Some parasites are also actually contagious, and they are a particular problem for children and for people who have a compromised immune function. Some symptoms of a parasite problem include a yellowish or pale face, dark circles under the eyes, damp lips at night or drooling while asleep, and eating that doesn't quench your hunger. Roundworms, tapeworms, and pinworms are more common than you would like to think. If you are experiencing unrelenting diarrhea, abdominal pain, vomiting, or an itchy anus and have ruled out other conditions, have your doctor check for parasites.

The best way to prevent a parasite infestation is to keep your immune system strong and your digestive system firing on all burners. Strong stomach function will destroy invaders, while a balanced intestinal system will crowd them out. Eating a high-fiber diet is essential, too, as this will improve colon function—and the nasty critters like to hang out in the colon. Alternative health practitioners recommend a parasite cleanse at least twice a year as a preventive measure—and perhaps more if you are well traveled. Your health products store likely carries parasite-cleanse products, which are typically a combination of medicinal herbs known to eliminate unwanted guests. Grapefruit seed extract, black walnut, garlic, and cloves are all beneficial as antiparasitic remedies.

Improving Your Digestion

Remember that the only fuel your body gets to keep you healthy—and by extension, gorgeous—is the food you eat. And problems with your digestion mean that you are not getting full value from those foods.

What is the point of eating all your vitamins and minerals if your body can't make use of them? You simply won't get all your nutrients if your digestive system is run down. Buildups, backups, inflammation, irritation, lost organs like the gall bladder or appendix, lack of enzymes, and lack of stomach acid all contribute to a sluggish system. You can put all the high-octane fuel in this engine that you want, but you may only get regular unleaded performance. You need a tune-up, and fortunately, there are many things you can do. Let's start with the easy ones, because after you try these, you might find that you have the energy to try the more drastic measures. (In this case, drastic is a good thing, but let's not jump ahead.)

In your pursuit of beauty, it's okay to start with baby steps: you will find that making a small lifestyle or dietary change makes you feel a little bit better. You might find that you have more energy or that you don't get a headache every afternoon. You might start to fall asleep moments after you go to bed or you might start to wake up refreshed instead of exhausted. You need to be conscious of the fact that these little improvements in the way you feel are a direct result of the small change that you made. When you realize that, you'll start to wonder what other small change you can make and how it will make you feel. That's what we're going for here: small changes that make a big difference in your life.

Let's Begin

Your digestion is very much like a combustion engine that needs a spark to get it started. But after years of neglect, that spark has started to fade, so we need to give it back some power. We'll do that by first going through a typical day. Some of these items may not apply to you, but read them all through because it's important to understand the impact of every decision you make.

The Nutrient Robbers

Okay, so your hideous alarm clock jolts you from your much-needed and probably unfinished sleep. No fear, you think, you wisely pre-filled and set the coffee maker last night before you went to bed, and that delicious aroma is already filling the house. But if this were a TV program, a big red

"X" would appear on your coffee pot, accompanied by the sound of a horn. The camera would cut to your stunned face, still lying in bed. The truth is, although you think you need caffeine's energy boost to get you through the day, coffee is actually an energy zapper. The caffeine does stimulate your nervous system, and in fact puts you on high alert, but it also does something you may not have realized. Caffeine shunts energy away from your digestion, causing it to slow down. Slowing down digestion means that you won't get all the nutrients from your food. You may also have food sitting around longer than it should, leading to unattractive bloating and painful gas.

So the first thing I want you to do is give up coffee. Take a deep breath! You're going to be okay! If you think there's no way on this green earth that you can give up coffee, try this. Have one less cup of coffee today. When you've made peace with that, have still one less cup every few days until the caffeine from the coffee is out of your system. If you actually try this, you can be done with coffee within three weeks. Look for an herbal substitute that you can mix half-and-half with your regular coffee brand as another way to help the weaning process.

If, however, the concept of giving up coffee scares you right now, try this. Don't put any sugar in your coffee. Refined sugar (the white stuff that's in everything from soup to ketchup to baked goods to anything that comes in a box) is toxic to your system. Much like coffee, it confuses you into thinking that it's giving you a boost when it's really robbing you of energy. As a way of gradually reducing the amount of sugar you eat, cut down on the sugar you add to your foods—a little each day.

And just to get it out of the way, I should mention that the third great energy robber is alcohol. Be aware of how much you drink and try to eliminate it from your life at least in the short term, so we can fix your digestion. I'm not saying you can't have a glass of wine to celebrate your birthday, but I am saying that if you can't commit to giving up alcohol for a while, then you need to do some real soul searching. If you can remove these nutrient robbers from your life, you'll find that you have more energy than what you "believe" they give you because you'll be getting everything your food is offering. But you won't know that until you do it. Weaning yourself from sugar and alcohol, like reducing your coffee intake, may give you withdrawal symptoms. That is perfectly normal. If you find you are experiencing uncomfortable headaches and nausea, slow down a bit. In the end, you'll be glad you persevered.

Ladies and Gentlemen, Start Your Engines

While working to clean and tone your digestive tract, start the day with a drink of freshly squeezed lemon juice in warm water. Add a dash of cayenne pepper or ginger to really get things warmed up. This is a beautiful substitute for the coffee you no longer drink. You should also ease into the day with some fruit. Fruit is easily digested, and since your stomach has been out of commission for about 12 hours, it appreciates a slow start to the day as much as you do. Fruit has another great feature: it's portable, so you no longer have the excuse that you don't have time for breakfast. Throw a banana or apple into your bag or briefcase before you rush out the door, and you can eat it in the car or on the bus—or better yet on your walk to work! About an hour later, you can have something more substantial like sugar-free yoghurt with almonds, a handful of trail-mix, or a homemade muffin. As you go through your day, it's best to let your stomach empty before you start filling it up again. Unless you suffer from hypoglycemia or other blood sugar issues, wait until you feel real hunger before you eat. This not only allows your body to burn up the extra bits and pieces in your system as it waits for more food; it also helps to teach you about hunger versus boredom, and may help with any weight issues you have.

> **Green Tea Bonus**
>
> Three cups of green tea (750 mg) contain 240–320 mg of immune-boosting antioxidant polyphenolic compounds.

How to Eat

Earlier in this chapter, we discussed some of the different enzymes that are used to help digest food. You will recall that specific enzymes break down specific food types: protease breaks down protein and amylase breaks down carbohydrates, for instance. In addition to requiring different mechanisms to break them down, different foods take varying lengths of time to be digested in the stomach. Fruit, for example, is digested in about an hour. Protein, like chicken or a rice and bean meal, can take up to three or four hours to digest. If you were to eat a chicken sandwich and follow it immediately with an apple, you would have the remnants of your apple stewing alongside your chicken for at least two hours. The wait causes the apple to start fermenting in your stomach. You might feel the effects of this concoction as gas or bloating.

While you are trying to clean your system, focus on the following guidelines for how to combine your food, so it is digested as easily as possible. That will bring you maximum digestion and minimum upset:

- Because it is most easily digested, always eat fruit alone, at least half an hour before and two hours after other food. Particularly avoid combining fruit with protein.

- Avoid mixing high-starch carbohydrates with protein. That means that you should replace your meat-and-potatoes dinner with another option.

- It is okay to eat high-starch vegetables (potatoes) with non-starch vegetables (broccoli). You can also combine protein with non-starch vegetables, so your chicken and vegetable stir-fry should be fine.

Remember that these are guidelines to help you heal your digestive system, and they may not be beneficial for everyone all the time. Those who burn calories very quickly or suffer from underactive adrenal glands may be better off using combinations that slow down the digestive process (such as combining starches with protein).

What to Eat

Improving your digestion will free up extra energy that can be sent to other parts of your body to provide the healing that makes you glow from the inside. To bring about this happy state of affairs, there's a very simple rule to follow in food selection: the farther it is from its natural state, the worse it is for you and the more potential it has to age you. For example, an apple is an excellent choice. Imitation apple-flavored fruit beverage is a bad choice. Steamed fish good; breaded deep-fried fish sticks not good. Potatoes are an excellent source of vital nutrients, but use those dehydrated instant mashed potatoes as wallpaper paste.

Eat more like a caveman or woman and you'll be well on your way to getting the nutrients you need to heal all the cells in your body—including the ones you can see. By eating this way, you'll also avoid the damaging preservatives and other chemicals that your body does not recognize as food, which are therefore processed as toxins. You can ease the burden on your liver and watch many skin conditions disappear. I understand how difficult it is to make some of these changes. You must accept that every small move you make in the right direction is a big victory. Falling off the wagon and enjoying a chocolate-covered donut every once in a while doesn't mean you should throw in the towel and go back to your old ways. What it means is you ate a chocolate-covered donut. The key is to not eat the whole box. As I tell my kids, when you're having a "treat," make sure you savor it. And don't be surprised if eventually those treats lose their appeal.

As you shift toward a natural diet based on eating a variety of fresh fruits and vegetables (eaten raw when possible), whole grains, nuts, seeds, legumes, and organic meat and fish, you'll start to notice

Falling off the wagon and enjoying a chocolate-covered donut every once in a while doesn't mean you should throw in the towel and go back to your old ways.

things "moving" a little better. This is a direct result of how much easier these foods are for your body to digest, along with the increased fiber in your system. Despite what you might have been told in the past, although it may be *normal* for some people in our current culture to have one bowel movement per day or every couple of days, it is not in any way healthy. In fact, a person with a healthy colon should have two to three bowel movements per day to correspond roughly with the three meals they've eaten.

The length of time that food stays in your body is called the "transit time." From bite to bathroom, a healthy transit time is about 12 to 18 hours. Any less than that means you might not be getting adequate nutrients from your food; any more means your food is likely fermenting and producing toxins along the way. Blood capillaries lining the colon absorb these poisons into the bloodstream, exposing the rest of your body to the toxins. These toxins damage all the cells in your body, and it shows on your face. To determine how long it takes for your food to take the journey, have a meal containing corn, then look at the clock.

Look at the clock again when you see the corn in the toilet. (I know. Not the most sophisticated test, but it works!)

Fiber Facts

Much misunderstood, fiber is basically the stuff that's left over after your body has taken all the nutrients out of it—that is, the indigestible cell walls of plant foods. There are two types of fiber: soluble and insoluble. Insoluble does not dissolve in digestive juices, but absorbs water, adding bulk and weight to the stool so it passes quickly through your body. A diet high in insoluble fiber can help prevent diverticulosis, a condition involving the presence of sac-like out-pouchings called diverticula anywhere in the digestive tract. If diverticula become inflamed, painful cramping and diarrhea can result in a condition called diverticulitis. Insoluble fiber is found in such things as celery, whole grains, and leafy green vegetables.

Soluble fiber dissolves in fluids in the large intestine and forms a gel. A diet high in soluble fiber helps lower blood cholesterol levels because it binds intestinal bile acids that contain fat and cholesterol, removing them with the stool. Soluble fiber is found in apples, broccoli, and strawberries—and in other fruits and vegetables. If you are experiencing some difficulty getting things moving, try natural psyllium husks. (They come from a plant often grown in India and are readily available at health products stores.) Taken with plenty of water, this soluble fiber is gentle on the system.

Digestive Aids

We've already considered the value of enzymes in your new beauty regimen because they work to repair cells, but I'm going to repeat the advice again. Everyone who is no longer exclusively breastfed has some level of enzyme depletion and should be taking supplemental enzymes with every non-raw meal. But there are other supplements you should also consider taking to improve your ability to digest food. Aged Garlic Extract, for example, enhances growth of friendly intestinal bacteria while inhibiting the proliferation of the unwanted *Candida albicans*. You'll learn more about that in the *Candida* chapter (Chapter 5).

Aged Garlic Extract also improves transit time throughout the digestive tract, which is essential if you want to prevent toxins from getting into the bloodstream and appearing on your face as acne, pimples, and generally unappealing skin quality. Studies also show that aged garlic protects the liver from damage by certain toxins and promotes the activity of detoxifying and antioxidant enzymes in the liver. Remember: any time you reduce the workload of the liver, you're allowing this important organ to get on with other activities—like clearing up your skin. And before you start to think that you'll be trading in one set of ugly problems for a different set of smelly problems, Aged Garlic Extract does not give you an odor! Unlike fresh garlic, which is nevertheless a delicious addition to your diet, aged garlic does not cause stomach upset or a bad smell.

Essential Fatty Acids

Essential Fatty Acids (EFAs) are also important for their ability to help assimilate food and lessen absorption problems. EFAs are a vital component of all the membranes in your body, from the individual cell to the outer layer of your skin. The evidence? Often dry skin patches or eczema start to clear immediately upon supplementation of EFAs. You'll recall from the last chapter that the word "essential" attached to any nutrient explains that the nutrient is not produced inside the body, so it's essential for us to get it from our diet. As a review, there are two types of EFAs: Omega-3s and Omega-6s, and they should be consumed in the ratio of approximately 1:3 (Omega-3: Omega-6).

Omega-6 is available in sunflower, safflower, and corn oil, as well as in meat and animal products. With our standard Western diet, most people get enough of that one. In fact, it's likely that you consume too much Omega-6 in relation to Omega-3, and an oversupply of potentially harmful Omega-6 acids such has linoleic acid (LA) and arachidonic acid (AA) can trigger inflammation, like that associated with allergies and arthritis.

Omega-3 acids, on the other hand, counteract inflammation, allergies, and arthritis and help with numerous other conditions. Omega-3s are the neglected Essential Fatty Acids because we no longer eat enough nuts, seeds, and cold-water fish (such as salmon). One of the best sources of Omega-3 fats is flax oil, which you can find at your local health products store. Look for a brand packaged in a dark bottle and kept in the refrigerator. (The problem with EFAs is that they immediately start to break down when exposed to light and heat, so opened bottles should be kept in the refrigerator.)

Pour flax oil on rice, use it in your salad dressing, include it in your smoothie, or take it directly from the spoon. Be sure to have a minimum of 1 to 2 tablespoons per day. And don't forget to include fish and fish oil, as these contain the Omega-3s EPA and DHA. If you have trouble swallowing oils, look at the variety of EFA supplements available in capsule form at the health products store. You can also get the benefits of fiber by grinding your own flaxseeds in a nut or coffee grinder and using them as a topping for your cereals and salads. The hard outer shell is too difficult for our digestive systems to break down, so we need to crack open the seeds mechanically to get to the Omega-3. Aim for 2 tablespoons of ground flaxseed every day.

> **You can also get the benefits of fiber by grinding your own flaxseeds in a nut or coffee grinder and using them as a topping for your cereals and salads. The hard outer shell is too difficult for our digestive systems to break down, so we need to crack open the seeds mechanically to get to the Omega-3.**

You may notice an improvement in your skin, an increased shine in your hair, a decrease in thirst, and a possible drop in weight because the fats help you feel full and they also boost your metabolism. You'll be reading about EFAs repeatedly throughout this book.

Probiotics

Earlier in this chapter, when discussing your intestines, I mentioned that you are host to trillions of naturally occurring bacteria. Many of them serve a useful purpose, as they help to break down our foods, and some even help form vitamins that our bodies need for optimal health. Some of them, however, serve us no useful purpose whatsoever. They are actually freeloaders. But if their numbers are kept low enough, we don't even notice that they've hitched a ride—that is, until something tips the balance of power in their favor.

Some foods, lifestyle choices, and medications quash the good bacteria, so the freeloaders gain power. The antibiotics we take to fight an infection, for example, can contribute to the problem. These drugs are not highly trained snipers that seek out and destroy only the bacteria that are causing a problem in your body. Instead, they're more like bombs that blast everything in their path. So while the antibiotics may help speed your recovery from an infection, they leave your body unprotected because the antibiotic bombs have also destroyed the beneficial bacteria in your body. And the freeloading bacteria are better at restoring their numbers after the antibiotic bomb has exploded. If you are having a hard time accepting this explanation, look to your own body for proof. The side effects of taking oral antibiotics often include upset stomach and diarrhea. What do those symptoms indicate if not a problem in your digestive system? And ladies, I'm sure that many of you are aware of the high incidence of vaginal yeast infection as a result of antibiotic use.

One of the invasive bacteria that are really good at taking advantage of a reduction in beneficial bacteria is called *Candida albicans*. Most people who've taken antibiotics (and who hasn't?) likely have some experience with *Candida* gone wild. *Candida* is a factor in everything from eczema to food cravings and allergies to migraine headache (see Chapter 5). Whether or not you have a problem with *Candida*, you likely have experience with chlorinated water, refined foods, or a diet that lacks fiber—all factors that contribute to a decline in the numbers of beneficial bacteria. Fortunately, however, you can boost the ranks of good guys and restore order to your intestines by using probiotic supplementation.

Probiotic capsules contain live bacteria such as *Lactobacillis acidophilus* that help re-establish bacterial crowd control and prevent harmful bacteria from causing so many problems throughout your body. Probiotics are also useful in preventing parasites from making a home in your intestines. Although probiotics occur naturally in some fermented foods like yoghurt and sauerkraut, supplementation through powders or capsules is recommended for therapeutic and preventive dosages. Prebiotics, on the other hand, are such things as fructo-oligo-saccharides (FOS). FOS are a group of naturally occurring carbohydrates found in vegetables that are indigestible by humans but feed the existing friendly flora in the intestines, including *Lactobacillis acidophilus,* helping them to grow and multiply. Aged Garlic Extract is one source of FOS known to enhance growth of the friendly intestinal bacteria *Bifidobacterium bifidum.*

Multiple studies have shown that in helping to return our intestines to a balanced state, prebiotics and probiotics also play important roles in a number of other areas: controlling cholesterol; preventing colon disease, including cancer; maintaining hormone balance; promoting mineral absorption and bone formation; and boosting the immune system to fight disease. Everyone should be sure to get their probiotics daily.

The Drastic Measures

A long, long time ago when a guaranteed meal was not available on a nearby street corner, our ancestors sometimes went hungry. As horrific as that sounds to us in the Western world, it actually wasn't all bad. Going without food for an extended period of time allowed the digestive system to burn out the "gunk," leading to improved efficiency. Eventually, our wise foreparents began to see the value of this cleanout, and some of the most ancient religions adopted the "fast" as an important part of the spiritual-mind-body journey. There are a number of different versions of the fast. Some of them allow only fresh juices, and the very strict versions allow only water.

In each instance, preparation is key. You need to gradually eliminate difficult-to-digest foods, working down to fruit only, and then finally only drinking liquid. Liquid, of course, is easy for the body to digest and does not add to the digestive burden as you are doing your cleanup. Water is essential to life, so you should always be sure to get enough. (In fact, simply increasing your water intake can help move toxins out of your body.) Your first fast will likely last one day. After that, you might move on to two, then three days. You must come out of a fast gradually, as well, adding first juices, then fruits, and then more substantial foods. I'm not suggesting that you're ready for a fast right now! In fact, if you are not already quite healthy, fasting is not a good idea at all. Although the purpose of a fast is to cleanse the body, if there are too many toxins released into the bloodstream at one time, you can make yourself very, very sick. So it's best to move at a more gradual rate. Pregnant or nursing women should not fast, nor should those with blood sugar conditions. When you are ready to fast for the first time, make sure that you do so under your physician's care—no matter how healthy you feel.

Other Cleansing Methods

Going without food is only one way of cleaning up your system—and some of the other methods may be a little easier to handle. These cleanses help move toxins out of specific organs so that organ is able to function better. Again, do not attempt these cleanses until after you've made significant strides in improving your diet and after you've eliminated the nutrient robbers from your menu. You do not want a tidal wave of toxins flooding your system.

Even when you carry out these cleanses in the right way, don't be surprised if you feel tired or have flu-like symptoms. This only means that the cleanses are working: poisons are leaving your organs, and they're being slowly neutralized and eliminated. The fatigue is an effect of the healing process, which takes a lot of energy. Also, if you are trying one of these cleanses to help clear up eczema or a skin rash, don't be surprised if the condition gets worse in the short term. Think of the expression "It's always darkest before the dawn" and remember that an increase in your symptoms is proof that toxins are leaving your body. Also, when you perform a cleanse, make sure that you do so under your physician's care.

Liver and Gall Bladder Cleanse

Keeping in mind that you're already eating a very natural diet and have banished boxed foods, many toxins have already started to leave the scene. Some blockages still need to be removed, however, if you want to look and feel your very best. Signs of liver and gall bladder trouble often appear on your skin as dryness, rashes, and eczema. Other signs include dizziness, headaches, tinnitus (ringing in the ears), mood swings, and anger.

> Traditional healers suggest that all cleanses should coincide with the full moon, as the pull of the moon helps to open our organs.

A number of cleanses are available for purchase at your local health products store. Simply follow the directions on the package. Look for products containing herbs that have been used traditionally for centuries to purify and strengthen the liver. Milk thistle, dandelion, and artichoke are good for cleansing, and licorice will help with inflammation.

Kidneys

As an organ of elimination, kidneys are also subject to blockage. Along with drinking adequate amounts of pure, filtered water, watch your salt intake if you are experiencing kidney trouble. Kidney cleanses are also available at your local health market, as are the kidney-strengthening gingko biloba and goldenseal. Uva ursi is good for pain and bloating, while vitamin C helps to relieve inflammation.

Colon

Headaches, skin blemishes, sallow or dull skin, bad breath, fatigue, constipation, bloating, and flatulence can all be linked to a congested colon. Colon and bowel problems are a big factor in early aging, too, as stagnant and fermenting foods allow toxins to enter the bloodstream and damage our cells. And if you need more encouragement for a cleanout, you could also lose several pounds by removing the "gunk" in your colon. Several cleanses are available to help loosen impacted feces from your bowel. Ask your health-care practitioner about colonic irrigation (colon hydrotherapy)—an effective method for cleansing the colon of waste material by repeated, gentle flushing with water. In a 45-minute session, approximately 15 gallons of water is used to gently flush the colon, eliminating far more toxic waste than in any other short-term technique.

With this method, there's no mess and no odor, and your privacy and potential embarrassment are respected throughout the process. Most people find the process quite relaxing and enjoy the feeling of "lightness" they experience afterwards.

Multiple products are also available on the market to help you create a clean slate. Follow your cleanse with a colon-friendly diet, including high-fiber fruits, vegetables, legumes, and whole grains. Absolutely avoid the "white foods" like white bread, white rice, white pasta, and white flour, which all become a pasty goo in your system.

As I was writing this section, I received an e-mail joke from my mother. Here it is: Why is it that when you mix water and flour together, you get glue, but when you add eggs and sugar, you get cake? Where did the glue go? Give up?

The glue is still there—it's what makes the cake stick to your thighs! It's also what makes it all stick to your insides.

The Keys to Your Own Sweet Ride

We've made it through most of the mucky bits on this journey. But remember, when it comes to your looks and your food choices, you can't make something amazing out of bad ingredients. The same holds true with choosing your supplements: all are not created equal. So do some research before you pick your brand. Focus on providing super-high-octane fuel, give your system regular maintenance, and don't blush when everyone starts looking at you with admiration!

Beauty Essentials for Digestion

Supplement	Amount	Nutrient Action
Digestive enzymes	Containing at least amylase, protease, lipase, and lactase. Follow label instructions	Everyone should take digestive enzymes to help digest cooked and prepared foods
Pancreatic enzymes and bile salts	Follow label instructions	Important additional requirement if your gall bladder has been removed
Essential Fatty Acids (EFAs): Flax Oil	1 to 2 tablespoons per day	Boost metabolism, improve digestion, promote cellular healing
Probiotics such as acidophilus/bifidus	5 to 10 billion viable units per day. Follow label instructions	Helpful for everyone to restore and maintain balance in intestines
Prebiotics (FOS)	1,000 mg per day	To nourish helpful bacteria

CHAPTER FOUR

Living Beauty Essentials at a Glance

Estranged from Beauty—none can be
For Beauty is Infinity
—Emily Dickinson

I've discussed the immune system and digestion in the first part of this book, because keeping these two systems strong will help melt away many of your health and beauty concerns:

1. You will build vitality with good antioxidant-filled foods and supplements, combined with adequate exercise and rest.

2. You will make the best use of your food by improving the efficiency of your digestion.

3. You will restore balance to your intestinal tract with food and lifestyle changes, coupled with digestion-boosting nutrients.

Living Beauty Essentials

In order to keep these systems in top working order—and to see the results in the mirror—be sure to take the following nutrients daily, in the amounts suggested at the ends of Chapters 2 and 3.

Multivitamin, Multimineral Formulation

Essential Fatty Acids (EFAs)

Probiotics

While I strongly encourage you to immediately avoid eating fried and sugary foods and focus your diet on fresh produce, lean protein, whole grains, nuts, and seeds, it's best if you gradually work into your new supplement regimen. Going slowly is particularly important if you're just starting out on your road to healthy beauty. I recommend adding supplements one at a time, giving your body a minimum of two weeks to adjust to one supplement before adding another. Start with the multivitamin/multimineral supplement first, then add probiotics or Essential Fatty Acids in the order that makes sense to you. Remember that no one knows your body as well as you do! After reading through this book, you should be able to identify symptoms that will guide your decision.

The Beauty Prescriptions: Therapeutic Use of Nutrients

As you learn more about your body systems, you will see that certain symptoms relate to nutrient deficiencies or imbalances. In order to correct these, you might require supplements in therapeutic doses. That simply means that you need more of a particular supplement than you get in your *Living Beauty Essentials*, in order for healing to occur. For some beauty concerns, for example, I will recommend that you take more Essential Fatty Acids (or vitamins/minerals or probiotics) than those suggested in the *Living Beauty Essentials* listed at the ends of Chapters 2 and 3. These extra amounts are shown in the *Beauty Prescriptions* that appear throughout the rest of this book. This, too, is to promote healing. Finally, in the *Beauty Prescriptions,* I also include herbs, minerals, and other nutrients that are *not* part of the *Living Beauty Essentials*.

In all cases, continue to take the *Living Beauty Essentials* (multivitamin/multimineral, EFAs, and probiotics) on a daily basis. But never exceed the amount shown for any nutrient listed in the *Beauty Prescriptions*. Use therapeutic amounts of a nutrient found in any given *Beauty Prescription* until you have achieved healing. Then reduce to the levels suggested in the *Living Beauty Essentials*. Before taking therapeutic doses of any nutrients or herbal preparations, however, always talk to your health-care provider about contraindications with any medications or conditions that you have.

Do note: If you are pregnant, or if you are breast feeding, remember the only safe levels of nutrients are those found in standard prenatal vitamins unless advised otherwise by your doctor for certain health conditions. Follow the Beauty Prescriptions only when you are not pregnant or when you are not breast feeding. Besides, with the maternal glow of pregnancy and new motherhood, you are already simply beautiful!

PART TWO
Beauty Prescriptions

CHAPTER FIVE

Facing *Candida* in the Mirror

That which is striking and beautiful is not always good; but that which is good is always beautiful.
—*Ninon De L'Enclos*

For years, I struggled with eczema. I would get it on my fingers, my lips, in and around my nostrils (I know, not so pretty!), and in spots on my arms and legs. One particular patch on my shin was about four inches long and two inches wide. It would often become infected from night-time scratching, and I would faithfully head to the doctor for a prescription cream that would make it go away. For two years I put those creams on that patch of skin and was amazed at how quickly they made my skin heal—until I stopped using them. As soon as I put the cream back in the drawer for what I thought should be the last time, the itchy tingling would start again, and in no time I would be looking at angry, red, oozing, and painful skin. I also noticed that using the creams to treat one patch seemed to cause a new spot of eczema to break out somewhere else. It was as if I were chasing eczema with the medication.

I tried "everything" to make it go away. Despite assurances from a dermatologist that food could not possibly be a factor in my eczema, I did start to pay attention to what foods made the condition worse. I cut wine and chocolate out of my diet, and yet the rashes wouldn't leave. I read up on alternative treatments for eczema and started taking therapeutic doses of Essential Fatty Acids (EFAs) and vitamins A, C, E, and B complex. (Therapeutic doses are those that exceed the minimal daily requirement that everyone should take each day.) After all this, there *was* an improvement in my general skin quality, yet the eczema persisted. In the meantime, I learned about *Candida,* which, you will recall from our chat about digestion, is a naturally present single-celled fungus in the digestive tract that can reproduce quickly in favorable circumstances. An overgrowth of *Candida* can lead to all sorts of problems that can appear far away from the digestive tract, including yeast infections, migraine, and even eczema. I had read about how to get rid of it, but it seemed like such an effort that I convinced myself that *Candida* wasn't my problem.

As most of us have been trained to do in North America, I kept looking for the fast, easy, one-stop solution. But as I faced yet another short Canadian summer with the lovely red patch clashing with my favorite skirts, I decided to bite the bullet and do the *Candida* cleanse. Within 30 days, the ugly red patch was gone. Not gone in the sense that it relocated to another place, but gone in the sense of "I don't have it anymore." I know what you might be thinking. If you had something as unpleasant-sounding as *Candida*, your doctor would know about it. Unfortunately, unless your doctor takes a "whole body" approach to healing, it's highly unlikely that he or she would associate your various symptoms and complaints with *Candida*. Western doctors aim to make your symptoms go away so you'll feel better, but they often do this without addressing the underlying cause of the symptoms.

> **Don't accept that your morning aches and pains, new-found forgetfulness, or lack of energy are an inescapable reality of growing older.**

Symptoms, however, have a purpose. They are the only way your body can tell you that things aren't quite right. So if you suppress those symptoms with medications, it won't take long for your body to come up with other symptoms to get your attention. If you ignore those, your body will then turn up the volume. By that time, however, a serious condition may be present. In all this, your body's goal, independent of your doctor and despite your possible neglect, is to be well. It's also important to understand that being healthy really means being symptom free. In other words, you can't claim that you're completely healthy just because the doctor gave you drugs for your various ailments and those symptoms no longer bother you. Don't accept that your morning aches and pains, new-found forgetfulness, or lack of energy are an inescapable reality of growing older. When you're 96 we can discuss that possibility! Right now, you are much too young.

So if you don't have a visible fungal infection on your body or an uncomfortable yeast infection, how could *Candida* possibly be your problem? I'm prepared to wager that, as you read this, the chances are very high that your body is struggling with *Candida* levels. *Candida* toxins travel to virtually all of your organs and tissues, and they've been associated with nearly every medical complaint known to man and woman, including headache, fatigue, and general aches and pains. *Candida* has also been associated with vague symptoms such as loss of memory, drowsiness, PMS, the inability to concentrate, confusion, and depression. It's often a factor in both hyper and hypothyroidism, as well as in adrenal gland function. If your body isn't sending you any of these signals of imbalance, it may be presenting you with acne, eczema, excessive sweating, hives, nail infections, flaky skin, or dandruff. Your body is sending you signals you can't ignore because some of them face you in the mirror.

> Are you troubled by sinus problems? A new study shows that 96% of sinus infections tested positive for fungus, and over 15% of the time, the fungus was produced by *Candida*.

Remember that your digestive system is an intricate process involving the right balance of acid and alkaline liquids, as well as a symbiotic relationship with the bacteria that reside in the intestines. Anything that disrupts the optimal functioning of your digestion opens the door for *Candida* to take over your bodily world. So coffee that diverts energy away from digestion may unlock the door, a sugar binge might nudge the door open, birth control pills or steroid medication for your eczema kick the door wide open, and drinking chlorinated water holds the door ajar.

The antibiotics we take to fight an infection can also contribute to the problem. As I mentioned in the previous chapter, these drugs do not just seek out and destroy the bacteria that are causing you difficulties; they blast away at everything in their path. So, while the antibiotics may help speed your recovery from an infection, they also leave your body unprotected by the bacterial police. If you are having a hard time accepting this explanation, look to your own body for proof. Often the side effects of taking oral antibiotics include upset stomach and diarrhea, problems linked with the digestive system. *Candida* is also given the green light by pregnancy, AIDS, high alcohol intake, refined (boxed) foods, pesticides, herbicides, or a diet lacking in fresh fruits and vegetables. Excess weight turns up the body heat—which yeast loves—and diabetes increases sugar levels, again a favorite of the yeasties. And, finally, if you don't recognize any of those as possible culprits, good old everyday stress plays havoc with our hormones, adrenal glands, thyroid, and digestion. Remember, the problem starts in your digestive tract. Take this test to see if *Candida* might be preventing you from looking and feeling your best. You might want to see how your family scores, as well.

Candida Questionnaire

In the following questionnaire, rate each of the possible effects of *Candida* that apply to you. In the column entitled **Week 1**, score yourself as follows: 3 for severe or frequently occurring; 2 for moderate or regularly occurring; and 1 for mild or rarely occurring. Leave blank any space that does not apply to you.

	Week 1	Week 3	Week 5	Week 7	Week 9
Acne					
Anger					
Anxiety					
Apathy					
Athlete's foot					
Bad breath					
Bed wetting					
Belching					
Birth control pill use					
Bloating					
Blurred vision					
Breast swelling					
Breathing difficulties					
Bruising					
Burning eyes					
Canker sores					
Circles under eyes					
Coated tongue (white)					
Cold hands and feet					
Confusion					

	Week 1	Week 3	Week 5	Week 7	Week 9
Constipation					
Crave alcohol, bread, sugars					
Dandruff					
Depression					
Diarrhea					
Dizziness					
Easy or unexpected weight gain					
Eczema					
Excessive ear wax					
Extreme fatigue					
Eyes dry, itchy, or watery					
Eyes sensitive to light					
Eyes have spots/floaters					
Fainting					
Feel worse on damp or snowy days					
Forgetfulness					
Frequent antibiotic use					
Frequent bladder infections					
Frequent sinus infections					
Fungal infections					
Fluid retention					
Flushing					
Gas					
Headache					
Hives					
Hyperactivity					
Impotence					
Increasing food sensitivities					
Insomnia					
Irritability					
Itchiness					
Itchy anus, ears, nose					
Joint aches					
Learning disorders					
Lethargy					
Liver spots (age spots)					

	Week 1	Week 3	Week 5	Week 7	Week 9
Loss of libido					
Low body temperature					
Low/high blood pressure					
Menstrual irregularities					
Migraine					
Mood swings					
Muscle aches					
Nasal congestion					
Nausea					
Night eating					
Numbness and tingling					
Pallor					
Poor concentration					
Pre-Menstrual Syndrome (PMS)					
Psoriasis					
Puffy eyes					
Rage					
Rash					
Red eyes					
Skin excessively dry or oily					
Sleepiness					
Spacey feelings					
Spontaneous bruising					
Thirst					
Thyroid problems					
Urgency to urinate					
Wheezing					
Yeast infections, recurrent					

(If you experience several of these symptoms you might be dealing with *Candida* overgrowth. Continue to use this chart to monitor your symptoms as you work to rebalance your system.)

Know Thine Enemy

If you've decided that a *Candida* imbalance may be affecting your life, it's time to learn what to do about it. Just as you can't fix a digestive problem until you understand how things are supposed to work, you won't be able to get rid of *Candida* without some advance knowledge of how it operates.

Let's pick up the digestion story at the intestines. Thousands of micro-organisms live here: some perform valuable services like food digestion, waste breakdown, and manufacture of vitamins. Others serve no useful purpose and have simply hitched on for the free ride. Because they don't bother us, we don't bother them, and we let them join the party. But like an obnoxious house guest who's had too much to drink, these little organisms sometimes get bold and start throwing their weight around.

Maybe, for example, your underactive stomach lets food pass that is not sufficiently broken down. That increases the burden on the other digestive organs like the pancreas, but it also starts to overwork the bacteria in our intestines that help with food breakdown. The result? Intestinal digestion slows to a crawl. You know this is going on if you experience gas, bloating, flatulence, and a foul-smelling stool. (With my apologies, again, for the graphic description!) The bacteria that came along for the free ride love this stagnant environment of decay, particularly if it's sweet, and they begin to multiply. They eventually outnumber the bacteria that are there to do some good. Then things start to get really ugly in the intestinal tract.

Leaky Gut

As these bacteria enjoy the banquet we've so graciously provided, they, too, release waste products, which happen to be toxic to us. These toxins eventually irritate the walls of our intestines, leading to inflammation. (Inflammation, you'll remember, triggers free radical production that causes much of the damage that we associate with aging.) To make matters worse, inflammation also causes tiny openings in the intestine to enlarge, leading to what is known as "porous bowel syndrome," or more commonly, "leaky gut." Having a leaky gut allows large, undigested food particles to pass undigested into the bloodstream. There, in an attempt to protect us from the food proteins that shouldn't be in our blood, the immune system launches an attack on the food particles, which, although harmless, shouldn't be floating around the bloodstream. This explains why leaky gut is often a factor in food sensitivities, particularly the ones that don't show up on standard allergy tests: when the immune system labels a particular food protein as a threat, it will attack whenever that protein is encountered in the body.

The *Candida* bacteria, still in the intestines, now grow extensions that act like feet, allowing them to grab on and root themselves there. By this point, they cease being known as harmless bacteria and are considered pathogenic. The newly formed yeasties exit the intestinal wall and enter the flow of the bloodstream, where they cruise along until they find an organ or tissue that looks like a nice place to raise a family. And like rabbits, they are prolific. Research shows that *Candida* has a competitive advantage over other fungal forms due to its ability to adapt to environmental stresses.

If you were to take the results of the *Candida* questionnaire to your GP and ask him for treatment, it's possible that, after an exaggerated roll of the eyes, he might offer you nystatin or some other drug to help kill the *Candida* fungus. The problem with this approach, however, is that unless you address the factors that allowed *Candida* to grow in the first place, the yeasties will be back. You can't continue to do the same things all the time and expect a different result.

The first step in saying a permanent goodbye to *Candida* is to make sure that your digestive system is firing on all burners. Partially digested foods that hang around too long are particular favorites of the yeasties. The next step is to starve the little critters by denying them their primary food source: sugar. If you've ever made bread the old-fashioned way, you know that yeast on its own does nothing to the mixture. When you add the sugar and keep the batter warm, however, the yeasties begin to multiply, creating gas that causes the bread to bloat—I mean rise. Well, the same scenario exists in your warm intestines. Without sugar, yeast doesn't function. So don't give the yeast any sugar.

The full-on *Candida* cleanse is intimidating. Some people are psychologically not ready for it, because it may involve changing some very comfortable habits. Others might have health challenges that would be worsened in the short term by jumping into the deep end of the cleansing pool. As the *Candida* dies, it releases toxins in your body that can cause your symptoms to become worse before they get better. I'm going to explain the complete protocol first, to show you where you might be heading, and then I'll backtrack to show you how to gain the benefits of the cleanse gradually.

If you are one of those people who are so frustrated with a skin condition or other problem listed in the *Candida* questionnaire that you plan to start the complete cleanse tomorrow, I caution you to obtain the guidance of a supportive health-care professional—particularly if you have an underlying health issue. For some people, it's much better to work into the cleanse gradually. If your medical doctor is not supportive or is unfamiliar with the strategy, look for a qualified naturopath or other medical adviser. A holistic nutritionist can also guide you through the process, but nutritionists are not qualified to give medical advice.

Although the goal is to starve the nasty critters virtually out of existence, you want to be sure that you're getting adequate nourishment yourself to support healing. Remember that the cleanse may last from three weeks to a few months. Of course, most people end up incorporating at least a few of these strategies into their lives after the formal "cleanse" ends. As you read the list of foods you'll have to give up, know that you will not have to eliminate them forever. All the same, the list is quite short, but powerful:

- **No sugar:** including refined white or brown sugar, glucose, fructose, malt sugar, etc.
- **No fruit:** contains too much sugar
- **No red meat:** digests too slowly
- **No dairy:** too much sugar. Unsweetened yogurt is allowed.
- **No alcohol:** diverts energy from digestion
- **No caffeine:** diverts energy from digestion
- **No fungus foods:** molds and mushrooms add fungus to your system
- **No nuts except almonds:** nuts often contain mold
- **No yeast:** we're trying to eliminate yeast!
- **No wheat:** difficult for many to digest

Are you already wondering what you're going to eat? Actually, you'll be surprised at your options. Think of this cleanse as an opportunity to try new foods. You can have as many of every single vegetable that you can possibly buy. Opt for fresh, not canned. (Canned produce is devoid of digestive enzymes and is often packed in sugar.) Eat raw foods when you can. Raw carrots, celery, and peppers are the perfect snack food. You can choose from chicken and turkey or fish if you enjoy meat. Eggs are fine too. Make sure that you buy *organic* meat, fish, and eggs to avoid antibiotics that will sabotage your cleansing effort. Instead of wheat, opt for rice, kamut, quinoa, or millet as your grain. My kids noticed the switch to rice pasta initially, but now it's all we eat. Look for yeast-free, sugar-free breads at the supermarket. You can often find them at the deli counter if they aren't in the bread aisle.

> ### Green Tea on the Grocery List
>
> Multiple studies show the benefits of drinking green tea, and protecting you from *Candida* is just one of them. Research done in Japan showed that plant nutrients called catechins in green tea have an anti-fungal effect against *Candida* and other fungal infections and may lead to a decreased need for anti-fungal medications. This is great news, particularly for those who experience side effects from these medications. Drink up!

For the purpose of this cleanse, tomatoes are a fruit, but you can have up to half a tomato per day. Do not eat canned tomatoes. If you think you can't live without fruit, opt for Granny Smith apples, as they are low in sugar. Again, allow yourself half an apple a day. And we certainly don't want to go to all the trouble of eliminating *Candida's* favorite foods and then give them leftovers to savor! Because foods break down at different rates, you can have a combination of partially digested food mixing with food that's starting to rot because it's broken down so quickly in your stomach. While the consequences of this are unpleasant and socially unacceptable to us, *Candida* loves the scenario. And whatever *Candida* loves has to go. To avoid fermentation, eat foods together only if they digest at a similar rate.

Food Combining Guidelines

How are you going to figure out what foods to eat together? Read on.

- Always eat fruit alone, at least half an hour before and two hours after other food.

• Be especially careful to avoid combining fruit with protein.

• Avoid mixing high-starch carbohydrates with protein. That means you should replace your meat-and-potatoes dinner with another option.

• You can eat high-starch vegetables (potatoes) with non-starch vegetables (broccoli). You can also combine protein with non-starch vegetables, so your chicken and vegetable stir-fry should be okay.

• Avoid eating at least three hours before going to bed.

As mentioned in Chapter 3, these are only *guidelines* to help you heal your digestive system, and they may not be beneficial for everyone all the time. If you burn calories very quickly, for instance, it would likely be better for you to use different combinations that slow down the digestive process, such as that meat and potatoes dinner. For the purposes of this cleanse, the point is to make sure any food that is in your digestive system in a given span of time will digest at about the same rate, so some isn't rotting away while the rest is taking its time to break down.

Portion Control

Getting optimal performance from the digestive system is not possible if it is overtaxed with extremely large portions. Use your own hand as a guide when filling your plate at mealtime:

• Complex carbohydrates in the form of whole grains: your entire hand, fingers closed.

• Complex carbohydrates in the form of vegetables: your entire hand, fingers outstretched.

• Protein (meat, fish): size of your palm.

Are You Still There?

I don't expect you to do this overnight. I know how hard it is to change so many food choices and habits at one time. So don't. Remember that it took me quite a while to get desperate enough to try the cleanse. But remember, as well, that it worked. What you need to do is make gradual changes so that eventually the full cleanse doesn't seem so painful.

Take the same approach that you did to improve your digestion. Change one or two habits or choices per week. If you drink double-double coffee, switch to double cream one sugar, then double cream no sugar, then just milk. Ask for half decaf and half regular. Go completely decaf. Go completely black. Have green tea. See how easy it is?

You'll learn two things in this process that you may not have known before. The first is that you don't "need" coffee to start, get through, or end the day. You may also make the distinction between what you think you want and "habit." You may learn, as I did, that it isn't so much the "thing" that you want; it's the comfort of the habit that you want. I used to have one cup of coffee every morning—just one—as I would sit with the kids at breakfast and then get them ready for school. I didn't want to give up the morning coffee because I didn't want to change my routine. I enjoyed it too much! But now that I've replaced coffee with green tea, the routine hasn't changed, just the beverage of choice. It's a similar challenge for those who smoke or drink. Aside from the obvious chemical dependencies that develop and must be broken if you want to quit, smoking and drinking have become behavioral habits for some people. When the phone rings, they'll reach for the cigarettes. Work ends; the gang heads to the bar. In the bar, the first sip of wine or beer suggests a cigarette, which is lit because it always has been. You have to find a new habit to replace the old habit. Believe it or not, your brain gets used to doing things a certain way. Shake things up a bit and get used to a new pattern of behavior. I'm not trying to say it's easy to break our behavioral addictions. I'm just pointing them out for those of us who have never considered ourselves to be addicted to anything. Like caffeine. Or sugar.

> If you drink double-double coffee, switch to double cream one sugar, then double cream no sugar, then just milk. Ask for half decaf and half regular. Go completely decaf. Go completely black. Have green tea. See how easy it is?

Sweet Addiction

You don't think it's possible to be addicted to sugar? That's probably because you haven't been "off" it long enough to go through withdrawal. The average adult consumes approximately 149 pounds of sugar per year, and it isn't always found in obvious locations. Take a look at the labels of the packaged foods in your cupboards. Soups, prepared foods, frozen dinners, sauces, salad dressings, canned vegetables, ketchup, salsa, pop—you name it, it likely contains sugar. Remember that fructose, glucose, maltose, dextrose (all the "ose" words), as well as corn syrup, rice syrup, maple syrup, barley malt, and honey are simple sugars with fancy names.

Eat more fresh produce and you'll cut down on your sugar. You can also ease out of refined sugar by eating more fruit. Full of natural sweetness, fruit will also give you vitamins, enzymes, and nutrients that will improve your energy levels and do amazing things for your complexion. Another easy step you can take is to stop eating white food: white flour, white bread, white pasta, and white rice are either full of sugar or empty of nutrients. Either way, you don't want them. Go for brown instead. Whole wheat breads or pasta, rice pasta, and brown rice are better choices. If you are the chief grocery buyer and chef in your home and "know" that your family will never eat these foods, I have a flash for you: they will. If they are hungry and there are no other choices in the house, they will eat. You may also slowly discover that you have less arguing in the house, easier bedtimes, easier wake-up times, and generally more pleasant children when sugar makes a gradual exit from your everyday lives.

Many of your favorite alcoholic beverages are also high in sugar. For a variety of reasons, you may want to consider reducing your alcohol intake: craving alcohol is a strong indicator of a *Candida* overgrowth, so you are on the right track with this cleanse if you are concerned about how much you drink. Alcohol use is associated with diabetes, high blood pressure, heart disease, and liver disease. It also dehydrates your cells, making your skin dry and prone to wrinkles. So, over a matter of weeks or months, you have prepared your body for the full *Candida* protocol. You have reduced your dependence on caffeine, cut back your intake of sugar, and hopefully strengthened your body through nutrients from the food choices above and the *Living Beauty Essentials* nutrients that you have now incorporated into your life. Despite your preparation, however, this cleanse might not be easy.

Nutrients

Starving *Candida* bacteria will bring them to a slow demise, but there are methods you can use to speed the die-off as well. Take cues from your own body and how you are feeling to determine how aggressive you should be in restoring *Candida* to harmless numbers. If you are in good health and do not have conditions that might be aggravated by the added stress of an aggressive cleanse, you can try the nutrients and herbs described below to help the process along. As always, talk to your health-care provider if you are uncertain. The nutrients are not harmful, but they are powerful. Since you aren't supposed to be drinking coffee, fruit teas, herbal teas, juices, or milk, you've probably realized by now that you will be drinking mostly good old water. This is probably a new situation for you, and the concept may not give you much joy. Remember, however, that you can add freshly squeezed lemon to your water to help with your digestive juices—but don't overdo it. Too much lemon juice may damage the enamel of your teeth. You can also try P'au D'arco tea. It's both antibacterial and anti-fungal, so it will promote cleansing, as well. It might take some getting used to, but after you've lost your dependence on sugar, you'll find P'au D'arco quite sweet. And clove tea is another tasty option.

> Don't be afraid that you'll lose a lot of friends if you start using Aged Garlic Extract. Aged garlic doesn't contribute to anti-social breath!

Garlic

Aged Garlic Extract is another powerful nutrient that you should include in your anti-fungal arsenal. Studies show that aged garlic is not only beneficial in the fight against *Candida*. It also enhances the growth of the beneficial bacteria *Lactobacillus acidophilus* and *Bifidobacterium bifidum*.

Don't be afraid that you'll lose a lot of friends if you start using Aged Garlic Extract. Aged garlic doesn't contribute to anti-social breath! When garlic is aged without heat, the sulfur-containing antioxidants are concentrated, and this diminishes garlic's signature smell. (Heated garlic supplements are also odor-free, as the heating process destroys many of the active ingredients.) Although garlic is a delicious and nutritious addition to any meal, you would have to eat 35 grams of raw garlic (approximately 10 cloves) to reproduce the effects of 1,800 milligrams of Aged Garlic Extract. Be sure that any product you buy is actually odorless and not treated with sugar or other coatings that simply mask the smell. Also look for a garlic product that is grown organically without chemical fertilizers or pesticides.

Caprylic acid is an anti-fungal agent derived from coconut butter that helps to destroy *Candida*. You can usually find it in either oil or capsule form. (Some people find the flavor of the oil hard to swallow, so if you have a delicate palate, you might want to choose the capsule!) Because all formulations are different, be sure to follow the label instructions. Also continue supplementing with your EFAs throughout your *Candida* cleanse. The Essential Fatty Acids will promote healing and help prevent damage to cells by pathogenic *Candida*. You may also consider using psyllium husk to boost your fiber intake. You want to be sure to eliminate debris from your bowel, and the psyllium husk will help you to do that. Remember that your goal is to have at least two bowel movements a day while on the cleanse—and always.

If you're using anti-fungal agents while cleansing, you may choose to stop using probiotic supplements, as they will be neutralized by the anti-fungal therapy. Using FOS (fructo-oligo-saccharides) prebiotic supplements might be more beneficial during the cleansing phase. You will recall that FOS are a group of naturally occurring carbohydrates that feed friendly flora, including *Lactobacillis acidophilus,* helping them to grow and multiply.

Cycles of Healing

The body is an amazing machine with one motivating goal: it wants to perform at peak levels all the time. But like any machine, it only works up to the capacity of the fuel that allows it to operate. Skimp on the quality of the fuel and you aren't going to achieve optimal performance. When you switch fuels from regular to high octane, however, changes are going to happen:

- **Caffeine Withdrawal:** Giving up this potent stimulating drug can cause headache, muscle ache, insomnia, fatigue, irritability, nausea, and a general feeling of unwellness. You will survive.

• **Sugar Withdrawal:** See previous page. This is the hardest one of all because you've likely never tried it before. You might feel as if you have the flu. Try not to take painkillers to cover the symptoms. Your body is releasing toxins, and over-the-counter medications can be toxic to your system. Use natural remedies when possible, including warm showers, cold eye compresses, and rest. For pain, herbal white willow bark (available at your health products store) is often effective.

You might question the sense of making yourself uncomfortable, but welcome to the irony of the *Candida* cleanse. Whatever symptoms of imbalance have driven you to try the cleanse (eczema, PMS, aching muscles, or fatigue, for instance) may worsen slightly in the short term. That's because your body will use the same avenues of symptomatic display it's always used to tell you that something weird is going on.

First, your body will process and eliminate the poisons that are easy to access—the ones in your digestive tract and bloodstream. As the toxins circulate through your body, you may not feel very well, and if you didn't know better, you'd think you had the flu. Then, as you continue to supply your body with the right nutrients, the repair process will kick up a notch. Cells that were pieced together with your old, inferior diet will gradually break down in a process called catabolism. So don't be surprised if you start to lose weight. If you're already thin or feel as if you are losing too much weight, consider increasing your intake of protein. It may be possible that you have a problem making use of protein or that you require more than others. Try adding a sugar-free protein supplement to your day. Although this diet takes a healthy approach to weight loss, remember to consult your medical adviser if you have concerns.

Continue feeding your body only good nutrients. Eventually, the inferior cells will be removed, and as a steady stream of optimal nutrition flows through your body, tissues will be rebuilt in a much stronger form. This rebuilding part of the cycle is called anabolism. You are on your way to feeling great and looking absolutely fabulous, but there will be rest-stops along the way. After your initial detox experience, you should feel better and have more energy than you did before you began.

Then you'll continue happily on your way, until one day you might feel a little flu-ish or under the weather. Perhaps you have a bout of diarrhea or a low-grade fever. This is a good thing! Your body is continuing its cleanup job. Try not to take any medications to suppress the symptoms. Again, white willow bark will help with aches, and rest is what your body really needs. This wave of discomfort will pass, and you will feel even better than you did before. Then you'll continue on your upward health climb until another cleansing phase sets in, and this time your symptoms may feel different. Again, do not treat the symptoms, as this can slow your progress. With proper nutrients, your body will start to heal and correct the imbalances that have developed over the years.

When Can I Stop?

Use the *Candida* questionnaire that appeared earlier in this chapter to track your progress in the cleanse. Continue to grade the severity of your symptoms every two weeks, and note when each symptom finally disappears. When most of the symptoms have decreased substantially or disappeared, you can lighten up on the rules. The cleanse will provide the best benefit if you pay attention to how you are feeling, both physically and mentally. Depending on the extent of your *Candida* problem, the cleanse will last from two or three weeks to several months. Your health-care adviser can help you decide when you are ready to reintroduce different foods.

Baby Yourself

If you are a mother, think back to when you started to give your little sunshine his or her first foods. (If you aren't a mother, trust me on this one.) Remember how you would introduce a new food every couple of days and watch to see if your baby had any reaction to the food? It's a good strategy, because it helps you try to isolate foods that might cause a problem. You have to take the same approach with yourself now, as you start to reintroduce foods into your diet. Many of the symptoms you were experiencing prior to the cleanse might have been caused by sensitivity to a certain food. If the sensitivity was caused by a food that you had eliminated for the purpose of cleansing, adding that food back

Food Diary

Week of:	1st Day	2nd Day	3rd Day	4th Day	5th Day	6th Day	7th Day
Morning							
Snack							
Lunch							
Snack							
Dinner							

to the menu might trigger the same symptom that it always has, but this time you will know which item in your diet is the culprit.

Make use of the food diary above to record what you eat and when and how you feel throughout the day. Mark any reactions (gas, bloating, headache) and the time when the symptom occurs. If a food causes any discomfort or a return of your symptoms, drop it from your menu for a while and try something else. After more time has passed, you can try the food again. If it still bothers you the next time, you've likely isolated a problem food that you should permanently remove from your menu.

After avoiding fruit for a month or more, you will absolutely marvel at its sweetness. (Who needs refined sugar, anyway?) Start expanding your diet with the addition of fruits, one at a time, in the morning, a few days apart. Pineapple is a good first choice, as it contains enzymes that will help you continue to clean out your system. Follow this a few days later with another low-sugar fruit, like Granny Smith apples. As the world of food opens up to you again, remember the consequences of overindulging and making unhealthy choices. That's how you got into this *Candida* predicament in the first place. And a funny thing may happen when the formal cleanse is finally over. You might like your glowing, rash-free, eczema-free skin. You may marvel at your energy—your ability to bounce out of bed in the morning and fall asleep quickly at night. You might even take a certain pleasure in the fact that your "thin clothes" fit. In the end, you may not want to lose the benefits you've gained by falling back into your old ways. So don't.

Continue to make *Candida*-unfriendly food choices, and keep the principles of food combining in mind as you start to put other foods back into your diet. Don't restart the coffee–sugar fast-food-late-night eating habits. Remember that sugar hides everywhere. Soup, ketchup, salsa, breads—even some brands of toothpaste—are sweetened with sugar. Become a label reader to be sure no refined sugar sneaks in.

I do still get eczema from time to time on my fingers and face, but I've learned that my skin is quite sensitive to the products I use. My skin even gets upset when I spend too much time in water. Stress can sometimes trigger a small spot, but when it occurs, I tighten up my diet for a few days and the eczema disappears.

Beauty Prescription for Eliminating *Candida*

Take your *Living Beauty Essentials* daily, as described in Chapters 2 and 3. You will see that, for this prescription, some of those nutrients should be taken in the higher daily-total amounts shown below, along with any extra nutrients listed in this table.

Caprylic acid	1,000–2,000 mg with meals
Aged Garlic Extract	2 capsules with each meal

Candida Sample Meal Plan and Recipes

Until your own imagination catches fire and you can create exciting *Candida*-free meals yourself, refer to the *Candida*-Free Menu Plan and Recipes appendix at the back of this book. You can use these recipes as a guide to healthy eating during and after the cleanse. The key to a successful cleanse lies in the variety of foods you can enjoy. Take the opportunity to try new foods and new ways of eating them.

Remember that eating foods raw preserves vital nutrients and precious enzymes, so try to think up tricks to avoid cooked and processed foods.

CHAPTER SIX

Hormones and Your Healthy Glow

Beauty—the adjustment of all parts proportionately so that one cannot add or subtract or change without impairing the harmony of the whole.

—*Leon Battista Alberti*

Okay, you don't want your *hormones* to glow, but healthy hormone function is important if you want to look and feel your best. Hormones are substances that are released from a gland or organ into the bloodstream and can be composed of amino acid chains, steroids, or fatty substances derived from cholesterol. They're the messengers in our bodies, telling our cells what to do, when to do it, and how quickly. Tiny quantities of a hormone can cause huge changes in the body. Among other duties, hormones control metabolism, blood pressure, bone formation, levels of sugar and salt in the blood, development and growth, sexual functions and characteristics, and reproduction. Although they work inside us, the effects of good (or bad) hormone function are visible on the outside. Hormones work in a delicate balance with one another, and too much or too little of one can have serious repercussions. Anyone who has experienced puberty knows first hand what a hormonal roller-coaster feels like. Any woman who transforms into a different person in the days or weeks before her period also has intimate knowledge of hormone swings. And menopause, well, that's just puberty in reverse. But there are other, non-natural factors that can, in fact, cause serious consequences. In this chapter I will focus on some of the major hormones, how they affect the smooth operation of our bodies, and how to support your hormonal system so that you can be the picture of health and beauty.

The Thyroid

You probably had no idea that thyroid health can affect your appearance, but alas, it can, in more ways than one. Let's start at the beginning. The thyroid is part of the team responsible for your metabolism, which involves such things as controlling body temperature, the synthesis of protein, and energy release from the cells. These functions are controlled by hormones T4 and the active form, T3. The liver manufactures about 80% of our T3 by converting it from T4, and the thyroid is responsible for the rest. The thyroid also secretes the hormone calcitonin, which works along with parathyroid hormone to control the balance of calcium in our blood and bones. This means that thyroid health is a factor in osteoporosis. Very simply, in the case of hyperthyroidism, or too *much* thyroid hormone, your metabolism becomes hyperactive and everything speeds up. In the case of too *little* thyroid hormone, or hypothyroidism, everything slows down. Look at the following chart for some of the common signs and symptoms of thyroid imbalance:

Symptoms of Thyroid Imbalance

Hyperthyroid	*Hypothyroid*
Increased sweat and moist skin	Dry, scaly, or wrinkled skin
Increased appetite and weight loss	Loss of appetite and weight gain
Frequent bowel movements	Constipation
Bulging, swollen eyes	Droopy eyelids
Eyes sensitive to light	Yellow bumps on eyelids
Hair loss	Dry, dull hair or hair loss (including eyebrows)
Trouble sleeping	Fatigue
Racing pulse	Slow pulse
Feel overheated	Intolerance to cold
Flushed skin	Yellow/orange skin coloration, especially on palms
Nails separating from nail bed	Face puffy
Decreased frequency of menstruation and flow	Fertility problems
Restlessness, irritability	Depression

Hypoglycemia is also a common result of thyroid hormone imbalance. If you are a woman who is approaching menopause, note that many symptoms of thyroid imbalance are similar to common menopausal symptoms. Don't simply assume that your symptoms indicate that you are perimenopausal or menopausal. Check it out. Low thyroid function is quite common, with approximately 25% of the population affected. In fact, those who are experiencing symptoms of hyperthyroidism often eventually find themselves dealing with an *underactive* thyroid, due to either thyroid exhaustion or treatment for hyperthyroidism. Women make up the majority of those with low thyroid function. If you suspect that you are experiencing thyroid imbalance, talk to your health-care practitioner.

> **Low thyroid function is quite common, with approximately 25% of the population affected. Women make up the majority of those affected.**

Know in advance, however, that the tests used to determine whether your thyroid is functioning properly may not accurately gauge your thyroid function. Let's assume for a moment that you recognize several of the symptoms in the column suggesting a hypothyroid condition. You take the list to your doctor, who respectfully orders up a blood test to see if you do have a hypothyroid condition. This test might only measure levels of T4 in your blood, but you will recall that T4 must be converted to T3 in order to be used by the body. It's possible that your circulating T4 levels are in a healthy range, but you might have a problem converting T4 to T3. Be sure to ask the doctor to test levels of both hormones. Remember, as well, that test results are judged by a standard based on averages: if you are in a certain range, you are diagnosed with a thyroid condition. If you fall outside that range, you are told that there is no problem. But a thyroid condition does not develop overnight.

Consider this: thyroid scores will be on the low-normal side in the case of hypothyroidism or on the high-normal side in the case of hyperthyroidism, but problems begin long before they eventually become evident through a blood test. Indeed, by the time the lab confirms an imbalance, it may be too late to try non-prescription drug alternatives to fix the problem. But you do have non-drug options for treating the problem if it is detected early. Few people would choose to be on prescription medications for the rest of their lives if they didn't have to be.

In alternative-treatment circles, thyroid imbalances that come in just under the laboratory radar are called "functional thyroid imbalances," and the great news is that, in cases like this, you can do plenty to support your thyroid.

Basal Metabolic Test

To test yourself for a functional thyroid imbalance, all you have to do is take your temperature twice a day for at least 10 days. Due to their normal hormonal fluctuations during the month, women should start recording their temperature on the first day of menstruation. Put the thermometer on your bedside table so you can take your temperature in the morning before you get up. Normal body temperature at rest falls between 97.8 and 98.2 degrees Fahrenheit. Then, sometime during the day, take your temperature again. Normal body temperature when you are active is 98.6 degrees Fahrenheit. The results are simple to decipher: a below-average body temperature suggests low thyroid function, while a higher-than-normal body temperature might indicate an overactive thyroid. You could also put some iodine on your skin, cover the area lightly with a bandage, and leave it overnight. Iodine is an essential nutrient in the manufacture of thyroid hormone. If the iodine disappears by morning (and isn't visible on the bandage!), assume that it has been absorbed by your body due to underactive thyroid function. Talk to your health-care practitioner about the results of your self-tests. If your medical doctor is not receptive to alternative methods of treatment, find one who is or locate a naturopath who can guide you with your healing.

Supporting the Thyroid

People with thyroid imbalance generally benefit from consuming more high-quality protein. If you have an imbalance, eat your largest meal at breakfast, and include protein with the meal. Avoid coffee, caffeine, alcohol, and nicotine. Avoid processed foods, and eat as many fresh, organic foods as you can. If you are concerned about an overactive thyroid, you must immediately seek medical attention. To support an overproductive gland, make sure that you improve your digestion by eating smaller, more frequent meals and by using digestive enzymes. Eat plenty of raw broccoli, cabbage, and other members of the *Brassica* family of vegetables, as well as peaches, pears, turnip, soybeans, pine nuts, peanuts, and millet. These foods contain goitrogens that can inhibit the absorption of iodine. Astragalus, a Chinese herb, helps support the immune system, as well as the thyroid and the adrenals. We'll talk more about the adrenals shortly. You might also try passion flower—an herbal tonic that may help to alleviate symptoms like anxiety and nervousness, without having a sedating effect.

You can support low thyroid function by making sure that you don't have a *Candida* overgrowth, as hypothyroid and *Candida* often go hand in hand. Re-read Chapter 5 if you suspect *Candida* to be a factor in your thyroid function. Since vitamin D is a co-factor in manufacturing thyroid hormone, a deficiency in this nutrient may also be connected with hypothyroidism. So if you live in a northern area, be sure that you get adequate sunlight or take supplemental vitamin D. If you have mercury fillings in your teeth, consider having them replaced, as research shows that mercury inhibits the liver's conversion of T4 to the active thyroid hormone T3. Mercury also displaces iodine in the body, and iodine is an essential nutrient in the manufacture of thyroid hormone. (Read Chapter 11, A Healthy, Beautiful Smile, for more information about replacing fillings.)

If you are diagnosed with hypothyroidism, eat plenty of iodine-rich foods, including beef, eggs, nuts and seeds, raisins, apricots, parsley, prunes, and chicken. Seafood and sea vegetables such as kelp, nori, and wakame are also excellent sources of iodine. In contrast to those who have hyperthyroid, if you have underactive thyroid function, you should limit or avoid food containing raw goitrogens. Heat helps to deactivate goitrogens, so cook your broccoli, cabbage, Brussels sprouts, and other *Brassica*-family vegetables before eating them. And don't forget your garlic. Studies show that Aged Garlic Extract can protect your blood cells against mercury in your system, so anyone with mercury amalgams should be sure to take supplemental garlic every day.

Certain herbs and nutrients have been used traditionally to support thyroid function. Supplemental iodine is helpful, of course. Ashwagandha is a traditional medicine that helps to increases levels of T4, while guggal extract helps to convert T4 to T3. L-Tyrosine, an amino acid, is necessary to produce thyroid hormones and is naturally present in bananas, almonds, and sesame seeds. The B vitamins, particularly pantothenic acid (B5), also help to ensure thyroid health by supporting adrenal gland function. For now, simply remember that when a thyroid hormone imbalance is suspected or confirmed, the thyroid is just one part of your body—and when it comes to your body, everything is related.

The Mysterious Adrenals

Western medicine pays very little attention to the adrenal glands—a surprising situation, considering that they produce our stress hormones. We have two adrenal glands, each consisting of two parts. The adrenal *cortex* produces hormones involved in regulating metabolism, reproduction, and mineral balancing, as well as excretory and immune-system functions. The *medulla*, on the other hand, triggers the "flight or fight" response and secretes adrenaline. You know what that feels like: racing heart, shallow breathing, dry throat, and tightness in the pit of your stomach. Blood flow to the brain, lungs, and muscles are all affected, as is cardiac output.

Corticosteroids, also secreted by the cortex, help us deal with long-term stressors, well after the initial threat and "flight or fight" response subsides. Chronic stress eventually causes adrenal exhaustion and can lead to chronic fatigue syndrome. Left untreated, low adrenal function can lead to Addison's disease—a potentially life-threatening illness. Anyone who has been prescribed corticosteroid drugs as part of their treatment for any condition is likely experiencing reduced adrenal gland function, simply due to the fact that the supplementation

Symptoms of Adrenal Exhaustion

- Loss of skin pigment
- Swollen extremities
- Puffy face
- Dark undereye circles
- Hair dry and thinning
- Beau's lines (depressions) on fingernails
- Skin conditions (eczema, psoriasis, rosacea)
- Muscle twitching
- Low energy
- Shortness of breath
- Heart palpitations
- Rapid pulse
- Neck or shoulder tension
- Frequent headaches
- Knee problems
- Cold feet
- Tightness in throat when upset
- Short temper
- Digestion problems
- Cravings for coffee, salt, sugar, junk food
- Dizziness upon rising
- Hypoglycemia
- Weight gain around middle

is required. Anyone suffering from a chronic disease commonly has under-functioning adrenals as a result of stress to the body. But you don't have to be sick (yet!) to show signs of adrenal exhaustion.

Here's a simple test of your adrenal gland function. It involves comparing your blood pressure while lying down to your standing blood pressure. For a healthy individual, the act of lying down involves little energy, so blood pressure is typically lower when you are in that posture. Since standing up requires more effort, the heart has to work harder, and logically, blood pressure should increase slightly. For someone with adrenal exhaustion, however, standing up causes blood pressure to drop. To see how your adrenal function rates, take your blood pressure while lying down. Then stand up and immediately measure your blood pressure again. Suspect adrenal exhaustion if your blood pressure drops when you stand.

> **Tooth Truth**
>
> Tooth infections, damaged or decayed teeth, problems with root canals, gingivitis, and other gum infections can also lead to adrenal exhaustion because they cause you stress. And research shows that the mercury from the fillings in your mouth can affect your adrenal gland function, leading to fatigue and possibly chronic fatigue syndrome. If you've started to experience fatigue since having dental work done or have simply tried every other option to combat unrelenting weariness, you might want to talk to a holistic dentist who could possibly make a few changes in your mouth. (Read Chapter 11, A Healthy, Beautiful Smile, for more information.)

Supporting the Adrenals

The best way to give your adrenals a rest is to decrease the stress in your life. You know what stress is. It's the traffic jam on the way to the airport, the workaholic boss with one little favor to ask, or your two-year-old—on his back in the cereal aisle screaming for the colorful frosted kind while everyone for miles passes judgment on your parenting skills. Frankly, if you thought you could fit "relaxing" into the remaining six seconds that you have to yourself in a day, you'd do it! Don't worry, I'll give you a few suggestions for making peace a reality in your life, but first let's see if you recognize any of these signs of stress:

> **Chronic stress eventually causes adrenal exhaustion and can lead to chronic fatigue syndrome. Left untreated, low adrenal function can lead to Addison's disease—a potentially life-threatening illness.**

Stress Test

Give yourself one point for each item that applies to you:

Poor concentration	Impatient with people
Shortness of breath	Make a "big deal" of everything
Fail to get a break from noise	Tightness in the stomach
Have few supportive relationships	Frequent colds or illnesses
Procrastinate	Itchy skin or skin rashes
Try to do everything yourself	Feel overwhelmed
Gossip	Decreased libido
Skip meals	Fatigue
Eat junk food	Fitful sleep
Neglect exercise	Prolonged or intense anger

If you score between **0** *and* **4**, *your life is relatively hassle free. Do not shy away from interesting challenges!*

5–10 *means that you have your priorities in order. Continue to find ways to relax and limit stress.*

11–15 *puts you in the danger zone. Find time to de-stress or your relationships might start to suffer!*

16+ *denotes a serious level of stress in your life that may lead to health problems! Focus on improving your diet, exercising for a few minutes per day, and schedule time to relax.*

Coping Strategies

There are tried-and-true stress-busters to reduce the pressure in your life without adding more to your "to do" list! First of all, ditch the "to do" list and replace it with a good daily planner to record your daily, weekly, and monthly goals. Use the same book for both business and social-family commitments, so there will be less likelihood of forgetting to pick up your daughter at ballet class. You'll also know at a glance if your boss has asked for one favor too many, and what weekend is good for out-of-town guests.

You should also find a "calmness" trigger word or phrase. It's the word that you will repeat to yourself, quietly or out loud, whenever you feel that familiar tightening in your stomach. Make it a word that you associate with feelings of tranquility. Practice repeating the phrase whenever you have a few free minutes, like in your morning shower.

Gradually, you will feel your breath becoming slower and deeper, your muscles unclenching, and your mind coming to a point of rest. Believe it or not, this is meditating. Daily practice of relaxation techniques can reduce your body's reaction to stress hormones, not only for the length of time that you spend soaking in the tub or doing yoga, but for the entire day. You'll see benefits with as little as 10 minutes of relaxation time per day! Try yoga, art class, or even therapy if you think it will help you deal with the stresses in your life. Consider working with a life coach, who can help you focus on your priorities and minimize your extra burdens. And don't underestimate the power of a time-out when you feel your tension levels rising. It worked for your two-year-old after that horrifying grocery store incident, so why wouldn't it work for you? Removing yourself from the stress for as little as five minutes will give you the ability to switch your focus from worrying about the problem to creating possible solutions.

Since stress is a natural (and sometimes life-saving!) reaction to a perceived threat, your body prepares for action when you are in a stressful situation. In the time of our ancestors, this response put blood in a person's extremities so they could run or fight to save themselves from predators. Most of us don't often face such threats anymore, but our bodies still react to stress with an ancient instinct that provides us with tons of energy. It makes sense, then, that one of the best ways to de-stress is to give your body what it is expecting. Move! Exercise will give you the ultimate relief, and you should find a way to fit a cardiovascular workout into your schedule at least four times a week for about half an hour each session. During the workday, use the stairs instead of the elevator. Get up off your chair and stretch. Walk around the block before you eat lunch. In fact, walk to the video store and rent a comedy to watch with your family after dinner—because laughter lowers levels of the stress hormone cortisol, which can be so damaging to your immune system and which ultimately leads to poor health and disease.

Time with your loved ones and time spent in spiritual pursuits will help you keep your stress levels in check, as well. Spirituality does not necessary imply meditation and prayer, though they are powerful tools. You can experience spirituality in many ways: absorbing the fragrance of a flower, losing yourself in some beautiful music, taking a hike in the woods. In fact, any activity that brings you joy—gardening, cooking, dancing, grooming your dog—can decrease stress and help to bring peace.

Don't think you have extra time in the day to relax? Sing in the car on the way to work. No one can hear you—and so what if they can! Buy some flowers for the dinner table when you stop at the grocery store on the way home and get lost in their beauty as you enjoy your meal. And stop thinking that life is supposed to be easy. If we accept that a few rough patches are inevitable, they won't be as hard to deal with when we face them. Even beautiful roses have thorns.

The most important change you need to make is to remove bad coping strategies from your life. Cigarettes, alcohol, and poor diet are detrimental in so many ways, but when you are stressed, your body uses up more vitamins and minerals so you are at even greater risk if you are consuming the wrong things. You must make sure that you're getting enough vitamins and minerals in your diet or through supplementation. Otherwise, when stressed out, you're going to get sick. Eat a balanced diet that includes plenty of fresh, organic fruits and vegetables, including rich sources of vitamins C, E, and B complex. If you suspect that your liver has also been overworked (and this is true for most people), a liver cleanse will help your adrenals as well.

Because you don't want to be stressed *and* irritable, aim for eight hours of sleep each night. Avoid adding to your problems by worrying about your stress level; remember that the only way to be totally stress free involves a flat line on a cardiogram! And don't forget the easiest de-stressing strategy of all: filling your lungs with a deep breath puts more oxygen into your bloodstream and gives your body the tools it needs to cope. Remember that chronic stress has a significant effect on your health. It affects virtually every part of the body, leading to physical, mental, and emotional symptoms. Stress causes our adrenal glands to secrete an excess amount of a hormone called cortisol, and high levels of cortisol cause cell death in organs involved in our immune system—including the thymus, the spleen, and the lymph nodes. Don't forget that the immune system is our defense against everything from the common cold to big guns like cancer. So don't let stress take over. It can have a powerful impact on your body, but only if you allow it to.

Nutrients

Nutrients known for their ability to support adrenal gland function are called adaptogens, because they help the body adapt to stress and maintain balance. Ashwagandha has been used in traditional Indian medicine for thousands of years and is starting to become popular in the West as an adaptogen. Siberian ginseng is also known to provide support for the immune system, as well as for adrenal function. Another powerful adaptogen is Aged Garlic Extract. Clinical studies show that Aged Garlic Extract not only works to prevent the elevation of the stress hormone cortisol, but also increases levels of the neurotransmitter serotonin, which is often depleted by stress. Serotonin helps to elevate mood, improve sleep, and increase energy.

Hypoglycemia

Hypoglycemia results from a pancreas that is working overtime to keep up with the body's requirements for the hormone insulin, typically because the diet is too high in concentrated sugars and starches. Insulin is necessary to allow glucose (sugar) to enter our cells. Hypoglycemia is also linked with adrenal exhaustion, thyroid imbalance, *Candida* overgrowth, and PMS. Do you believe me yet when I say that everything is related?

The antidote to hypoglycemia is to limit your intake of refined carbohydrates (such as sugary snacks and boxed foods). Eat small, frequent meals, and focus on choosing fresh, raw fruits and vegetables. Avoid caffeine, alcohol, and cigarettes, as these can affect blood sugar levels. Be sure to take your multivitamin/multimineral supplement every day.

> ### Symptoms of Hypoglycemia
> • Strong cravings for alcohol, coffee, or desserts
> • Heavy consumption of alcohol, coffee, or desserts
> • Anxiety relieved by eating
> • Irritable if meal is late or missed
> • Shakiness or trembling if meal is late
> • Overweight
> • Family history of diabetes
> • Frequent headache
> • Short temper

The Sex Hormones

The term "estrogen" is used to classify a group of hormones that contains two dozen estrogens at least. The most important ones are estrone, estradiol, and estriol. Estriol is considered to be the safest form of estrogen, as the other two have the potential to become dangerous in our bodies. Along with their familiar roles in development, menstruation, and reproduction, estrogens are also important for both women and men in bone development and in keeping our skin looking healthy and youthful. Unfortunately, estrogen also has a dark side. Having too much estrogen in relation to other hormones is called estrogen imbalance, or estrogen dominance. Excess estrogen in relation to other hormones like progesterone leads to PMS, including symptoms such as bloating, swollen breasts, irritability, depression, and insomnia. Estrogen dominance can also lead to increased blood pressure, endometriosis, and other conditions of the reproductive system, as well as decreased thyroid function—to name but a few consequences. Too much of the wrong type of estrogen can also lead to breast cancer.

In the appearance department, you can also sometimes blame an estrogen imbalance for your weight gain, acne, hair loss, increased facial hair, or accelerated aging. You might be surprised to learn that estrogen dominance is not necessarily a result of having too much estrogen: the key is how much estrogen a woman has in relation to progesterone. Ovulation is the term used for the release of an egg, and this triggers the production of progesterone. Less progesterone means excess estrogen in some women. For instance, if progesterone levels fall further or faster than estrogen levels, estrogen dominates. Several factors contribute to estrogen dominance, including diet, congested liver, alcohol consumption, or the length of time a woman may go without ovulating.

The diet and liver work hand in hand in the case of estrogen dominance. The liver is charged with detoxifying our bodies, including removing excess estrogen. A clogged liver can't detoxify anything properly, including natural hormones. But when the system is working efficiently, the liver sends excess estrogen to the intestines for elimination from the body. Here is where diet comes into play. Women who don't eat enough fiber typically have more problems with estrogen dominance. Fiber, in the form of fruits, vegetables, and whole grains, acts as a broom that helps to sweep the bowel clean. Without the broom, debris lingers too long in the intestinal tract, causing estrogen to be reabsorbed into the bloodstream. Our dietary choices also affect estrogen levels in our bodies, because some foods contain xenoestrogens (pronounced "zeeno"-estrogens), or estrogen-mimics.

Unfortunately, we eat a lot of xenoestrogens if we regularly consume non-organice foods, as pesticides and fertilizers are well-known estrogen-mimics. Although DDT has been banned for use in North America for decades, it is still readily found in the fat stores of wildlife worldwide. PBBs, PCBs, and the DDT metabolite DDE are all found in our food supply and have estrogen-like properties. We also meet up with xenoestrogens in our personal care products, but those will be discussed in Chapter 13, If Looks Could Kill.

How Do Xenoestrogens Work?

As I mentioned earlier in this chapter, tiny quantities of a hormone can cause huge changes in the body. But how do they make those changes? They get right in there and alter cellular function by binding to a cell at the hormone receptor site. Think of the receptor sites as the gameboard of the children's game Perfection®. In this game, players must try to fit differently shaped game pieces into the matching space on the gameboard. A star shape, for example, will only fit into the star-shaped hole. The star-shaped piece won't fit into a square hole no matter how clever you try to be. The same is supposed to be true of hormones, where only the right fit should match up. This is how the body tries to guarantee that the right things occur—but things don't always happen as they should.

In the hormonal "Perfection" game, the hormones match up (or bind) to the appropriate receptor site and affect the cell's function by slowing down or speeding up the cell and opening or closing it to other substances. The hormone, in effect, tells the cell what to do. This is a normal part of our body's function, but when xenoestrogens come onto the scene, things start to go haywire because these estrogen-mimics *look* like, *walk* like, and *act* like the real thing. They fit right into the hormonal gameboard, binding easily with the estrogen receptor sites on our cells. Unlike our natural hormones that do their job and move on, however, estrogen-mimics aren't as easy to turn off. They cause cellular functions to change, often with undesirable results. False estrogens, for example, have been found to trigger breast cancer cell lines, and have been associated with other forms of estrogen-related cancers, as well.

Because, our hormones are designed to operate in a delicate balance with each other, when xenoestrogens attach to our cellular receptor sites and hang around for a while, they can lead to estrogen dominance. (That's why these mimics are also called hormone disruptors.) We only need to think back to the 1950s and 1960s to see the results of hormone disruptors at work. In those years, women were given the synthetic estrogen diethylstilbestrol (DES) to prevent miscarriages. Not only did DES not work as intended, but when the daughters of these women reached their teens, it became evident that the girls had been born with birth defects of the ovaries and uterus. They also experienced high rates of unusual vaginal cancers. We need to be aware of the potential threat associated with these false estrogens.

Take Control of Your Estrogen

Premenstrual Syndrome (PMS) has become the subject of many jokes, and most people, unfortunately, believe that PMS is a necessary evil. The truth is that women can make changes in their diets and lifestyles that will virtually eliminate the monthly joke-spawning cycle. Many of these recommendations will help women dealing with menopause, as well, because estrogen imbalance is at the root of both conditions. Be sure to eat as many organic foods as you can, to limit your dietary intake of xenoestrogens. Try giving up non-organic dairy products, as cows on non-organic farms may eat food that has been treated with artificial fertilizers and pesticides. Although you may think that organic products are more expensive, in the long run, you may be saving your health—and avoiding the expenses that come with illness. Bulk up on the fiber in your diet with fruits, vegetables, and whole grains (not white bread!) to keep things moving through your intestinal tract. Avoid alcohol, as it is known to raise estrogen levels in women. Follow the *Candida* diet outlined in Chapter 5. Even if you don't think you have

Candida, you might notice some of your PMS or menopause symptoms disappearing when you follow a more natural diet. You may also want to use your food choices to beat estrogen at its own game. Some plant foods contain healthy estrogen-mimics called phytoestrogens. ("Phyto" simply means "plant.") Phytoestrogens have estrogenic and anti-estrogenic effects, acting to provide hormonal balance. These dietary estrogens latch onto our receptor sites, effectively blocking the effects of both our natural estrogens and the xenoestrogens that may be circulating in our bodies.

The excess estrogens and xenoestrogens then make their way to the liver to be detoxified and escorted to the intestines for removal. Phytoestrogens have other advantages too: they exert a much weaker estrogenic effect than other forms, are not stored in the body, and can be easily dismantled and removed. Phytoestrogens are found in herbs, grains, and fruits. Among them are isoflavones (such as the daidzein and genistein found in soybeans and fermented soy products). Lignans are another form of phystoestrogen, typically found in legumes, cereal bran, and flaxseed. Flax is the richest known plant source of lignans, containing up to hundreds of times more lignans than other sources. The third grouping of phytoestrogens is known as the coumestans, and these are found in alfalfa and clover. Research shows that adding a small amount of phytoestrogens to your diet may help restore estrogen balance. Talk to your health-care provider about using phytoestrogens to help with your PMS or menopausal symptoms.

> **Fabulous Flax**
>
> Grind two tablespoons of flaxseed daily and add it to your cereal, yoghurt, or salad. Flax is an excellent source of lignan precursors. And lignans are now being studied for their potential to prevent the development of breast cancer and other cancers. Flax is also a source of Omega-3 fatty acids!

Nutrients for PMS, Perimenopause, and Menopause

Many women experience hormone surges either around the time of their period or during the perimenopausal and menopausal years. (Perimenopause is the time leading up to the menopause, which is the permanent cessation of menstruation.) It's important to understand that, throughout the month and throughout a woman's life, estrogen levels might rise or progesterone levels might be on the upswing. Alternatively, fluctuations can also cause either estrogen or progesterone levels to fall, and even if estrogen levels are on the decline as menopause approaches, a woman could be estrogen-dominant if progesterone levels are too low. Although you might not know what is going on inside your body, you might be familiar with how hormone fluctuation can make you feel. If you experience premenstrual syndrome (PMS) or the symptoms of perimenopause or menopause, you'll be interested in some herbs that have been used for centuries to ease female complaints!

Black cohosh exerts a mild estrogenic effect and has been used to treat mood swings, fatigue, and hot flashes caused by low estrogen levels. There are no known drug interactions with this herb. Vitex, or chasteberry, encourages the production of progesterone, thereby balancing estrogen. It has been used extensively for PMS, breast swelling, and acne. It is also useful for symptoms of perimenopause. The phytoestrogens daidzein and genistein are ample in soybeans and are used for menopausal symptoms and to prevent bone loss. They are typically listed as soy isoflavones on product labels, in case you are searching at the health products store for herbal relief of your symptoms. And don't forget the phytoestrogen lignans found in flax! Essential Fatty Acids (EFAs), particularly gamma-linolenic acid (GLA), found in borage oil (20–22% GLA) and evening primrose oil (8–10% GLA) are especially helpful for women who experience PMS.

Not for Women Only

Many people don't realize that estrogen is a naturally occurring hormone in men's bodies, as well. Males create their estrogen through the mechanism of aromatase enzymes, which actually convert male androgens to estrogen in gonadal and other tissues. Although there are still many unanswered questions about the impact of estrogen on men, so far science has discovered that the hormone is beneficial in bone development, coordination, and cognitive function—and it may even help prevent Alzheimer's disease. Yet too much estrogen leads to the feminization of males, including excessive development of breasts.

Estrogen dominance in men frequently occurs due to a decrease in the male hormone testosterone, which often accompanies aging. Age also causes testosterone to bind with sex-hormone-binding-globulin (SHBG), which inactivates the testosterone. At the same time, SHBG increases estrogen production, leading to estrogen dominance. Most notably, a drop in testosterone leads to a decline in sex drive. The interelationship with our hormones becomes significant when we consider that the adrenal gland also helps produce the androgens that are converted to estrogen. This production tends to decline with age, and as we have already discussed, many people are walking around with exhausted adrenals! It also appears that men with hyperthyroidism have increased levels of the estrogen estradiol in their blood.

And then there's the effect of alcohol consumption. Studies show that alcohol intake encourages the conversion of androgens to estrogens in the liver. That is why alcoholic men are known to develop breasts. Animal studies have also indicated that alcohol consumption causes gonads to shrink and sperm production to diminish. Other lifestyle choices also affect hormone balance in men. As with women, extra body fat in males encourages estrogen dominance. In men, fat cells produce the aromatase enzymes that convert androgen into estrogen. Low-fiber diets are also associated with higher estrogen levels, as estrogen is not eliminated from the bowel fast enough and becomes reabsorbed. And we can't underestimate the power of xenoestrogens in our men.

> A 1995 review studying the fate of the endangered Florida panther indicated that environmental hormone disruptors, including DDE, mercury, and polychlorinated biphenyls (PCBs) has caused feminization of the male panther.

Chemicals in fertilizers and pesticides produce undesirable estrogenic effects for our males; we need only look at our wildlife to see the dangers this entails. A 1995 review studying the fate of the endangered Florida panther indicated that environmental hormone disruptors, including DDE, mercury, and polychlorinated biphenyls (PCBs) has caused feminization of the male panther. Results show that there is no longer a significant difference in estradiol levels between the male and female panthers and that males have been demasculinized as a result of exposure to these xenoestrogens. The researchers concluded that environmental contaminants might be a major factor contributing to reproductive problems for the Florida panther. And what's bad for panthers may also be bad for humans. Remember that these contaminants are the same ones that coat many parts of our food supply as well.

Shifting the Balance of Power

But, gentlemen, there is some good news. You can do many things to help put estrogen in its proper and healthy place. Limit alcohol consumption, and be sure to eat more fiber to help eliminate excess estrogen from your body. Focus your diet on organic fruits, vegetables, meats, and fish to limit exposure to dietary estrogens from fertilizers and pesticides. Re-read the section on cleansing and supporting the liver in Chapter 3. (When the liver is functioning optimally, estrogen is more readily cleared out of the system.) Be sure to support your adrenal glands to promote the healthy production of androgens, and address any thyroid imbalance. I've said it before and I don't mind repeating it, everything in our bodies is connected! Mothers of young boys should be cautious about the amount of soy that could sneak into their diets. Studies suggest that we are getting too many of the phytoestrogens found in soy, not only in products like soy milk and tofu, but also in soy oils used in prepared foods. No food is a perfect food, and we must remember this about soy as well. Remember to read labels and keep a tally! All things in moderation.

Beauty Prescription for Healthy Hormones

Take your *Living Beauty Essentials* daily, as described in Chapters 2 and 3. You will see that, for this prescription, some of those nutrients should be taken in the higher daily-total amounts shown below, along with any extra nutrients listed in this table.

Thyroid health		*Total Daily Amount*
Hyperthyroid	Siberian ginseng	100–300 mg extract, once or twice per day (max. 600 mg daily)
	Vitamin B complex	50 mg, 2 times per day (max. 100 mg daily)
	Vitamin C with bioflavonoids	3,000–5,000 mg or to bowel tolerance, in 2–3 equally divided doses.

Thyroid health		Total Daily Amount
Hyperthyroid (cont.)	Vitamin E	Do not exceed 400 IU
Hypothyroid	Siberian ginseng	100–300 mg extract, once or twice per day (max. 600 mg)
	Vitamin B complex	50 mg, 2 times per day (max. 100 mg daily)
	Vitamin C with bioflavonoids	Do not exceed 2,000 mg; in 1–2 equally divided doses
Adrenal gland support	Siberian ginseng	100–300 mg extract, once or twice per day (max. 600 mg)
	Ashwagandha	300 mg standardized extract, 2–4 times per day (max. 1,200 mg daily)
PMS To stabilize mood	Borage oil	Increase to 1,000–3,000mg
Anxiety, sadness	St. John's Wort	300 mg extract (standardized to 0.3% hypericin)
Irritability	Black cohosh	40 mg
Menopause Irritability / Night sweats	Black cohosh	40 mg
Anxiety / sadness	St. John's Wort	300 mg extract (standardized to 0.3% hypericin)

CHAPTER SEVEN

All About Skin

Wrinkles should merely indicate where smiles have been.
—*Mark Twain*

Our skin is probably the most underappreciated, abused, and misunderstood part of our bodies. As our largest organ, it makes up between 12% and 15% of our total body weight and covers a surface area of approximately 1 to 2 meters. Skin is our first line of defense against the outside world. As a physical barrier, skin keeps our insides from getting out, and it keeps the outside from getting in. It's involved in touch, pressure, absorption, elimination, and detoxification. It plays a large role in regulating our body temperature and in the manufacture of vitamin D. Specialized skin cells also determine what color we are and how deeply we will tan. With such a long list of chores, it's remarkable to consider that our skin is only about half a millimeter thick on our eyelids and only three millimeters thick on our palms and the soles of our feet. In fact, skin depth is often compared to the thickness of tissue paper.

Just the Facts

The *epidermis* is the skin that you can see and touch. The bottom layer of the epidermis is known, appropriately enough, as the basal layer, and this is where new skin cells are formed. As the new cells are pushed upward toward the surface, they flatten, and when you can finally see them, they are already dead. The skin cycle takes approximately two weeks when we are young, but slows to a month or more as we age. This is one explanation why older skins are slower to heal than younger ones. Although the epidermis houses our melanin (pigment) and some nerve endings, there are no blood vessels in this layer. The second layer of the skin is called the *dermis*, and this layer provides structure and strength to the skin. Contained in the dermis are the collagen and

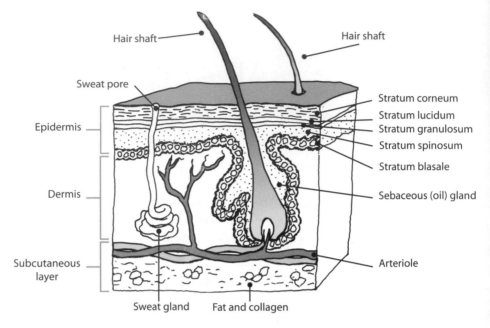

Hair shaft

Hair shaft

Sweat pore

Stratum corneum
Stratum lucidum
Stratum granulosum

Epidermis

Stratum spinosum

Stratum blasale

Dermis

Sebaceous (oil) gland

Subcutaneous
layer

Arteriole

Sweat gland   Fat and collagen

Anatomy of the Skin

elastin fibers you've likely heard about in television commercials for skin-care products.

Collagen is a strong, fibrous protein that accounts for 70% of the dry weight of our skin. Elastin, like a rubber band, gives our skin some snap and keeps it in place. Hair follicles, oil glands, and sweat glands are located in the dermis. Immediately below the dermis is a layer of insulating fat. Oil glands generally open into the hair follicle, and they manufacture fats and oils known as sebum. Sebum is used to keep skin soft and pliable, to control moisture retention, and to prevent excess water absorption. Sebum also helps prevent heat loss from the skin, as fats are poor conductors of heat. Sweat glands, on the other hand, regulate heat by secreting moisture, which evaporates and helps us stay cool. These glands are also a major exit point for toxins and waste, and that is why they should be kept clean and clear. (See Chapter 8, Your Skin Doesn't Stop at Your Neck, for more discussion about this topic.) Meanwhile, dead skin cells are shed regularly as enzymes dissolve the structures that bind cells together. Loss of dead and contaminated cells triggers the dermis to create more collagen and elastin and inspires the epidermis to produce more skin cells.

Skin Nutrient A, B, Cs

When we talked earlier about the immune system (you remember Big Burly Mike?), we discussed free radicals and how they cause aging and damage by stealing a little bit from every cell they touch. The antidotes to free radicals, you'll remember, are antioxidants. These vitamins and other nutrients give the temperamental free radicals what they want, so that they stop pillaging cells. As if there were a divine plan guiding the workings of our cells, many of these antioxidants come from our food and arrive in the form of vitamins. Interestingly, these are the same vitamins we need to keep our skin strong and healthy! What a coincidence ... As a brief review, our bodies need a variety of antioxidants not only for our health, but also for good-looking skin:

> As if there were a divine plan guiding the workings of our cells, many of these antioxidants come from our food and arrive in the form of vitamins.

- **Vitamin A** is necessary for new cell growth, and it's essential for the mucous membranes that line your mouth, throat, and stomach.

- The **B vitamins** in a complex formulation are required for the maintenance of healthy skin and hair. B vitamins also help maintain healthy blood, metabolize carbohydrates, and support immune function.

- **Vitamin C** helps keep our blood from clotting abnormally and protects against bruising. This vitamin is a crucial component in the formation of collagen.

- **Vitamin D** promotes the healthy development of immature skin cells as they journey from the lower epidermis to the outer layers. It also helps to slow cell division—a trait that is useful for cancer prevention and psoriasis treatments.

- **Vitamin E** is a fat-soluble vitamin that prevents free radical damage to the fats that make up cell membranes. It is also vital for tissue repair, wound healing, and scar reduction.

- **Selenium** is a very powerful antioxidant that is essential for the integrity of our skin.

- **Essential Fatty Acids** (EFAs) make the skin moist, smooth, and supple. These fats also help to create anti-inflammatory chemicals in the body. The most important beneficial fatty acids are alpha-linolenic acid (ALA) from flaxseed, gamma linolenic acid (GLA) from borage oil, eicosapentaenoic acid (EPA) and docosahexaenoic acid (DHA) from fish oils. For infant growth and development, arachidonic acid (AA) is also crucial, but the North American adult diet typically provides more AA than our bodies require. Excess AA from eggs, fish, and meat produces inflammatory mediators and contributes to inflammation, chronic disease, and aging.

And you'll be happy to learn that all of these nutrients also help protect you from the sun.

Here Comes the Sun

I don't know if it's because I live in a northern climate and never get enough summer for my liking or if it's because I'm part cat and really need to soak up the sun, but I'm telling you, nothing says "life" to me so much as the heat of the sun on my skin. I was a "baby oil in the backyard with a book" sunbather until I reached the ripe old age of 18. Fortunately for me, I realized that the hobby was probably not a good one, and I've tried to avoid overexposure ever since. Only time will tell what effect my early, unrestrained love affair with the sun will have on my skin. Since most of us get 50–80% of our lifetime exposure to the sun before the age of 18, I'm a little concerned about my facial future! I'm sharing this with you, however, so that you know I feel your pain when you hear that you have to stay out the sun for the sake of your skin.

For convenience, ultraviolet rays from the sun are categorized as either A or B. When you lie out in the sun—or walk or work in the sun—UVB light penetrates the second layer of your skin and neutralizes its natural antioxidant protection. By depleting the skin of immune-defense cells and damaging DNA, B-Rays are notorious for burning your skin. UVB rays also cause skin cancer. UVB rays are at their most intense between the hours of 10 AM and 4 PM, so try to stay in the shade or covered up with light-weight cotton during those hours.

UVA rays, on the other hand, can get to us all the time and are therefore responsible for much of our skin's aging. UVA rays are equally intense from dawn to dusk, summer to winter, and they can penetrate glass. So if you wisely decide to stay in the house during the noon hour but position yourself in your glass sunroom, the UVA rays will find you anyway. If you drive a lot for work or for leisure, the UVA rays will come through your windows even in mid-January. In fact, studies show that most facial skin cancers occur on the left side of the face—where the rays reach the driver. Remember the "A" in UVA. It could stand for "always" and "aging."

What Happens When You Lie Out in the Sun?

While we are out lounging by the pool or weeding the garden, those delicious sunny rays are penetrating our skin, burning our cells and damaging our DNA. Enzymes get to work removing damaged bits, and these are quickly replaced. This triggers our melanocytes to produce melanin, and our evidence of this is the "tan." Obviously, then, since tanning occurs because cells have been damaged, there really is no such thing as a safe tan. The tan's job is to protect your DNA by deflecting the sun's rays. And melanin is a free radical scavenger, which is good because sunlight triggers lots of free radicals. Unfortunately, as we age, the number of melanin-producing cells diminishes, and we are at increased risk of sun damage. The adorable freckles of our youth become the dreaded age spots of our not-so-youth.

Overexposure to the sun also leads to dry, rough, leathery skin, wrinkles, and of course, skin cancer. So too much sun can contribute to premature aging of your skin in more ways than one. Ironically, however, more and more research is linking a *deficiency* of sunlight with several diseases, including colon cancer, prostate cancer, rickets, and even dental decay. Rates of Parkinson's disease and multiple sclerosis also seem to be higher in northern locations that don't experience as much sunlight. And we know our skin needs a good daily dose of sunlight in order to manufacture vitamin D. This seeming contradiction begs the question: How can we have our sun and protect ourselves too?

Mother Nature to the Rescue

You will remember from our discussion about the immune system that antioxidants help our skin remain strong and healthy by fighting the free radicals that cause so much damage—and this includes sun damage.

Perhaps not surprisingly, many of the sun-protective nutrients are the same ones that help build healthy skin in the first place. And studies are now showing that these nutrients might help prevent sun damage as we are drinking in the rays. Selenium, for example, is an essential skin nutrient, and recent studies show that a deficiency in selenium hampers the skin's ability to prevent damage from UVA rays. Beta carotene and lycopene are also proving to be effective edible sunscreen agents. (Lycopene is the bioflavonoid that gives tomatoes their redness, while beta carotene makes carrots orange.) In one study, a group who ate lycopene-rich tomato paste for 10 weeks experienced less sunburn than the group who did not eat the tomato paste. It seems that the concentrated form of lycopene found in the paste is more beneficial than that found in raw tomatoes.

> **Many sun-protective nutrients (like vitamin C and selenium) are the same ones that help build healthy skin in the first place. And studies are now showing that these nutrients might help prevent sun damage as we are drinking in the rays.**

Beta carotene has been used for over 30 years to repair sun-damaged skin, and more recently, it's been shown to prevent the DNA mutations triggered by sun exposure. The major antioxidants vitamins C and E have also been extensively studied for their sun-protective abilities, particularly in preventing the development of sun-induced free radicals. One study concluded that vitamin E in combination with vitamin C produced the best photo-protective effect. The genestein found in soy has also demonstrated an ability to inhibit the development of sun-induced skin cancer. And don't forget the fish. The Essential Fatty Acids (EFAs) found in fish improve cellular health and prevent sun damage, as does the gamma linolenic acid in borage oil. Cells also seem to use Essential Fatty Acids to control the inflammation and pain associated with a sunburn.

Other research indicates that the dietary combination of vitamins E and C, along with carotenoids, selenium, and flavonoids, prevent sunburn, as well as subsequent chronic skin damage. Flavonoids are responsible for the pigments found in plants, and the flavonoid quercetin provides excellent protection against UV light. Look for quercetin in apples, berries, black tea, grapefruit, and onions.

Since our natural sun defense comes from melanin in our skin, it is not surprising that scientists have tested the melanin-type pigments in foods for sun-protective effects. The dark pigments in grapes and black tea intensively absorb sun radiation, and one study has shown that black tea can also help repair damage from sunburn. Then there is green tea. Its wonders are seemingly endless. Studies confirm that EGCG polyphenols in green tea have antioxidant, anti-inflammatory, and anticarcinogenic effects, and now are showing an ability to prevent sun-induced aging, melanoma, and non-melanoma skin cancers. If you haven't yet jumped onto the green tea bandwagon, try cooling green tea with lemon to quench your summer thirst.

Foods to Avoid

There are also certain foods you should avoid before you head for the great outdoors. Citrus fruits and figs, along with some wild herbs and plants (including fennel, dill, celery, and buttercup) contain psoralens, which actually amplify the effects of a sunburn. Likewise, some medications trigger photosensitivities, causing toxic or allergic reactions. Always read package-insert information or ask your pharmacist about possible interactions with the sun before taking diuretics, antihistamines, arthritis medication, and antibiotics. Remember that some ingredients in shampoos, cosmetics, perfumes, after-shaves, hair sprays, and even contact lens solutions may react with sunlight.

You should also save your favorite frosty alcoholic beverage for a time when you're out of the sun's reach, as alcohol dehydrates the skin, making it more susceptible to burning. Instead, remember that keeping your skin adequately hydrated with pure, filtered water will help to prevent damage and improve healing whether you are in the sun or not.

And What about Sunscreen?

First of all, you need to know that some commercial sunscreens contain ingredients that are shown in some studies to contain chemicals that may be unhealthy. You will read about that in Chapter 13, If Looks Could Kill. Also, because some mutagens could be carcinogenic, various sunscreen options may protect against sunburn while increasing the risk of sunlight-related cancers. This puts us between

Sunblocks are the only form of sunscreen that are effective against UVA rays, and they usually contain zinc oxide or titanium dioxide. When you are shopping for sunscreen, be sure that your choice protects against both UVA and UVB rays.

the proverbial rock and the hard place. What's more, while most products broadcast their ability to protect against burning UVB rays, be aware that UVA rays also burn and are responsible for skin aging.

Sunblocks versus Sunscreens

Sunscreens rely on chemicals to absorb harmful UVB rays, while sunblocks form a physical barrier that prevents the rays of the sun from penetrating the skin. Sunblocks are the only form of sunscreen that are effective against UVA rays, and they usually contain zinc oxide or titanium dioxide. It is possible that a combination of the newer ingredient Parsol 1789 with either zinc oxide or titanium dioxide can block up to 80% of A-Rays. When you are shopping for sunscreen, be sure that your choice is a "broad spectrum" one, meaning that it protects against both UVA and UVB rays. You'll want to do some homework, and learn to read labels.

By now it probably won't surprise you to learn that some antioxidants are proving to be powerful topical agents in the fight against sun damage. Check to see if your favorite sunscreen brand contains any of these! Studies confirm that applying vitamin E (alpha-tocopherol acetate) to the skin protects against UVB radiation, decreases the development of cancer, and helps to reverse signs of skin photo-aging. Vitamin C (L-ascorbic acid) applied topically has proven to protect against sunburn, limit sun-induced DNA damage, and speed healing of sunburned skin. It's also useful in delaying the onset of skin tumors, as well as in reducing wrinkling caused by UVB rays. Research confirms that the green tea polyphenol epigallacatechin-3-gallate protects against oxidative cellular and genotoxic damage from UVA radiation. A 2003 study also supports the topical application of zinc, silymarin, and soy

---

Sunscreen Tips

Remember your ears, the back of your neck, and since bald heads are in vogue nowadays, the uncovered areas of your scalp. Your nose gets a double-whammy, since your sunglasses can reflect rays back to your skin, so be sure to really cover your nose well.

When using foundations and creams with Sun Protection Factor (SPF) protection, don't count on the full protection quoted on the box because chances are quite good that you won't apply them thickly enough to achieve that level of coverage. Use a separate sunscreen under your make-up.

Sunscreens break down over time. If your sunscreen doesn't look right, smell right, or feel right, throw it away. Products that make an SPF claim must also include an expiry date.

isoflavones to boost sunscreen's ability to protect your skin against rays and cancer.

You can also follow the lead of Hawaiians who have been using the natural sunscreen properties of coconut oil to protect their skin from the sun's harmful rays for centuries! Peruse the label of your sun product to see if it contains any of these beneficial ingredients. But whatever potion you choose, don't fall into the trap of believing that sunscreen allows you unlimited time in the sun or that reapplying extends the length of time you can soak up the rays—because it does not.

Beach Safety

Experts suggest that the reason sunscreens don't work as they should is that we either don't put enough on or we fail to reapply them after sweating or swimming. Be sure to use an ounce of sunscreen on your body—and another teaspoonful to cover your face and neck. Some advocates suggest applying your first coat of protection 20 minutes before heading outdoors and following that with another coat 20 minutes after you are outside. The theory is that the second coat will cover the spots you missed the first time around. Whether or not you apply a second coat soon after heading outside, you should reapply every two hours when you are in the sun. After exercise or bathing, pat yourself dry and cover yourself with sunscreen again. I'm sure you've quickly realized that your 8-ounce tube of sunscreen should last about as long as your week at the beach. Being economical with your application may save you some money, but in the long run it won't be saving your skin.

The Condition of the Skin You're In

Stress, worry, tension, anxiety—my parents call it "nerves." Whatever name you use for it, stress causes chemical changes in your body that can jump-start or aggravate existing skin conditions, including acne, eczema, hives, psoriasis, and rosacea. Stress can also cause you to make horribly unhappy facial expressions and—just as your mother warned—your face will freeze that way in the form of lines and wrinkles. In Chapter 6 (Hormones and Your Healthy Glow), we've already considered the effects of stress and how to cope. But go back and take another look if you find yourself locked in a facial clench as you read this!

When you're feeling relaxed again, you can learn a few other tricks to overcome skin conditions that may be bothering you.

What's Your Type?

The first thing you have to do is determine your skin type. It's essential that you take an honest look at your skin before you do this, and don't hold onto the diagnosis that you made 20 or 30 years ago. Your skin changes over time, and if you had oily skin in your 20s, for example, it's quite possible that conditions have changed. It is also possible that your skin may not be dehydrated after all: you might actually have healthy skin that you are unintentionally stripping of moisture with the products you are using to clean it. Please take the time to do a current assessment of your skin type.

For simplicity, three names have been given to the skin types: Normal, Dry, and Oily. In reality, however, there are myriad combinations of skin types, and different locations on your face are oilier or drier than others. It's best to assume that your skin type is the one that represents the majority of the skin on your face. To determine that type, gently cleanse your face, but do not put moisturizer on it. After at least 30 minutes, examine your face in the mirror and follow the guidelines below to make your assessment.

Dry Skin

Dry skin feels tight and has no slick areas, and its pores are barely visible. Severe dryness can lead to skin that flakes. Quite often those who have fair coloring have this skin type. Dry skin also heightens the appearance of fine lines and wrinkles.

Oily Skin

If you have oily skin, you probably know it already. Excessive production of sebum (oil) causes the outer layer of the epidermis to become inflamed, while enlarged pores give the skin a coarse appearance. Oily skin is shiny, feels greasy, and is prone to pimples and blackheads. There are 20,000 oil-producing sebaceous glands on the face, and most of them are found on the forehead, nose, and chin—fondly known as the T-Zone. Approximately 43% of women aged 21–64 have oily skin, or combination skin that includes an oily T-Zone.

Normal Skin

The term "normal" seems to be a misnomer, because it is actually quite rare to have skin that has no overtly dry or oily areas. That said, normal skin has medium-sized pores and has a balance of moisture and suppleness.

Sensitive Skin

Complaints about sensitive skin often come from those with dry skin, and the result is stinging and redness after the use of topical preparations. Sensitive skin often occurs after years of using products that break down the skin's natural defenses, leaving it vulnerable to irritants.

Healthy Skin

Healthy skin is naturally acidic, with a pH balance of around 5.5, to prevent bacterial overgrowth. Whatever your skin color, healthy skin is clear, soft, and smooth. Find a picture of yourself when you were five years old, and chances are pretty good that it will show you what healthy skin looks like! If you have troubled skin, along with the *Living Beauty Essentials*, you might find it helpful to supplement with dietary silicon. Next to oxygen, silicon is the most plentiful element in the crust of the earth, and on average, our bodies contain seven grams of silicon in various tissues and fluids. It's surprising that we don't hear more about dietary silicon as an essential nutrient, as it plays a significant role in our health.

> Healthy skin is naturally acidic, with a pH balance of around 5.5, to prevent bacterial overgrowth.

Studies show that we need dietary silicon for proper bone development and maintenance. In fact, a deficiency in dietary silicon can cause skeletal deformities, including abnormal skull formation. Because dietary silicon provides structural integrity for bone and connective tissues, including the connective tissues that produce collagen and elastin, it can help prevent and treat osteoporosis while at the same time giving you better skin and fewer wrinkles.

Sources of dietary silicon include fruits, vegetables, and whole grains. The silicon in these foods is converted by stomach acid into its active form (orthosilicic acid), which is directly absorbed into the blood through the stomach and intestinal walls. Unfortunately, low levels of stomach acid caused by dietary choices, illness, or aging make this transformation and absorption difficult. So if you have skin problems, you might benefit from silicon supplementation.

Although horsetail extract and colloidal silicic acid are common forms of supplementation, these must also be converted by stomach acid into the active form of dietary silicon. So you are better off supplementing with orthosilicic acid directly. Studies show that choline-stabilized, concentrated orthosilicic acid is absorbed two and a half times better than either horsetail extract or the colloidal form. Keep this in mind, particularly if your digestion is weak.

What Does It All Mean?

Underlying the quality of your skin is the truth about how you are looking after yourself. Your skin also offers clues about what nutrients your diet may be lacking, as well as more advanced signs of ill health. Read the following recommendations with an eye to improving your nutrient intake, changing some habits, and pursuing medical advice when necessary.

As you continue reading, you will see that therapeutic levels of certain nutrients have been used in the *Beauty Prescriptions* in order to promote healing. Therapeutic levels are higher than those typically used for health maintenance and are often taken for a short period of time until improvements are made. Note that these levels indicate *total* nutrient requirements, including those taken as part of the *Living Beauty Essentials*. They should not be taken in addition to those nutrients. For example, if a *Beauty Prescription* recommends that you supplement with B complex 100 mg daily and your multivitamin already contains 50 mg, you would supplement with an additional 50 mg to equal the 100 mg total.

Acne

Acne is a common skin disorder, affecting as many as 95% of adolescents and young adults, and it's not something you necessarily grow out of. More than 40% of adults over the age of 25 experience acne, and between 3% and 12% of adults bring acne into their middle age. There is a familial tendency to develop acne, and typically the condition begins around puberty. Some studies suggest that acne is, in fact, the first outward indication of puberty in females. Hormonal changes, hormone disorders, stress, tumors, and extreme weather changes are all factors in triggering acne, so if you have this condition, you might have to do a little detective work to figure out its cause.

When the sebaceous (oil) glands in our hair follicles become more active at puberty or during the menstrual cycle, they can easily become clogged with excess oil, dirt, and skin cells. This plug causes the follicle to bulge, forming what is called a comedo. A whitehead is an open comedo, and a blackhead is a closed comedo. If the wall of the follicle ruptures from the pressure, dead skin cells, bacteria, and oil typically found on the skin's surface are able to enter the pore and form small, infected areas known as pimples. A nodule is a bump that extends deep into the skin, often destroying nearby tissue. Often painful, nodules lead to scarring. Cysts are similar to nodules, but they are filled with liquid. Eventually, acne lesions heal, forming a red spot called a macule, but several macules together make the skin look inflamed. Acne is painful on many levels, as research shows that acne also scars the self-esteem of those who experience it.

Physicians, scientists, and Moms and Dads have been disagreeing for years about the impact of food choices on acne and pimples. But finally, Dr. Loren Cordain has found evidence that the Moms and Dads have been right all along. According to the University of Colorado's Dr. Cordain, a diet that is high in refined carbohydrates (like pizza and pop) permanently boosts the hormone insulin. We know that our hormones work in tandem, so it shouldn't surprise us that sustained insulin levels elevate our other hormone levels, and this stimulates the production of pore-clogging oil. Dr. Cordain discovered that in societies in New Guinea and the Amazon where fruits and vegetables are the main food sources, acne is virtually unknown. Of course, in North America, we all know what "pizza face" means. Now we know what triggers it.

> In societies in New Guinea and the Amazon where fruits and vegetables are the main food sources, acne is virtually unknown.

If you have acne, be conscious of foods that are your personal triggers and simply avoid them. Focus your diet on fresh, organic fruits and vegetables while avoiding refined carbohydrates and saturated fats. A dietary deficiency in Essential Fatty Acids (EFAs) will also encourage the production of sebum, and a deficiency in vitamin A is linked to acne. Zinc is also essential to control acne. If you are female and you experience worse acne around the time of menstruation, investigate a deficiency in vitamin B6 (pyridoxine). Be cautious in choosing your multivitamin, however, as huge doses of B, particularly B12, can aggravate the condition. You should also check the strength of your stomach acid. Acne is associated with low acidity, suggesting a problem breaking down food, as well as imbalances in the digestive tract. Revisit Chapter 3, The Beauty of Digestion, to learn how to check your acid levels. If you discover that your stomach is functioning at below optimal levels, be sure to use a hydrochloric acid capsule and digestive enzymes with your meals. And remember that *Candida* is also often a factor in acne.

Be cautious about using synthetic hormones for birth control, endometriosis, or menopausal symptoms, as these have been linked to the development of acne. Various other prescription medications such as steroids are also known to cause this condition. And be watchful of your personal care and make-up products, as these can block your pores.

Avoid waterproof make-up that cannot be removed without scrubbing, since added friction and rubbing can stimulate oil glands. When washing your face, use lukewarm water—never hot or cold. Use nonirritating, fragrance-free skin-hydrating products that do not block pores. (That is, they are non-comedogenic.) A few drops of essential oil (either calendula, lavender, or German chamomile) can be added to your rinse water or moisturizing products to help calm inflammation and redness.

Beauty Prescription for Acne

Take your *Living Beauty Essentials* daily, as described in Chapters 2 and 3. You will see that, for this prescription, some of those nutrients should be taken in the higher daily-total amounts shown below, along with any extra nutrients listed in this table.

	Total Daily Amount
Vitamin A	15,000 IU daily until healed; then 5,000 IU daily
Beta carotene	25,000 IU
Vitamin B complex	100 mg

	Total Daily Amount
Vitamin C	**3,000 mg in divided doses**
Vitamin E	**800 IU**
Dietary silicon	**3 mg choline-stabilized, concentrated orthosilicic acid, once or twice per day (max 6 mg)**
Borage oil	**1,000–3,000 mg**
Selenium	**200 mcg**
Zinc	**50–100 mg. Do not exceed 100 mg daily from all sources.**
Tea tree oil	**5% solution applied topically, to kill bacteria**

Age Spots

Also known as liver spots, these flat brown spots can appear anywhere on the body but are most troubling when they appear on the face. While the spots themselves are harmless, they may indicate a buildup of byproducts of free radical damage, and this accumulation is an exterior signal to you that free radical intoxication may also be damaging internal organs such as the heart muscle, liver, and retina. Remember that what happens on the outside of your body is an indication of what is going on inside, as well. Age spots are very common in those who live in sunny climates and in those who consume excessive amounts of alcohol. They have also been linked to deficiencies in vitamin E, selenium, glutathione, and chromium.

The best defense against age spots is prevention. Keep your liver clean and strong and limit alcohol consumption. Probiotics will help to improve digestion and restore balance to the intestines. Eat a diet that is at least 50% fruits and vegetables, plus fresh whole grains, seeds, and nuts. Avoid caffeine, fried foods, red meat, processed foods, saturated fats, sugar, and tobacco—and stay out of the sun.

Beauty Prescription for Age Spots

Take your *Living Beauty Essentials* daily, as described in Chapters 2 and 3. You will see that, for this prescription, some of those nutrients should be taken in the higher daily-total amounts shown below, along with any extra nutrients listed in this table.

	Total Daily Amount
Vitamin B complex	100 mg
Vitamin C with bioflavonoid	3,000–6,000 mg daily, in divided doses
Vitamin E	600–800 IU
Co-Enzyme Q10	50–60 mg, with food
Milk thistle	Taken as tea

Dry Skin

This may seem obvious, but dry skin is lacking moisture. Boost your moisture retention by drinking at least eight glasses of pure, filtered water per day. Dry skin is also an indication of hypothyroidism, so if you are bothered by dryness, you might want to investigate that possibility. See Chapter 6 to learn about this condition. Dry skin around the lips and nose is linked to a deficiency in vitamin B2 (riboflavin), and those with dry skin should definitely be concerned about a deficiency of Essential Fatty Acids. Avoid washing your face or bathing in hot water, as this effectively "melts" the lipids in your skin that help retain moisture! There is also no rule about bathing your body daily. If you are clean and have no body odor, try showering every *other* day. Trust those close to you to be honest about whether or not you are a candidate for this approach!

Remember that chlorine in your water can be very dehydrating and irritating, so you should purchase a shower-head chlorine filter. You can purchase one for under a hundred dollars at the hardware store, and you won't believe the difference a good filter can make to your skin. After showering or washing your face, pat your skin dry and immediately apply a moisturizer. Allowing your skin to "air dry" can actually cause more moisture to evaporate from the skin surface. You should also make sure that you use a humidifier in your home and use it whenever the furnace is on, so that precious water can stay in your skin. Be sure to rehydrate with at least eight daily glasses of pure, filtered water.

Beauty Prescription for Dry Skin

Take your *Living Beauty Essentials* daily, as described in Chapters 2 and 3. You will see that, for this prescription, some of those nutrients should be taken in the higher daily-total amounts shown below, along with any extra nutrients listed in this table.

	Total Daily Amount
Vitamin A	10,000 IU daily for 2 or 3 months
Vitamin B complex	100 mg
Selenium	200 mcg
Vitamin C	3,000–5,000 mg
Vitamin E	800 IU
Dietary silicon	3 mg choline-stabilized, concentrated orthosilicic acid), once or twice per day (max 6 mg daily)
Zinc	50–100 mg. Do not exceed 100 mg daily from all sources.
Borage oil	1,000–2,000 mg daily

Eczema

Eczema is also known as "atopic dermatitis" and causes dry and sometimes red and cracked skin that is extremely itchy. It is an immune response in the skin, set off by an allergen. The allergen could be something used on the outside of the body, but it's just as likely to be caused by a food allergy. Eczema is often associated with *Candida*, the overgrowth of an unfriendly yeast in the digestive system. Conventional treatments make use of steroid creams, but these can thin the skin and should therefore be used with extreme caution on the face. In circular fashion, steroid creams also encourage growth of *Candida* and may trigger another flare-up. If you have struggled with conventional treatments for your eczema but it keeps returning, work with your health-care professional to try to isolate food triggers. Your body will also benefit from a cleanse that will give your system a fresh start. See Chapter 5, Facing *Candida* in the Mirror, for instructions.

It's also crucial that you continue supplementing with probiotics if you have eczema. As early as 1930, researchers established that a deficiency of the Essential Fatty Acid (EFA) Omega-6 leads to inflammatory skin conditions. More recently, scientists have determined that those with eczema are unable to adequately convert the Omega-6 EFA linoleic acid to gamma linolenic acid (GLA)—the acid responsible for soothing inflammation. Studies suggest that GLA improves symptoms of eczema and skin roughness. *The American Journal of Clinical Nutrition* reports that a deficiency in linoleic acid also results in excessive water loss through the skin and recommends including vegetable oils such as flaxseed oil in the diet.

Because your body might have trouble converting linoleic acid to soothing GLA, you absolutely must supplement with GLA directly if you have eczema. Borage oil is the best source. Since you also want to be sure that you have adequate antioxidant protection, you should increase your intake of vitamins A and E. And zinc and vitamin C are needed, as well, to encourage healing. Aged Garlic Extract (AGE) will help to cleanse and support the liver, and it's essential if you are battling *Candida*. AGE also helps reduce inflammation.

For topical relief, try chamomile ointment or apply GLA evening primrose oil directly to the affected area. You can also combine one cup Epsom salt with 1/4 cup olive oil and add this to a warm bath. Soak for no more than 15 minutes. Alternatively, if you don't like a slippery bath, soak in the Epsom salts and massage the olive oil into your body skin when you come out of the tub. Filling the toe of an old nylon stocking with oatmeal and adding it to your bathwater is also an effective method of soothing the itch associated with eczema. Be sure to come out of the bath after 15 minutes. If you stay longer, you will only cause your skin to dehydrate more! As I mentioned in Chapter 5, Facing *Candida* in the Mirror, I suffer from eczema as well. That's why I know these treatments work.

Beauty Prescription for Eczema

Take your *Living Beauty Essentials* daily, as described in Chapters 2 and 3. You will see that, for this prescription, some of those nutrients should be taken in the higher daily-total amounts shown below, along with any extra nutrients listed in this table.

	Total Daily Amount
Vitamin A	10,000 IU
Vitamin B complex	100 mg
Beta carotene	25,000 IU

Total Daily Amount

Vitamin C with bioflavonoids	3,000 mg in divided doses
Vitamin E	800 IU
Selenium	200 mcg
Zinc	50–100 mg. Do not exceed 100 mg daily from all sources.
Borage oil	Increase from 1,000–4,000 mg daily
Dietary silicon	3 mg choline-stabilized, concentrated orthosilicic acid), once or twice per day (max 6 mg daily)
Grapeseed extract	50–200 mg, 3 times per day (max 600 mg daily)

Oily Skin

Oily skin results from overactive sebaceous glands in the dermis. To a degree, oily skin is inherited, but hormones and diet can also play a role. Skin tends to be oiliest in the teen years, and drier as we age. On the plus side, those with oily skin tend to have fewer lines and wrinkles! The caveat, however, is that oily skin is prone to breakouts.

> Drink at least eight glasses of water per day to flush out toxins and keep your skin hydrated. It may seem strange, but oily skin can also be dehydrated—often because of the harsh products we sometimes use on our faces.

Studies show that a deficiency in Essential Fatty Acids can trigger oil production, so make sure your diet or supplements are giving you enough EFAs. Avoid saturated fats like those found in dairy foods and red meat, as well as processed carbohydrates—and focus your diet on fresh organic fruits and vegetables, lean meats, whole grains, nuts, and seeds. Drink at least eight glasses of water per day to flush out toxins and keep your skin hydrated. It may seem strange, but oily skin can also be dehydrated—often because of the harsh products we sometimes use on our faces. Oily skin must be kept clean to limit its collaboration with dirt and bacteria (which causes acne).

When washing your face, be sure to use warm water and gentle pressure with your face cloth because rubbing can stimulate sebaceous glands to produce more oil. Use a cleansing wash specifically designed for oily skin, since creams and milks are usually formulated for dry skin and may be too greasy. Masques that absorb oil may be useful, but limit the use of exfoliating facial scrubs to once or twice per week. Note that these scrubs can also stimulate oil production. And avoid products formulated with alcohol to "dry" out the oil, as these also remove precious water from your skin. You don't want to be oily and wrinkly too!

Beauty Prescription for Oily Skin

Take your *Living Beauty Essentials* daily, as described in Chapters 2 and 3. You will see that, for this prescription, some of those nutrients should be taken in the higher daily-total amounts shown below, along with any extra nutrients listed in this table.

	Total Daily Amount
Vitamin A	15,000 IU
Vitamin B complex	100 mg
Vitamin C	3,000 mg in divided doses
Dietary silicon	3 mg choline-stabilized, concentrated orthosilicic acid, once or twice per day (max. 6 mg daily)
Zinc	50–100 mg. Do not exceed 100 mg daily from all sources.

Psoriasis

Psoriasis appears as thick red skin patches that are covered in silvery scales. In this condition, lesions frequently appear on the chest, stomach, and back, and the outsides of the arms and legs, particularly on the knees and elbows. They can also appear on the scalp and cause flaking similar to dandruff. About 25% of those with psoriasis experience nail problems, including pitting or ridges and scales on the free edge of the nail. Nails may also become thick, yellow, or opaque. Women are slightly more susceptible than men, and fair-skinned people are more likely to be affected.

Psoriasis occurs when the production of skin cells outpaces the body's ability to shed them normally. While it typically takes a month for new skin cells to be produced, for those with psoriasis, the sequence is shortened to four or five days.

Psoriasis is also linked to absorption problems, coupled with the inability to properly digest fat. If you have some of the symptoms described above, ask your health-care provider to help you determine whether you have low stomach acid. Eliminate foods that are high in saturated fats (such as those found in fried food, dairy products, and fatty meats), since they promote inflammation. Focus your diet on

> If you want to get rid of psoriasis, butt out. Research shows that people who smoke have a higher risk of psoriasis. And the association is higher for women than for men.

fresh, organic fruits, vegetables, whole grains, nuts, and seeds. The fiber in these foods will help to prevent stagnation in the bowel and speed elimination of toxins. Choose turkey and fish if you enjoy meats, and be sure to continue with probiotic supplementation.

Excess alcohol and a deficiency of Essential Fatty Acids (EFAs) are also psoriasis triggers. Be sure to take at least a full tablespoon of flax oil daily, combined with supplemental borage or evening primrose oil. Fish oil has also been found useful. Evidence also suggests a connection between psoriasis and a compromised immune system, so be sure to give your security team adequate antioxidant support. You may also benefit from a liver cleanse. Finally, be sure to drink at least eight glasses of pure, filtered water each day to help with hydration and to flush out toxins. For topical relief, try anti-inflammatory capsaicin or licorice cream, or apply borage oil directly on the lesions. Cranberry oil may also give you some relief. Research also shows that minerals found in water from the Dead Sea help to slow skin cell proliferation in psoriatic skin. Soak for no more than 15–20 minutes in a warm bath with Dead Sea salts.

Beauty Prescription for Psoriasis

Take your *Living Beauty Essentials* daily, as described in Chapters 2 and 3. You will see that, for this prescription, some of those nutrients should be taken in the higher daily-total amounts shown below, along with any extra nutrients listed in this table.

	Total Daily Amount
Vitamin A	10,000–25,000 IU daily until healed
Vitamin B complex	100 mg
Beta carotene	25,000 IU

	Total Daily Amount
Vitamin C	3,000–6,000 mg or to bowel tolerance
Borage oil	2,000–12,000 mg daily
Fish oil	1,000–6,000 mg daily
Dietary silicon	3 mg choline-stabilized, concentrated orthosilicic acid, once or twice per day (max. 6 mg daily)
Selenium	200 mcg
Glutathione	500 mg
Zinc	50–100 mg. Do not exceed 100 mg daily from all sources.
Grapeseed extract	50–200 mg, 3 times per day (max. 600 mg daily)
Milk thistle	(as silymarin) 300 mg, 3 times per day (max 900 mg daily)

Rosacea

Rosacea is a chronic skin condition involving acute inflammation and skin redness. It affects about 13 million people in the United States. Women are three times more likely to suffer from rosacea, though men tend to have a more severe version. Rosacea typically appears after age 30 and is most common in those with fair skin.

Rosacea often begins with a tendency to flush easily, and this leads to persistent redness and enlarged blood vessels. Acne-type lesions then appear (commonly on the central face and sometimes on the chest, neck, back, or scalp). Serious cases involve the eyes, causing them to become gritty and red. The nose can also become enlarged, red, and bumpy. Those with rosacea should avoid stimulants that can induce flushing, like spicy foods, caffeine, and alcohol. Temperature extremes and stress are also triggers.

Recent studies have found a significant link between rosacea and *Helicobacter pylori* bacteria. *H. pylori* are usually acquired during childhood, and they live in the lining of the stomach, where they attach to the mucous and epithelial cells. Most people with *H. pylori* demonstrate no symptoms, but they are six times more likely than others to develop ulcers. Ulcers can cause stomach burning or pain, particularly after eating and in the evening. *H. pylori* has also been linked to stomach cancer. If you have rosacea, even if you have no symptoms of digestive troubles, ask your doctor to test for *H. pylori*. A round of antibiotics will eliminate it. Of course, you'll want to follow the antibiotics with a boost in your probiotics supplementation! As a double bonus, researchers have found that probiotic supplementation may help to reduce inflammation and control the reproduction of *H. pylori* bacteria.

> **A few drops of either calendula, lavender, or German chamomile essential oil added to your rinse water or moisturizing products may help to calm inflammation and redness.**

Use the same skin-care strategies for rosacea as you would for acne. Avoid hot water and be gentle with your skin. When washing your face, use lukewarm water—never hot or cold. Use nonirritating, fragrance-free skin hydrating products that do not block pores (non-comedogenic products). A few drops of either calendula, lavender, or German chamomile essential oil added to your rinse water or moisturizing products may help to calm inflammation and redness.

Beauty Prescription for Rosacea

Take your *Living Beauty Essentials* daily, as described in Chapters 2 and 3. You will see that, for this prescription, some of those nutrients should be taken in the higher daily-total amounts shown below, along with any extra nutrients listed in this table.

	Total Daily Amount
Vitamin A	10,000 IU
Vitamin B complex	100 mg
Vitamin C	3,000–5,000 mg
Vitamin E	800 IU
Selenium	200 mcg
Dietary silicon	3 mg choline-stablilized, concentrated orthosilicic acid, once or twice per day (max 6 mg daily)
Zinc	50–100 mg. Do not exceed 100 mg daily from all sources.

Wrinkles and Wrinkle Delay

I remember my grade seven geography teacher telling the class one day that she never bought any clothes that might need ironing, because she tended to iron in more wrinkles than she took out. Sometimes our skin seems to be just like my teacher's clothes—or like raw silk. After a certain age, it seems to wrinkle more every time you look at it. The key, then, is to choose where the wrinkles will rest and what they will look like. Opt for laugh lines rather than scowl marks and you'll look younger no matter what your age.

Two things cause wrinkles: lack of moisture and repetitive facial expressions. You can influence the impact of each.

> ### You Give Me More Than Gray Hairs!
>
> Parents often blame the graying of their hair on their children. Although we can offer sympathy about those silver locks, there is no scientific evidence to support the offspring connection. It does seem, however, that our kids are not entirely blameless when it comes to our aging appearance. A 2003 Seoul, Korea, study found that the risk of facial wrinkling increased significantly with each full-term pregnancy a woman experienced. While researchers concluded that the wrinkling was influenced by estrogen levels, the result is still the same: the kids did it!

• When it comes to cigarettes, don't smoke 'em if you've still got 'em. Smoking robs your skin of vital nutrients and chokes the oxygen supply to the skin—and the constant squint and pucker will eventually engrave themselves into your face.

• Be sure to wear sunglasses outside and reading glasses if you need them to cut down on the eyestrain. This will also slow the development of the crow's feet you get from squinting. And whenever possible, stay out of the sun.

• When you catch yourself in a frown of concentration, replace the stress with a smooth forehead and relaxed eyes. Try to avoid facial expressions that make you look mean or angry. And laugh. Laughter is always good.

• Avoid caffeinated, carbonated, and alcoholic beverages and drink lots and lots of water. Remember that EFAs from salmon or flax oil help keep water in your cells.

Beauty Prescription for Wrinkles

Take your *Living Beauty Essentials* daily, as described in Chapters 2 and 3. You will see that, for this prescription, some of those nutrients should be taken in the higher daily-total amounts shown below, along with any extra nutrients listed in this table.

	Total Daily Amount
Vitamin A	10,000 IU
Vitamin B complex	100 mg
Vitamin C	3,000–5,000 mg, in divided doses
Vitamin E	800 IU
Selenium	200 mcg
Dietary silicon	3 mg choline-stabilized, concentrated orthosilicic acid, once or twice per day (max 6 mg daily)
Zinc	50–100 mg. Do not exceed 100 mg daily from all sources.

A New Perspective on the Appearance of Aging

Our relationship with gravity is another example of life's little balancing acts. While we need gravity to keep our feet planted firmly on the ground, the trade-off of this constant pulling is that our internal organs start to sink, breasts lose their perkiness, and after years of downward pressure, we can even shrink an inch or more in height. And we need only look in the mirror to find more evidence of the power of gravity: eyelids and brows start to droop, earlobes and nose elongate, chin migrates floor-ward, and the upper lip disappears into the mouth. Bags or hollows under our eyes give the impression that we are constantly tired, while bone and muscle loss associated with aging leaves us with loose skin that eventually starts to drape at our necks and dangle unattractively from our arms. Yes, it appears that we pay a high price to avoid floating into space.

Turnabout Is Fair Play

Despite the fact that we are at the mercy of gravity for about 16 upright hours per day, we don't have to throw in the towel. Although you can't change gravity, you can change the influence it has on your body. All you need to do is change your perspective. Literally. Turning yourself upside down allows you to harness the power of gravity to prevent and undo some of its nasty body damage.

When your feet are higher than your head, you can help move blood away from your legs, feet, and lower body. As gravity starts to pull in a different direction, the space between the vertebrae increases, repositioning organs upwards. More blood circulates to your brain, as well as to your face, neck, and scalp. This new circulation leads to firmer muscles, giving a bit of a natural facelift. Studies show that improved circulation in the face may prevent the formation of some types of wrinkles. And anecdotal reports even claim that turning upside down can stimulate healthy hair growth and possibly delay or reverse graying of the hair!

> **Over 2,400 years ago, Hippocrates created the first inversion therapy device to ease the suffering of back pain with a system of ropes and pulleys, and for centuries yoga practitioners have recognized that inverted postures release muscle tension and promote relaxation.**

This isn't a newfangled concept. Over 2,400 years ago, Hippocrates created the first inversion therapy device to ease the suffering of back pain with a system of ropes and pulleys, and for centuries yoga practitioners have recognized that inverted postures release muscle tension and promote relaxation. But you don't have to stand on your head to make gravity your friend. Try the bending-forward yoga posture. Stand straight, keeping your feet together and your arms hanging at your sides. Inhale deeply as you raise your arms above your head. Be sure to keep your elbows straight. Exhale as you bend over and grasp your toes, ankles, or calves—as far as you can go! After exhaling, move your head as close to your knees as possible while keeping your knees straight but not locked. Hold for a few seconds, then slowly stand. Inhale. Repeat this process twice.

Getting inverted increases oxygen supply to the brain, and this leads to increased physical and mental energy, improved lymphatic drainage of toxins, and reduced tension and stress. It is also a scientifically proven treatment for many back conditions. Studies show that a slant board—a table that tilts the head toward the ground—improved severe back pain enough for participants to return to their fulltime employment after pain caused them to be absent from their jobs.

Another study showed that muscle pain decreased 35% for participants within 10 seconds of inverting on the board. And despite questions raised in the past about blood pressure, research shows that the inversion table is not a concern for those with normal blood pressure. Talk to your doctor to see if inverting is an option for you. Slant boards are readily available at fitness stores and on the Internet.

Going in Another Direction

If just thinking about turning upside down gives you a head-rush, consider going against gravity for some cell-nourishing exercise. Rebounding, the new term for jumping on a trampoline, uses gravity in a different way. When you're at the top of your bounce, you actually pause in the air for a split second, exerting pressure on your cells in the opposite direction of the pull of gravity. The downward bounce works with gravity, exerting pressure on your cells again. This pushing and pulling on your cells strengthens fibers, muscles, and tissues throughout your body. Rebounding also helps to move enzymes, hormones, nutrients, and oxygen into the cells as it sends debris out. Rebounding is gentle on the joints, and some proponents consider it to be the ultimate fountain of youth.

> ### The Shoulder Stand
>
> Do try this at home if you have normal blood pressure: lie flat on your back. Inhale deeply while raising your legs and spine until your toes point to the ceiling and your body rests on your shoulders and the back of your neck. Place your hands at your waist for balance. Keep your spine and legs straight. Breathe deeply, and work up to holding the position for about two minutes. When you're finished, bend your knees, curve your spine, and slowly unroll until your back is flat on the floor. Take a deep breath before slowly lowering and straightening your legs.

As we get older, we learn that it's okay to break a few rules. The law of gravity should be no exception!

Beauty at a Glance

Eat a minimum of five servings of fruits and vegetables daily. Choose the vibrant dark greens, oranges, yellows, and reds. These foods are rich in antioxidants and bioflavonoids that help protect and nourish your skin. Nurture your skin with Essential Fatty Acids, including Omega-3 oils from fresh, deep-sea, cold-water fish and flaxseed, and gamma linolenic acid from borage seeds. Remember to hydrate with at least eight cups of fresh, pure water per day to help cleanse and refresh your outer layer. Because skin cells replicate about every 28 days, you have repeated opportunities for refreshment. It's never too late for more beautiful skin!

CHAPTER EIGHT

Your Skin Doesn't Stop at Your Neck

Some people, no matter how old they get, never lose their beauty—they merely move it from their faces into their hearts.
—*Martin Buxbaum*

Most of us spend a great deal of money on our faces and don't give our body skin a second thought. It's as if there were some invisible dividing line between the neck and the shoulders—and anything south of the line is expected to miraculously fend for itself. Until today. I'm going to let you in on a few beauty secrets that will have your skin glowing from head to toe—and you might be surprised to discover that paying more attention to the skin below your neck might lead to amazing improvements in your face!

Food for Thought

Of course, your complexion has already gone through remarkable changes because of your new diet and the *Living Beauty Essentials* (multivitamins/multiminerals, EFAs, and probiotics) you're taking every day. But have you noticed that your body skin has also improved? Tiny bumps on the backs of your arms may have disappeared because you now have adequate vitamin A in your diet. The pinpoint red dots known as petechiae, may be gone, too, since you've increased your vitamin C intake. And have you noticed that you don't bruise as easily, or that cuts and burns are starting to heal faster and better? You can thank vitamins C and E, along with silicon and zinc, for that. And what about skin dryness and flakiness? Is your skin softer and more supple? That's because of the Essential Fatty Acids. If you haven't noticed improvements yet, you will. You didn't become deficient in these nutrients overnight, and it may take a while for the improvements to show.

You can also improve the quality of your skin by boosting your circulation and helping it eliminate toxins. Remember that one of the skin's major responsibilities is to get rid of wastes, and more than a pound of waste products exits our bodies through the skin every day! If our skin is clogged with debris, however, impurities remain in the body, causing our other cleansing organs to work harder. Eventually, our kidneys, liver, and colon become exhausted, and disease is likely to follow. Along the pathway to full-blown illness, of course, is the reality that clogged and dirty skin can't possibly look its best. To remedy that problem, make sure that dead cells and debris are removed from the surface of your body skin, in the same way that you exfoliate your facial skin.

> **One of the skin's major responsibilities is to get rid of wastes, and more than a pound of waste products exits our bodies through the skin every day!**

Waste Management

Our skin cells are cleansed and nourished with a sea of fluid called lymph. Although we have far more lymph fluid than blood in our bodies, lymph systems lack the powerful pumps used to circulate our blood (our hearts). Instead, lymph relies on active and passive motion such as massage and exercise to make its way around our bodies. But nowadays, unfortunately, most people don't get enough of either. Enter skin brushing. Also known as "dry brushing," this extraordinarily powerful technique is incredibly fast, simple, and inexpensive to perform in the comfort of your very own home. Skin brushing stimulates circulation and glands and tones the skin. With only five minutes a day, you should see improved circulation, softer skin, fewer skin irritations and infections, and an increase in your overall level of stimulation and health.

To start your skin-brushing enterprise, buy a brush suitable for the purpose. You should be able to find one at your local health products store. Look for a natural-bristle brush with a long handle, so you can get to those hard-to-reach places. While you're at it, buy one for each member of your family, as they all will benefit, whatever their age. For hygienic reasons, you don't want to share.

After you wake up in the morning, go into the bathroom five minutes earlier than you normally would. While you (and the brush) are completely dry, start at your feet, and with long, firm strokes, brush upward toward your heart, front and back. Brush across your buttocks, and use a counterclockwise motion on your stomach and abdomen. Finish with your arms and each hand. Don't forget your palms and the soles of your feet. Your scalp and the back of your neck will also enjoy the attention, but avoid your face. Cover each area only once. Your skin will let you know how firmly you should press, but start with a light touch at first. As your skin becomes more fit and firm, you'll be able to work more vigorously. Follow the routine with a rinse in the tub or shower.

Contrast Showers

I know you've been bathing yourself for decades, so you might not be able to imagine how to improve that routine. But, yes, there's even a way to boost the benefits of taking a shower. The contrast between warm and cold water promotes detoxification by increasing circulation, and improved circulation is what you want. It brings nutrients, oxygen, and immune cells to damaged tissues and helps eliminate inflammatory byproducts and other toxins. This all leads to better-looking skin.

Start with three minutes of warm (never boiling hot!) water, followed by one minute of cold water. Repeat the pattern as many times as you like. It's quite invigorating!

A New Kind of Bath

Our tendency to bathe in hot water, especially to take the bite out of a cold winter night, actually causes lipids to melt away and decreases the protective barrier of our outer skin. Studies show that soaking in a tepid bath for no more than 20 minutes is most beneficial to dry skin. (Longer than 20 minutes causes the skin to lose moisture.) Add Epsom salts or olive oil to soothe and moisturize. And if you suffer

> **Our tendency to bathe in hot water, especially to take the bite out of a cold winter night, actually causes lipids to melt away and decreases the protective barrier of our outer skin.**

from dry skin all over, baths are preferable to showers because hot water should not touch your face and we're inclined to use hotter water when we shower.

Is "Clean Water" Really Clean?

Throughout our history, microbes and biological contaminants have caused waterborne disease, often with fatal consequences. In North America we chose to address this problem by adding chlorine to our tap water, but this decision has created other problems. Chlorinated water, for instance, can irritate your eyes and skin, and studies show that chlorination of drinking water may lead to harmful chemical byproducts such as chloroform, trihalomethanes, and haloacetic acids. These are produced when chlorine reacts with organic material in the water, and they have been blamed for increasing the risk of cancer, miscarriage, neural tube defects, birth defects, respiratory problems, and reduced fetal growth. According to the Environmental Protection Agency (EPA), over 9,300 Americans suffer from bladder cancers every year as a result of chlorine in the water.

You don't even have to drink it to feel the sting of chlorine. A study carried out at University of North Carolina's Chapel Hill School of Public Health showed that the use of chlorinated water, particularly in showering, boosted blood levels of trihalomethanes in women. We don't have much choice about accepting chlorine in our water if we don't live out in the country with our own supply of non-chlorinated well water. But if like me, you are sensitive to chlorine—or if you simply want to reduce your exposure to potentially dangerous toxins— buy yourself a water filter. You can have a full-home system installed where the water enters your home from the municipal supply. Look for suppliers in the yellow pages.

If finances are an issue, buy a shower-head filter that will remove most of the chlorine from your shower water. They're readily available at your local hardware store. Also be sure to buy filters for your faucets if your skin comes into contact with the water they deliver. And if you bathe babies, particularly those with dry skin or eczema, run the bathwater through your shower-head filter so junior isn't soaking in irritating chlorine.

Bathing in Sweat

You might think perspiration stinks, but it's actually vitally important to keeping your body at a safe temperature. And when you perspire, your body is throwing off lots of toxins. In fact, sweating is so essential to our health that various cultures around the world have used sweat baths, steam baths, and saunas as methods of relaxation and therapy. And exercise, of course, promotes perspiration that's good for your body. It only follows, then, that any exit point for sweat should be kept clear, to make it easy for you and your toxins to part company. We don't want to block our sweat pores, and we don't want to shut them down. Doing so traps toxins, causing them to circulate throughout the body and wreak unspeakable havoc.

That's why you need to throw away your antiperspirant. Yes, you read that correctly. Antiperspirants are not body friendly. Now, I know what you're thinking. You don't want to stink. Believe me, I don't want anyone to stink either, especially the person I'm sitting next to on a crowded bus. But antiperspirants may not be the answer.

First of all, sweating is important. The average person has 2.6 million sweat glands in their skin. Adults lose approximately three-quarters of a liter of perspiration per day, but in extreme heat a grown person can produce as much as two and a half liters per hour. We have two types of sweat glands; the apocrine glands and the eccrine glands. The apocrine glands are located mostly in the armpits and the anal-genital area and don't become active until puberty. Their primary function is to generate pheromones, the subtle odors that help us attract a mate—whether we like that idea or not! They tend to open into hair follicles, and sweat from apocrine glands contains proteins and fatty acids. Eccrine glands, on the other hand, are smaller, open into a pore, and are fully operational from birth. Perspiration from eccrine glands consists of 99% water and 1% sodium, chloride, potassium, calcium, urea, ammonia, uric acid, and phosphorus. Sweat on its own does not have an odor, but when bacteria on the skin and hair metabolize the proteins and fatty acids from apocrine perspiration, you can smell the results.

> Sweat blockers, or antiperspirants, work by causing sweat ducts to close so the perspiration can't escape. But trapping sweat in your body may not be such a good idea. Where will the toxins go?

Sweat blockers, or antiperspirants, work by causing sweat ducts to close so the perspiration can't escape. If you've been following the discussion about the importance of releasing toxins, you'll see that trapping sweat in your body may not be such a good idea. Where will the toxins go? Some antiperspirants bring another potential health problem, as well. This one comes in the form of the active ingredient used to close the sweat duct. If you do some label reading, you'll likely see some type of aluminum-based compound (such as aluminum chloride, aluminum chlorohydrate, or aluminum hydroxybromide) in your antiperspirant, and as you may already know, aluminum is the subject of a controversy regarding Alzheimer's disease (AD). A 2002 review of studies suggested that there was insufficient data to establish that exposure to aluminum was a cause of the debilitating disease. Nevertheless, it recommended that because the toxic effect of aluminum on human health cannot be ruled out, exposure to aluminum should be limited as much as possible. Since that review, new studies have shed more light on the topic. An animal study found that long-term exposure to aluminum caused behavioral and neuropathological changes similar to those observed in AD. A more recent (2004) study indicated that chronic exposure to metals such as aluminum may promote the development of AD and other neurodegenerative disorders. I would consider daily contact with an antiperspirant containing an aluminium-based compound to be chronic exposure.

Concerns have also been raised about cancer and the use of antiperspirants. One study (in the *Journal of the National Cancer Institute*) concluded that there is no proof that the use of antiperspirants or deodorants causes breast cancer. However, a more recent study suggested that frequency and earlier onset of antiperspirant/deodorant usage with underarm shaving were associated with an earlier age of breast cancer diagnosis. Researchers concluded that underarm shaving with antiperspirant/deodorant use might, in fact, play a role in breast cancer, and that absorption of aluminum salts was increased by the act of shaving. Scientists were unable to determine whether it was the shaving or the antiperspirant that was responsible, but if someone insisted on using antiperspirant, I'd recommend they do one of two things: shave their underarm hair or use antiperspirant, not both.

And to be extra safe, you don't need to use antiperspirant at all. You can use other methods to keep you smelling fresh as a daisy. Of course, you can't underestimate the power of a daily shower. The aroma associated with sweat is actually caused by bacteria, so you have to limit the bacteria, and a daily shower can help you do that. You can also opt for natural fabrics like cotton that not only prevent moisture from being trapped next to your body, but dry quickly as well. And you can use a deodorant product that prevents bacterial growth. Note that I am not referring to the aforementioned antiperspirant. You will still perspire when you use a deodorant; you just won't stink. Look for non-aluminum-based deodorants at your health products store.

Since you've started to make dietary changes in your life, there's another important point to consider. You'll find that giving up certain foods and eating a more healthy diet will allow your body to focus on the business of detoxifying your system. But as toxins leave your body, you might notice a stronger aroma than you had when you were keeping toxins in your system. This, too, shall pass as your system clears up. Your personal smell might also provide you with vital clues as to foods you might want to avoid. Remember that food sensitivities do not always show up as a rash or hives. A friend of mine, for instance, noticed that she didn't have body odor unless she ate wheat. No wheat in her diet, no smell. She was astute enough to make the connection and has since given up wheat.

Heavy Sweater

Approximately 1 in 25 people experiences hyperhydrosis, a condition marked by excessive sweating. If you suffer from this disorder, make sure that your doctors have ruled out all underlying conditions that may be leading to your perspiration problem. Autoimmune disorders, malignancy, endocrine disorders, psychiatric disorders, obesity, menopause, and hyperthyroidism can all lead to hyperhydrosis. (See the discussion of hyperthyroidism in Chapter 6.)

Foot Job

Our feet take a lot of abuse. We wrap them in suffocating socks, we cram them into boots, we lace them into shoes, and on occasion, we torture them with straps and three-inch heels. Not factoring in exercise, most people walk about 3,000 steps just with daily activity. The average person walks about 1,000 miles in a year, and according to the American Academy of Orthopaedic Surgeons, every step puts about 1.5 times a person's body weight on their feet. In one hour of vigorous exercise, the feet withstand and cushion up to one million pounds of pressure. Our feet become blistered, calloused, and sore—and then when summer comes, we break out the sandals and expose other people to our neglected feet. (Okay, looking at abused feet gives me the willies, but I figure I have two choices: I can look the other way or I can point out the importance of proper foot care. I've chosen the latter.)

> The average person walks about 1,000 miles in a year, and according to the American Academy of Orthopaedic Surgeons, every step puts about 1.5 times a person's body weight on their feet. In one hour of vigorous exercise, the feet withstand and cushion up to one million pounds of pressure.

Many people don't consider the fact that, as an exit point for toxins, our feet are quite valuable. With more that 250,000 sweat glands per foot, each one can put out a pint of sweat daily. That sweat contains innumerable toxins, and when they leave our bodies, our skin quality improves. But how can the toxins go anywhere if their exit is barred by a thick layer of dead, calloused skin? I'm guessing that the toxins back up and try to find another port of exit—maybe on your face or back. It also makes sense that toxins could be trapped in the dead layer of skin on your feet, just sitting there, being toxic. It's time to get rid of them and improve the appearance of your feet with a good pedicure.

The All-Natural Pedicure

Soak your feet in warm water for 10 minutes; for an invigorating soak, add peppermint or rosemary essential oil to the water. If you want a relaxing end to your day, opt instead for lavender or rose oil. Use a nailbrush to clean under and around your nails and to scrub the bottoms of your feet. Gently exfoliate with a pumice stone or foot scrub, taking care not to remove too much of the protective outer layer. Regular exfoliation should help remove painful corns and calluses. When you've had your soak, thoroughly dry your feet. Then carefully push back your cuticles with an orange stick. Never cut your cuticles, as doing so can lead to infection. Using straight-edge clippers, trim your toenails to a length near the end of your toes to prevent the nail from growing painfully into the skin around it. Give yourself a well-deserved foot massage with coconut, olive, or avocado oil, and slip on a pair of cotton socks.

Corns and Calluses

Excessive pressure or friction causes skin to thicken or harden over a bony prominence on a foot. These areas are called calluses when they develop on the bottom of the foot and corns when they appear on the sides, tops, and tips of the toes. Common causes are ill-fitting footwear (either too tight or too loose), high-heeled footwear, tight socks, or a deformity of the foot. Untreated corns can lead to ulcers and bursitis. Treatment involves removing the source of pressure or friction, usually by modifying the shoe. Corn pads are sometimes too difficult to position properly to be effective. Never try to cut away the hardened corn, as this can lead to infection. To prevent the development of these painful foot conditions, wear properly fitting shoes with extra room at the toe and avoid hosiery that is too tight.

Cracked Heels

Cracked heels, or heel fissures, are not only unattractive to look at, but can also lead to more serious problems if they become deep, or if infection sets in. Those with compromised immune function or diabetes are particularly at risk from complications. Although anyone can develop cracked heels, the people most likely to suffer from this condition are those who tend to go barefoot or wear open-backed shoes, are overweight, live in a dry environment, or have inactive sweat glands. Cracks can occur when skin on the bottom and outer edges of the heel becomes dry and hard—and deep fissures can be painful and bleed. These poor heels are crying out for moisturizer, which should be applied at least twice a day. Wearing cotton socks after applying a moisture cream before bed will be very helpful. Gently use a pumice stone to remove the thickened layer of dead skin. Do not go barefoot or wear open-backed sandals or thin-soled shoes. And continue taking your Essential Fatty Acids to moisturize from the inside.

Plantar Warts

These warts result from a virus, and they differ from other warts because they grow inward through the sole, or "plantar" of the foot. Walking might become painful if you have one or more of these lesions.

Home remedies include repeated applications of salicylic acid. I treated my daughter's plantar wart with Thuja oil, which is available at the health products store. Make sure that you continue to take your regular multivitamin containing vitamins A, C, E, and zinc to help with the healing.

Athlete's Foot

Tinea pedis, or athlete's foot, is a common and contagious fungal infection of the feet that can also thrive in footwear. Symptoms include blisters, open sores, redness, and scaling—and a persistent burning itch, particularly between the toes. Often, this infection also gives feet a

> **If you have athlete's foot, you can put antifungal tea tree oil directly on affected areas. And take Aged Garlic Extract daily for internal antifungal support.**

strong smell. To treat athlete's foot, the skin should be kept clean and dry. Wash in warm, soapy water and be sure to pat your feet dry. Use the towel only once before laundering, and wash it in hot water. Try a footsoak with tea tree oil in a tub of warm water. You can also put antifungal tea tree oil directly on affected areas. If you've run out of Aged Garlic Extract, make sure you replenish your supply and take it daily for internal antifungal support.

Paronychia

Paronychia is another a fungal infection. This one is caused by organisms entering the skin in the gap between the nail and the surrounding skin. The infection may be the result of aggressive manicuring or an injury, and it may be caused by a variety of bacteria, including *Candida*. Make sure to read Chapter 5, about *Candida*, if you suspect or know that your infection is caused by those bacteria. If no abscess has formed, a warm-water soak with tea tree oil will often help. Otherwise, you should seek medical attention. Hot compresses can also provide some relief, often encouraging the draining of pus. Left untreated, you could lose your infected toenail.

Smelly Feet

Those 250,000 sweat glands in our feet can really cause some social problems if we don't stay on top of the situation! As mentioned before, sweat doesn't stink, but we need to be sure that the bacteria that thrive on our perspiration and excrete their own foul waste products don't get the better of us—or our noses! To prevent malodorous feet, be sure to bathe your feet daily in lukewarm water and mild soap, and be sure to dry them thoroughly. Change your socks every day. You should also be sure that shoes are given 24 hours to air out after wearing. If your shoes start a chronic stinking routine, throw them away! Wear natural materials like cotton socks instead of nylon hosiery, and wear leather or canvas that allow your feet to "breathe" instead of plastic shoes. And as I've told my daughter a hundred times: when you wear closed shoes, always, always, always wear socks!

If you can't rid yourself of foot smell, check for fungus between your toes and seek treatment if you find redness or patchy skin. Be aware that a persistent odor can indicate a low-grade infection.

Treat Yourself to Sweet Feet

Try this at-home remedy for odiferous feet. Boil two bags of black tea for 15 minutes, then add 2 quarts of cool water. Soak your feet for half an hour. The tannic acid in the tea will kill any bacteria that are hanging around.

Once you've beautified your feet (and depending on how long you've ignored them, this might take a while!), your new foot-care regimen is really quite simple: a few times per week, after your bath or shower, use a pumice stone to gently exfoliate the outer layer of dead skin. Massage in your favorite body oil or cream, and you're done. Two minutes tops. Just be sure that you have a cozy pair of slippers or cotton socks to put on afterwards if there's a chance that you could slip on your floors. And from the tip of my toes, thank you for taking one small step to improve the beauty of the world's feet!

Head-to-Toe Skin

Most people have a few moles and continue to develop them until about the age of 20. Women might find that pregnancy adds a few as well. Happily, most moles pose no health risk. On the other hand, with escalating deaths from melanoma reaching nearly eight thousand in America yearly, it's important to know something about moles.

Moles can be round, oval, flat, or raised. Most are brown, but colors can range from flesh tones to yellow, dark blue, or black, and they can appear on any part of the body. Pigment-producing cells, called melanocytes, sometimes gather together to become benign moles. Unfortunately, however, sun-induced DNA damage can cause melanocyte production to go haywire, leading to melanoma. Have your moles "read" by a specialist to determine their baseline appearance. Then use the ABCDs of moles to keep track of changes that could signal a problem:

A. Asymmetry: If the two halves of the mole are not identical, have the mole checked.

B. Borders: Irregular mole borders or borders that are indistinct may be a sign of trouble.

C. Color: Report any change of color to your doctor immediately.

D. Diameter: Watch for any changes in the size of your mole. If you have young children in your life, make sure that their moles grow at the same pace as their overall growth. Report any moles—your own or your child's—that are larger than the eraser on a pencil.

Pay attention to any mole that develops after the age of 20. Immediately report any mole that bleeds, itches, or looks unusual. And have your doctor check all moles—your own or your child's—at every regularly scheduled medical checkup

CHAPTER NINE

The Story of Hair

Life is an endless struggle full of frustrations and challenges,
but eventually you find a hair stylist you like.
—*Author Unknown*

So many things about your appearance were decided before you were born—and your hair future may be one of them. Three months before you made your first appearance in this world, you already had all the hair follicles that you would ever own. Whether male or female, blondes are blessed with approximately 140,000 follicles, followed by brunettes with about 108,000, and redheads with 90,000.

> Researchers have recently determined that scalp-hair growth patterns in newborns are closely linked with the development of the central nervous system. In fact, numerous metabolic, genetic, and neurological disorders are associated noticeable scalp-hair abnormalities.

The hair follicle is the shaft through which hair leaves your body and becomes visible. The hair root, root muscles, and sebaceous glands reside in the epidermis and draw nutrients from the lower layers. Within the hair bulb, dead cells are filled with a type of protein called keratin and are sent up as hair. The outer portion of a hair is called the cuticle, and the inside is known as the cortex. Our tresses grow at an average pace of half an inch per month. Each individual hair grows for two to six years, after which time it rests. Then it falls out, and the cycle begins again. About 85% of our hair is growing and 15% is resting at any time.

Hair Food

If you've made the dietary and lifestyle changes I've described up to this point in the book, it won't be long before you notice that your hair, along with your skin and nails, is healthy and vibrant. Remember that hair is essentially protein, so be sure that you're taking in an adequate supply of that nutrient. Look to legumes for a nutrient-rich protein source. Beans, peas, lentils, and beans such as adzuki, lima, and pinto are delicious in a variety of recipes and can add to your intake of vitamin A, folic acid, and calcium. But since legumes must be combined with a grain to make a complete protein, eat them with brown rice and spelt or whole wheat pasta. Soybeans are the only bean that are a complete protein, and they can be enjoyed as miso, tamari, or tofu. Fermented soy is often used to make protein supplements. Of course, meat and fish also provide protein in your diet.

It's important to keep your immune system strong, because hair growth is a low priority on the survival totem pole and tends to suffer when you are fighting an illness. Be sure that you are getting a variety of antioxidants from colorful fruits and vegetables, and boost your intake with a daily multivitamin. Reread the recommendations in Chapter 2, Protecting the Body Beautiful, if you think your hair health has been affected by a weakened immune system. To prevent your hair from becoming dry and brittle, ensure that you are getting enough of the Essential Fatty Acids, as well as adequate vitamin E. Limit the refined sugar found in cereals, boxed and bagged snacks, and fast foods. Avoid harmful hydrogenated fats.

Sulfur is an amino acid used to make hair, and it's readily available in onions, garlic, and turnips. And if you want to give your hair a real boost, be sure that you include dietary silicon in your diet. Your hair's cuticle is rich in silicon, which provides elasticity and strength. Increasing silicon intake brings another advantage, as well: it may help prevent the buildup of aluminum in the brain. In some studies, high levels of aluminum have been associated with Alzheimer's disease. Researchers believe that silicon bonds with the aluminum and prevents it from being absorbed by the gastrointestinal tract. Cabbage, cauliflower, celery, leeks, onions, and rhubarb are excellent sources of dietary silicon.

Because dietary silicon is difficult to absorb, however, you may be better off using the supplemental version, particularly if you have weakened digestion. Dietary silicon is broken down in the stomach to create orthosilicic acid, which is then absorbed directly into the blood through the stomach and intestinal walls. Supplementing with orthosilicic acid directly improves the amount absorbed and boosts the benefits from the silicon.

Beauty Prescription for Beautiful Hair

Take your *Living Beauty Essentials* daily, as described in Chapters 2 and 3. You will see that, for this prescription, some of those nutrients should be taken in the higher daily-total amounts shown below, along with any extra nutrients listed in this table.

	Total Daily Amount
Vitamin B complex	100 mg
Vitamin C	3,000 mg, in 2–3 equally divided doses
Vitamin E	400–800 IU
Zinc	50–100 mg. Do not exceed 100 mg daily from all sources
Dietary silicon	3 mg choline-stabilized, concentrated orthosilicic acid, once or twice per day (max. 6 mg daily)

The Colors of Your Life

Just as our skin pigment is determined by melanin, so is our hair color. Produced in the melanocytes, eumelanin creates light brown to deep black hair, while pheomelanin orchestrates blondes, golden browns, and reds. When we are first born, the melanocytes are less active, so many people come into the world with blonde or lighter hair that darkens with the years as the melanocytes kick into high gear. Of course, this process reverses as time goes on, with melanocytes starting to shut down production. Hair the color of protein begins to appear (that is, white hair), and some hair grows out lacking pigment. Surrounded by other colored hairs, this new hair appears gray in comparison. But as more and more melanocytes become dormant, hair becomes obviously white.

> Premature graying has been linked to thinning of the bones. So if you're too young to go gray (and aren't we all?), you might be wise to have your doctor check your bone density.

I'm sure we all know someone who started to gray as a teenager, but graying typically begins in the 30s, starting at the temples and reaching to the top of the scalp. Forty percent of people have a few gray hairs by the age of 40. Other body hairs also turn gray, but this typically occurs after the scalp hairs change color. Caucasians seem to gray earlier than Asian races, and heredity is also a determining factor.

Certain health and lifestyle factors can also play a role in your gradual graying, and premature graying has been linked to thinning of the bones. So if you're too young to go gray (and aren't we all?), you might be wise to have your doctor check your bone density. Along with vitamin B12, a shortfall of the other B vitamins, including biotin and Para-Amino-Benzoic Acid (PABA), is also associated with going gray. Thyroid imbalances and anemia have both been linked to gray hair. See the chart at the beginning of Chapter 6 to determine whether your thyroid may be a factor for you. Anemia is a potentially serious condition, in which the number of red blood cells in the body decreases. Red blood cells carry oxygen to our various cells, providing them with energy. Without enough oxygen, cell formation and repair are severely hampered. Anemia is associated with many conditions, including peptic ulcers, thyroid imbalances, rheumatoid arthritis, and even cancer.

Deficiencies in vitamins B6, B12, folic acid, and iron can lead to anemia. To boost your iron intake, eat asparagus, nuts and seeds, fish, beef, whole grains, parsley, raisins, legumes, and eggs. Be sure to include a source of vitamin C with your iron foods to enhance absorption of the mineral. Eat plenty of brown rice, egg yolks, wheat germ, organ meats, and bananas for your B vitamins. You'll get folic acid from oranges and asparagus. Besides graying hair, some symptoms of anemia include loss of appetite, headaches, fatigue, cessation of menstruation, dizziness, and depression. If you suspect that you may be anemic, you must follow up with your health-care provider for proper treatment. As a final note, smokers go gray faster than non-smokers. So thank goodness you don't smoke!

Dandruff

Dandruff isn't life threatening, but it certainly can be a source of embarrassment and frustration. Like many of our cosmetic concerns, however, dandruff can also provide us with clues about what is going on in the body. Flakes result from an overgrowth of skin cells on the scalp. People with oily hair tend to be more prone to dandruff, and flakes seem to increase when we couple cold weather with indoor heating, and of course, times of stress. Hormone imbalances can also manifest themselves in annoying flakes, and a sensitivity reaction to hair products and styling tools like blow dryers may produce the white stuff.

But scalp flakes are not all bad. They may be a sign that you have food allergies. That's not good news, but it's better to know about and figure out a solution than to suffer from eating the wrong things. When trying to isolate food triggers, avoid animal proteins and dairy products, as these have been associated with dandruff. Citrus fruit is also a common problem. Because fast foods contain large quantities of salt, sugar, and hydrogenated and saturated fats, these should also be avoided. Focus on fresh, raw fruits and vegetables, whole grains, and legumes. Some research suggests that an overgrowth of the naturally occurring skin yeast *Pityrosporum ovale* may also be a trigger. Be sure that you have alleviated any fungal problem in your body and are including a source of beneficial probiotics in your daily regimen. Shampoos containing anti-fungal rosemary may be helpful, and thyme is also known to help eliminate the itching caused by fungal infections. See Chapter 5's discussion of *Candida* for more information about dealing with fungal infections.

Aged Garlic Extract (AGE) is a potent anti-fungal, and AGE supplements might be useful in treating your dandruff. Deficiencies of B complex vitamins, Essential Fatty Acids, and selenium have also been linked to dandruff, so be sure to include those in your diet.

Beauty Prescription for Dandruff

Take your *Living Beauty Essentials* daily, as described in Chapters 2 and 3. You will see that, for this prescription, some of those nutrients should be taken in the higher daily-total amounts shown below, along with any extra nutrients listed in this table.

	Total Daily Amount
Vitamin A	10,000 IU
Vitamin B complex	100 mg
Vitamin C	3,000–5,000 mg, in 2–3 equally divided doses
Vitamin E	800 IU
Zinc	50–100 mg. Do not exceed 100 mg daily from all sources

	Total Daily Amount
Dietary silicon	3 mg choline-stabilized, concentrated orthosilicic acid, once or twice per day (max 6 mg daily)

Dry, Damaged Hair

Dry hair can be the result of over-washing, using harsh styling products, or too much heat from your blow dryer or curling iron. Try using a milder shampoo and cut back on the frequency of your washing. If you need wet hair every day so you can fix your bed head, try skipping the shampoo and simply rinsing with water at least every other day. A deficiency in iodine can result in dry hair, so eat more sea vegetables and seafood. You also want to be sure to get enough Essential Fatty Acids (EFAs) and vitamin E.

Remember that your hair is already made up of dead cells, so you can't bring it back to life if you've overprocessed, burned, or otherwise destroyed it. Use conditioning products so you can hold onto your damaged hair until it's long enough to cut off into a style that you like. Then learn from your mistake and treat your hair with kindness. Hormones can affect almost anything, so don't be surprised if hormone fluctuations change your hair quality. My sister-in-law complained of dry "witch's hair" when she was pregnant, while my own went from short and straight to long and curly with my first pregnancy. (It didn't last!)

Beauty Prescription for Dry Hair

Take your *Living Beauty Essentials* daily, as described in Chapters 2 and 3. You will see that, for this prescription, some of those nutrients should be taken in the higher daily-total amounts shown below, along with any extra nutrients listed in this table.

	Total Daily Amount
Vitamin A	10,000 IU
Vitamin B complex	100 mg
Vitamin C	3,000–5,000 mg, in 2–3 equally divided doses
Vitamin E	800 IU
Zinc	50–100 mg. Do not exceed 100 mg daily from all sources

	Total Daily Amount
Dietary silicon	3 mg choline-stabilized, concentrated orthosilicic acid, once or twice per day (max 6 mg daily)

Oily Hair

If you have oily hair, try shampooing daily and leaving the suds on your head for a few minutes before rinsing. Use a non-irritating shampoo. Do not overbrush your hair, as this will carry oil from the scalp to the very tips of your hair. Be sure that you are getting your Essential Fatty Acids (EFAs) as well, because, as you learned in Chapter 7, All about Skin, a deficiency in EFA triggers oil production. See my comment above about hormones: hormones can affect practically everything including adding oil to hair.

Beauty Prescription for Oily Hair

Take your *Living Beauty Essentials* daily, as described in Chapters 2 and 3. You will see that, for this prescription, some of those nutrients should be taken in the higher daily-total amounts shown below, along with any extra nutrients listed in this table.

	Total Daily Amount
Vitamin A	10,000 IU
Vitamin B complex	100 mg
Vitamin C	3,000–5,000 mg, in 2–3 equally divided doses
Vitamin E	800 IU
Zinc	50–100 mg. Do not exceed 100 mg daily from all sources
Dietary silicon	3 mg choline-stabilized, concentrated orthosilicic acid, once or twice per day (max 6 mg daily)

Losing It

Shedding up to 125 hairs per day is considered normal. But hair loss problems occur when those hairs are not readily replaced or when the numbers start to creep over the 125 per day mark. This is a problem for men and women alike. The medical term for hair loss is alopecia, and there are several different forms. *Alopecia totalis*, for example, refers to total loss of the scalp hair, while *alopecia universalis* involves loss of all body hair. We'll look at the most common forms.

Gentlemen First

Twenty-five percent of men start to experience androgenetic alopecia (AGA), more commonly known as male pattern baldness, by the time they reach 30 years of age. Sixty-six percent of men either have a balding pattern or are bald by the age of 60. This form of balding typically starts with a receding hairline, on the sides, or at the top of the head. According to the American Hair Loss Council website, AGA accounts for 95% of all hair loss. The scientific name derives from the two components of male pattern baldness: the male hormone androgen and the inherited or *genetic* trait for losing hair. In the 1990s, researchers discovered that testosterone combines with an enzyme called 5-alpha-reductase in the hair follicle to produce another hormone called dihydrotestosterone (DHT). DHT suppresses the hair follicles, with the result that hair loss increases while fewer and thinner hairs are produced. When the follicle finally ceases to function, the hair is lost permanently. It's important to understand, despite what you may hear on late-night TV commercials, that when the follicle finally gives out, there is as yet no method to restart hair growth. But you can bet your bottom dollar that companies are pouring millions into research to find the answers so many people want to hear. Stay tuned.

> **Shedding up to 125 hairs per day is considered normal. But hair loss problems occur when those hairs are not readily replaced or when the numbers start to creep over the 125 per day mark. This is a problem for men and women alike.**

The Prostate Sidestep

Coincidentally, the DHT hormone responsible for male pattern baldness is the same one linked to benign prostatic enlargement, or BPE. Affecting millions of men, BPE and prostate cancer are a great concern, so it's important to pay attention to keeping the prostate healthy. Seventy-five percent of men 50 years of age and older have BPE symptoms, and one in six men will develop prostate cancer in his lifetime. An enlarged prostate leads to frequent nighttime visits to the bathroom, a sense of urgency, trouble getting urination started, and inadequate urinary flow. While all men should be aware that protecting prostate health is important, those who experience male pattern baldness already know that the DHT hormone is affecting them. And a recent study indicated that men with BPE are more likely to also be losing their hair. So, gentlemen, if your scalp is starting to show, it might be a good time to book an appointment with your doctor for a prostate exam.

Herbs and plant nutrients have been used for centuries for prostate problems, and we now know that they are effective due to their ability to block the enzyme 5-alpha reductase, which is responsible for the production of the DHT that suppresses hair follicles. Recently, some of these alternative therapies have been studied to determine their effectiveness against male pattern baldness. A double-blind, placebo-controlled study determined that *Serenoa repens* (saw palmetto) and beta-sitosterol from plants are both effective in treating this kind of baldness. Sixty percent of those in the study saw improvement by the end of the trial. Although native to North America, saw palmetto plant extract has a long history of use in Europe for the treatment of prostate enlargement. Numerous well-controlled scientific studies have shown that saw palmetto extract is very effective for relieving the symptoms of enlarged prostate, with few side effects. Aged Garlic Extract is also useful for preventing the conversion of testosterone to DHT. While we are on the subject of prostate, gentlemen might be interested to learn that drinking green tea also appears to be prostate protective. And you can reduce your risk of developing prostate cancer by consuming the bioflavonoid lycopene (which gives tomatoes their redness).

Meal plans that rely too heavily on saturated fats, such as those found in "manly" red meat, have also been associated with prostate problems. Remember from Chapter 2 that saturated fat promotes inflammatory PG-2 and that the resulting inflammation contributes to the process of aging. Not surprisingly, it is also a factor in hair follicles shutting down. Men: cut back on your saturated fats and focus on eating more vegetables. Rates of prostate cancer are much lower in Asian countries, and scientists have determined that the primarily vegetarian diet of the East is responsible. Because prostate conditions are hormone dependent, the phytoestrogens, or plant estrogens, found in the vegetables and fermented soy foods of Asian diets help to increase levels of the sex-hormone-binding globulin that inactivates testosterone. Reducing the impact of this male sex hormone seems to have a positive effect on the prevention and treatment of enlarged prostate. This is great for the prostate, but it has other far-reaching implications—including loss of libido. There is definitely a balancing act to consider as men add phytoestrogens from soy products to their diet.

A discussion of prostate health wouldn't be complete without talking about beta-sitosterols. Sterols and sterolins are plant fats found in fruits and vegetables, and they're readily available in a balanced diet. Multiple studies show the effectiveness of these nutrients in strengthening the immune system. Unfortunately, because phytosterols and sterolins are destroyed by processing, heating, and freezing and because many of us don't get the necessary 7 to 10 servings of fruit and vegetables every day, our diets are deficient in these vital nutrients. Research also shows that beta-sitosterol supplementation improves the symptoms of an enlarged prostate. In fact, it's possible that the effectiveness of herbal remedies such as saw palmetto and pumpkin seeds may well be due to the phytosterol content of the plants.

> ### The Thyroid Factor
>
> Thyroid function has been noted as a factor in hair loss affecting men, women, and children. If you are losing your hair, have your doctor check your thyroid function or try the Basal Metabolic Test described in Chapter 6.

And the wonders of vitamin C never cease. This powerful nutrient will not only boost your antioxidant status to keep your immune system strong; it may also increase circulation to the scalp. Continuing with your EFA supplementation in the form of fish oils will help to decrease the inflammation associated with the demise of the hair follicle. Whatever alternative aids you consider, the research definitely suggests that the use of nutritional supplements may both protect your prostate and help you hold onto your hair!

Now for the Ladies

Unfortunately for women, androgenetic alopecia (AGA), does not discriminate by sex, so women can also experience this form of hair loss. Unlike men, however, ladies typically don't encounter a receding hairline. Instead, they notice gradual thinning all over the head. Ladies may also notice that they lose some body hair, while facial hair might become more coarse. The causes are the same as for men. Family history is a strong indicator of your hair future, coupled with that pesky hair-follicle-suppressing DHT hormone.

Women usually notice hair thinning as estrogen levels start to drop at the approach of menopause and afterward. As mentioned in Chapter 6, estrogen and testosterone work in a delicate balance with each other, and for much of a woman's life, estrogen levels are high enough to protect her from the hair-loss potential of testosterone. But as estrogen starts to lag with the approach of menopause, its levels are no longer high enough for some women, and the thinning begins. Female androgenetic alopecia may also be present in women who have hyperandrogenism (too much of the hormone androgen), and it may also be a factor for those with polycystic ovarian syndrome (PCOS). PCOS involves high levels of male hormones, combined with multiple fluid-filled sacs on the ovaries, and it leads to gradual masculinization of females. PCOS tends to run in families. Complications include infertility and problems with miscarriage or gestational diabetes. Women with PCOS are also at higher risk for cardiovascular disease, hypertension, and adult-onset diabetes, and untreated PCOS can lead to cancer of the uterine lining. Studies also suggest that women experiencing insulin resistance are more likely to lose their hair. Insulin resistance is a factor in type 2 diabetes.

Other Forms of Alopecia

Alopecia Areata (AA)

This form of alopecia leads to patchy hair loss, as well as complete loss of hair on the head and body. The loss is normally temporary and typically does not lead to baldness. The cause of AA is not certain, but one theory is that this form of hair loss might be an autoimmune response, in which the body defense system mistakes the hair follicle as foreign and launches an attack. Stress may also be a factor, as some research links AA with anxiety and mood disorders. Supporting the immune system and learning to control stress in your life is a good idea for everyone, but it's especially important for those with AA.

Traction Alopecia

This form of hair loss is caused by excess and prolonged stress on the scalp from hairstyles such as corn rows and hair weaving. If you are sporting these styles and notice your hair falling out, it might be time to consider a new look!

More Hair Loss Triggers

Other factors that can result in hair loss include stress or trauma, rapid weight loss, and hormones. Research also indicates that women with androgenetic alopecia tend to have low levels of iron in their blood. This, of course, can lead to anemia. Some women notice that they lose hair when they stop using birth control pills or after a pregnancy. Hair loss due to hormones typically occurs three months after the hormone change takes place. Doses of vitamin A exceeding 100,000 IU daily can also trigger the loss of hair, as can the use of some drugs. Chemotherapy for cancer patients is a recognizable example. Women should always seek medical advice regarding hair loss.

Lost in a Puff of Smoke

Besides causing bad breath, cancer, wrinkles, and gray hair, a recent observational study has found a significant link between cigarette smoking and baldness. Researchers speculate that the free radicals triggered by smoking cause inflammation and DNA damage to the hair follicle. Smoke also seems to reduce estrogen levels, which allows testosterone and hair-loss promoting DHT to gain easier access to the follicle.

Ring around the ... Scalp?

Ringworm is the common name for a fungus called *Tinea capitis* that causes scaling of the scalp and leads to bald spots. It is a contagious condition that often spreads through schools. Be sure to boost the immune system if you are dealing with this fungus. Remember that Aged Garlic Extract is extremely powerful as an anti-fungal agent, and probiotics will help to restore levels of beneficial bacteria that may be deficient. Massage tea tree oil into the scalp to help eliminate the fungus.

Beauty Prescription for Reducing Hair Loss

Take your *Living Beauty Essentials* daily, as described in Chapters 2 and 3. You will see that, for this prescription, some of those nutrients should be taken in the higher daily-total amounts shown below, along with any extra nutrients listed in this table.

Total Daily Amount

Vitamin B complex	100 mg
Vitamin C	3,000–5,000 mg, in 2–3 equally divided doses
Vitamin E	800 IU
Zinc	50–100 mg. Do not exceed 100 mg daily from all sources.
Dietary silicon	3 mg choline-stabilized, concentrated orthosilicic acid, once or twice per day (max 6 mg daily)
Rosemary essential oil	Diluted and massaged into scalp
Beta sitosterols	Follow label directions
Saw palmetto	Men can take 1–2 g saw palmetto or 320 mg standardized hexane extract

Too Much of a Good Thing: Hirsutism

While some women lament the loss of hair, others would do anything to get rid of some. A 2004 survey in the *American Family Physician* determined that hirsutism, or excess hair growth, affects 5–15% of adult women. The male hormone androgen is typically responsible. Polycystic ovarian syndrome (PCOS), described earlier in the chapter, is commonly associated with hirsutism, but adrenal imbalances and thyroid problems can also be factors. Be sure to re-read the sections about these conditions if you think that they may be affecting you. (See Chapter 6 for a discussion of adrenal imbalances and thyroid problems.) Type 2 diabetes is also associated with excess hair growth. As you have probably already figured out, all of these conditions relate to hormone function. Be sure that you've discontinued use of products containing xenoestrogens, as these estrogen-mimics can exacerbate hormone conditions. And as in the case of hair loss, women should discuss concerns about hirsutism with their health-care providers.

CHAPTER TEN

The Nail File

Everybody needs beauty as well as bread, places to play in and pray in,
where nature may heal and give strength to body and soul.
—John Muir

There are two kinds of people: those who admire fingernails, and those who don't. This rule applies to both men and women. If you don't give much thought to your nails until the calendar screams that you are mere weeks away from some spectacular event that demands you look your very best from head to nail tips, this chapter will help remove the worry of whether your evening wear comes with matching gloves. If, on the other hand, you are one of those people who grow nice fingernails, you, too, may learn a thing or two about our miraculous nails.

Dunked in soaps, chemicals, and hot liquids; subjected to freezing temperatures, heat, and air conditioning; used as paint and pot scrapers, phone dialers, and tweezers; and essentially ignored until we have an important date—or worse, an infection—our nails really need a break!

Besides providing us with another source of admiration, our nails offer vital clues about our general health and well-being that should not be ignored. Composed mainly of the protein keratin, nails are essentially non-living material. They are strong and flexible and grow about 3/16 inch per month. Our nails protect our nerve-filled fingertips and toes, help us pick up small objects, and of course, are useful in taming an itch. And let's not forget that beautiful nails get noticed.

Nails grow from a semicircular white area near the base known as the "lunula," or half-moon. It's made up of a group of cells that manufacture keratin. Keratin then merges with the nail plate (the visible part of the nail) and pushes the nail up and out. The base of your nail is embedded into the skin, and some of the nail along the sides is also set into the fleshy part around your nail, called the nail fold. The rim of skin over the flat side of the lunula is called the cuticle, and its job is to prevent bacterial infection and to protect the nail from impact. Although healthy nails are actually transparent, a pink nail bed should be visible through them. This indicates a rich blood supply. The tips should be nearly translucent: opaque and white nail tips indicate that nails are severely lacking in oil and moisture.

> ### Fast Facts about Your Nails
>
> It takes more than six months for a lost nail to grow back completely. Nails grow faster in the summer, during pregnancy, and just after an illness. In normal circumstances, fingernails grow much faster than toenails, and men's nails generally grow faster than women's. And if a person is left-handed, the nails on their left hand will grow faster. For right-handed people, the reverse is true.

The appearance of your nails is also affected by the physical trauma of knocking or banging them. As we age, our nails grow more slowly and tend to become dull and brittle. The tips may start to fragment or our nails may harden and thicken. They may also change from translucent to opaque, with a definite yellowing. But these symptoms can be prevented or delayed by dietary and lifestyle choices.

Because of their never-ending growth cycle, nails provide an accurate record of our health. They can also signal internal problems before any other symptoms appear. Brittle nails, for example, might indicate that your diet is deficient in vitamin A, while dry nails suggest a lack of B vitamins. And insufficient protein, vitamin C, or folic acid might be causing hangnails. Your nails might also hold clues to more serious conditions, as well: a pale nail bed is associated with anemia, and white nails might suggest liver disease. Be sure not to underestimate these signals, and make your doctor aware of the clues.

What Are Your Nails Telling You?

Appearance	*Health Considerations*
Clubbing: Your nail looks like the back of a teaspoon.	Disorders that affect the amount of oxygen in the blood, such as abnormal heart anatomy, lung diseases
Spoon-shaped nails (tip turning upward)	Anemia or B12 deficiency
Downward-turning nail tip	Respiratory problems

Appearance	*Health Considerations*
Horizontal ridges (from side to side)	Severe physical or psychological stress
Vertical ridges (from tip to base)	A tendency towards arthritis; adrenal weakness; kidney weakness; hormone imbalance; protein deficiency
Horizontal depressions (called Beau's lines)	Severe illness or surgery
White lines and horizontal ridges	Arsenic poisoning
Black vertical lines or spots on the nails	Ulcer: digestive/intestinal or kidney ulcer
White horizontal lines	Can indicate urine protein and a kidney problem. Pellagra; Hodgkin's disease; Sickle Cell Anemia
Brittle nails, or nail plate splitting from nail bed	Thyroid disease or vitamin deficiency
Splinter hemorrhages (red streaks in the nail bed)	Internal infection, especially of the heart valve
Thick nails	Circulatory problems
Splitting nails	A lack of hydrochloric acid used for digestion
Flat nails	Reynaud's disease
Nail beading (bumpy nails)	Arthritis
Unusually wide, square nails	Hormonal disorder or thyroid disease
Red skin around cuticles	Poor metabolism of Essential Fatty Acids (EFAs)
Creamy, pale-ridged nails	Iron deficiency, anemia
Thin nails	Diet lacks sulfur-containing amino acids.
Yellow nails	Digestion problems; fungal nail infection
Brown nails	Chronic renal failure

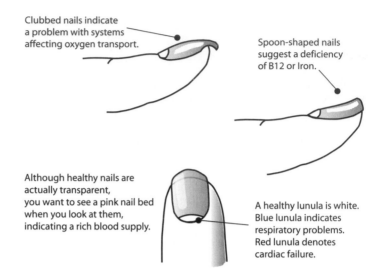

Clubbed nails indicate a problem with systems affecting oxygen transport.

Spoon-shaped nails suggest a deficiency of B12 or Iron.

Although healthy nails are actually transparent, you want to see a pink nail bed when you look at them, indicating a rich blood supply.

A healthy lunula is white. Blue lunula indicates respiratory problems. Red lunula denotes cardiac failure.

Appearance	*Health Considerations*
Bluish nails	**Circulatory, heart and lung problems**
Half-pink, half-white nails	**Kidney disease**
White nails	**Liver disease**
Yellowish nails with slight blush at base	**Diabetes**
Pale nail beds	**Anemia**

The chart "What Are Your Nails Telling You?" illustrates the important role your nails play in your overall health and well-being. Because the effects of these problems may take a long time to correct, you might not see the result in your fingernails for a year or two.

Side Effects of Prescription Drug Use

If you are receiving certain medical treatments, such as chemotherapy, be prepared for changes in the quality of your nails. Drug-induced complications from taxanes used in chemotherapy include such things as Beau's lines, fungal infections, nail pigmentation, splinter hemorrhages, infection of the nail fold, and pain and loss of the nail. Brimonidine, a potential therapy for certain forms of glaucoma, can result in lichen planus of the nail and contact dermatitis on the skin around the nail.

Lichen planus is a skin condition involving bumps on the skin. When the nail is affected, it can contain grooves, become thin, split, or be lost entirely. A more complete discussion of lichen planus will follow in the coming pages. These side effects gradually disappeared when use of brimonidine was discontinued. Beau's lines have been linked to the use of maxifloxacin for anaerobic pulmonary infection, while yellowed nails have resulted from the use of depakote for the treatment of convulsions, migraines, and bipolar disorder. Drug interactions usually involve all or several of the nails. Talk to your health-care provider if you are experiencing trouble-some nail reactions to prescription drugs you are using. In the mean-time, in the next few pages you'll learn what you can do to help your nails heal.

> **Age brings a loss of moisture to the nails that can leave them thinner and more brittle. Drastic dieting and eating disorders can also affect your nails, as can vitamin deficiencies. In fact, nail disorders comprise about 10% of all skin conditions.**

About Nail Trouble

Onychomocosis is the technical term for a fungal infection of the nail bed or nail plate, and it accounts for 50% of all nail diseases reported to health-care providers. The numbers rise to 60% in the elderly population. These fungal infections cause discolored, thickened, and damaged nails, and they affect 2% to 18.5% of adults. The infections pose major inconveniences, and it's not surprising that 25% of the people treated reported that the condition interfered with their professional lives due to discomfort or embarrassment. Because feet are often trapped inside shoes and socks, fungal infections are most common on the toenails. The most frequent cause of fungal nail infections, *Candida albicans,* is a factor in 60% of cases.

Mainstream medical treatment of fungal infections normally includes use of one of two potent anti-fungals, itraconazole or flucona-zole, but relapses after treatment are common. There are two possible explanations for this. First of all, *Candida* infection is always a sign of a depressed immune system, and it has the potential to return until the immune system is strong. Second, the use of antibiotics and anti-fungal treatments can become a vicious circle. While antibiotics may help speed your recovery from an infection, they also eliminate many beneficial bacteria, creating an environment where invasive bacteria like *Candida* can restore their numbers. So in circular fashion, any type of infection that is treated with antibiotics or anti-fungals has the potential to create a new fungal infection in a matter of time.

> ### At-Home Care for a Nail Infection
>
> If you would like to try a remedy for your infection at home before you head to the doctor for a prescription, take advantage of the healing properties of tea tree oil. Researchers at the University of Rochester School of Medicine found tea tree oil to be as effective as the prescription medication clotrimazole. Massage the nail bed with a drop of tea tree oil two or three times a day. Look for tea tree oil at your health products store.

If your fingernails are showing a *Candida* infection, it's likely that you already have a systemic infection, so you'll have to take a few more steps to get permanent relief. (See Chapter 5.) The key to a complete cure is to focus on the cause of the infection while you treat the uncomfortable symptoms. Make sure that you limit the burden on your immune system with proper diet, exercise, rest, and supplemental nutrients when necessary. Take advantage of the antioxidant power of grapeseed extract to speed healing. Remember that when it comes to any kind of infection, antibiotics should be used with discretion. Always support the proper functioning of your body by rebuilding your beneficial bacterial security team through the supplementation of probiotics.

Hammering Out Nail Problems

Problems with nails are not common in children, but they increase as we age due to a weakened immune system caused by poor dietary choices, circulatory problems, and the use of medications. Be sure that you consult your health-care provider if you suspect that you have any of the following six nail conditions.

Yellow Nail Syndrome

This syndrome is associated with yellow nails, excess fluid in tissues causing swelling (lymphedema), and excess fluid around the lungs (pleural effusion). Chronic sinusitis is often a factor, and such conditions as recurrent pneumonia and humoral immunity deficiencies can also be present. Along with medical treatment, vitamins A and E, in conjunction with zinc sulfate, have proven beneficial. Spontaneous healing is reported in 30% of the cases. (Do not assume, however, that because your nails are yellow, you have yellow nail syndrome. Dark nail polishes can also cause the nail to yellow.)

Tumors and Warts

Either cancerous or benign, these lesions can occur near any portion of the nail unit, and the actual nail can be destroyed as a result. Warts are painful viral infections that affect the skin underneath or around the nail. Treatment usually involves freezing or application of a chemical, but if the growth extends into the nail fold or under the nail plate, surgery may be necessary. Speak to your health-care practitioner if you think you have this problem.

Nail Psoriasis

Up to 50% of patients with psoriasis experience nail problems, and 80% of people who suffer from inflammatory arthritis associated with psoriasis show pitting and discoloration of the fingernails or toenails. The size, shape, and depth of the marks can vary, and affected nails may thicken, yellow, or crumble. The skin around the nail is sometimes inflamed, and the nail may peel away from the nail bed in a process called onycholysis.

Follow both your health-care practitioner's advice and the nutritional recommendations for psoriasis made in Chapter 6. Your nails will benefit especially from nutritional supplements, including folic acid, vitamin A, vitamin E, selenium, zinc, and dietary silicon.

Paronychia

If your hands are frequently immersed in water (as in the case of bartenders, dishwashers, and cooks) or if they often come into contact with chemicals, you are at risk for paronychia, another fungal infection. It results from organisms entering the skin when a gap occurs between the nail and the surrounding skin. Aggressive nail biters and children who suck their fingers are also susceptible. Often a warm-water soak with tea tree oil will help if no abscess has formed. Otherwise, you should seek medical attention. Left untreated, you could lose the nail. If your hands are regularly deep in water, wear a pair of cotton gloves under your rubber gloves for ultimate protection.

Lichen planus

Lichen planus is a non-contagious skin disease that often occurs in middle-aged adults. Its exact cause is unknown, but the condition has been linked to allergic reactions to medications for arthritis, heart disease, and high blood pressure. Some people with Lichen planus may also have Hepatitis C, so a dermatologist should check for this. Lichen planus is characterized by reddish-purple itchy bumps that favor the inside of wrists and ankles, although it can appear anywhere on the body. When it attacks nails, it may also cause thinning, brittleness, and exaggerated vertical ridges. In severe cases, the nail may be temporarily or permanently destroyed. Speak to your health-care practitioner if you have signs of this condition.

Artificial Nail Trouble

Resins used in artificial nails can cause allergic reactions, including pain, swelling, and redness in the nail bed, and they can also affect other parts of the body, such as the face and neck. Severe reactions can actually cause the nail to lift from the nail bed. If the root becomes damaged in the process, the replacement nail can be permanently malformed. Fungal infections are also common if moisture is trapped between the real nail and the artificial one. Studies show that nurses with artificial nails have more bacteria on their hands than those with real nails.

Prevention

Since many nail disorders result from poor nail care, developing good habits early will help keep them healthy. Make sure you keep nails clean and dry so that bacteria have no chance to grow. Take at least 15 seconds to wash your hands, using soap and water. Avoid biting your fingernails, pulling at hangnails, or digging out ingrown toenails. Do not remove or cut your cuticle, as this will invite infection. Instead, gently push the cuticle back with an orange stick. Researchers have discovered that artificial and natural nails extending farther than 3 millimeters beyond the tip of the finger harbor more harmful bacteria and yeast than short nails, so if you have a problem with infections, shorter nails are better. Regular supplementation of acidopholus should also help prevent recurrences of fungal infections.

Growing Healthy Nails

Your nail health depends on a varied and well-balanced diet that includes fresh fruits and veggies, whole grains, and plenty of protein from legumes (beans, peas, lentils, and soy products), seeds, nuts, low- or non-fat dairy if you eat diary, eggs, fish, and lean meats. Also include broccoli, onions, and sea vegetables, as they are excellent sources of sulfur and silicon.

> **Biotin-Rich Foods for Cracking and Splitting Nails**
>
> Egg yolks
> Fish
> Liver and other organ meats
> Soybeans
> Whole grains and cereals
> Yeast

Studies have proven that the B vitamin biotin can help remedy cracking or splitting nails, and this nutrient occurs naturally in cauliflower, lentils, and especially peanuts. Although biotin deficiency is rare, it might be a problem if you are on a long-term regimen of antibiotics or a long-term calorie-reduced diet. A diet too high in citrus fruits, salt, or vinegar can also adversely affect your nails.

Home Remedies for Common Nail Problems

Nail Biting

Along with the obvious fact that you will never have beautiful fingernails if you keep chewing them off, biting nails easily transmits germs and infection from your mouth to your fingertips and vice versa. And biting down to the "quick" usually involves the skin around the nail, inviting yet another entry point for infection. Coating your nails with something distasteful may help you break the habit. Look for safe, all-natural products that contain no harmful chemicals like acetone or lacquer. Remember, the problem is that your fingers are in your mouth! You don't want to be swallowing toxic chemicals. Try to determine what triggers your need to nibble, and refocus your energy on a more productive pursuit.

Ingrown Toenails

Ingrown toenails are an extremely painful condition in which the nail grows directly into the flesh beside the nail. Most common in males between the ages of 10 and 30, ingrown nails often result from cutting toenails too short, from wearing shoes that cramp the toes, or from a poor, leaning-forward posture (which causes a corner of the nail to curve downward toward the skin). To avoid getting ingrown toenails in the first place, trim your nails straight across, but with a slight curve at the tip for maximum strength. Leave them longer than the nail fold and be sure to wear shoes with ample toe room. Ingrown toenails can lead to infection if not properly treated, but be sure to consult your health-care practitioner for an accurate diagnosis. Do not try to dig out the problem nail yourself! That could add an infection to your original problem.

Hangnails

Those tiny pieces of skin that break near the side of your nail are most often the result of dehydrated cuticles. They have no nerve endings, but they can still hurt because they affect the "live" part of the nearby skin. Avoid biting or picking the hangnails, as this can lead to tearing and infection. Instead, use nail scissors to snip off the part that is no longer "live." But be careful not to cut to the quick. And if your hangnails become infected, give your fingers a soak in tea tree oil. As always, an ounce of prevention is worth a pound of cure, so keep your cuticles properly moisturized by massaging them nightly with jojoba or vitamin E oil. And to protect your nails, don't use them as tools for scraping, picking, or turning screws!

> **Like skin, our nails are permeable. That means that whatever you put on them soaks into them, and by extension, you. In fact, medical treatments for certain nail conditions involve applying medication as you would a nail polish.**

The Cosmetic Conundrum

Like skin, our nails are permeable. That means that whatever you put on them soaks into them, and by extension, you. In fact, medical treatments for certain nail conditions involve applying medication as you would a nail polish. Because chemicals enter our bodies through our nails, it's important to give some thought to what we are using on them. Unfortunately, many of the products found in your local drugstore or cosmetics counter may contain dangerous and potentially lethal chemicals.

Of course, allergic reactions are the most common complication associated with nail products, and these can result in itching, burning, and pain in the nail bed and cuticle. This pain can even extend to other parts of the body, including the face and neck. Eyelids are also a common site of allergic reactions to nail care products. But more serious issues need to be considered before you empty your wallet at the cosmetics counter.

Acetone, ethanol, limonene, and tolulene are common ingredients in nail products, and all have been linked to allergic and toxic reactions. Formaldehyde is another ingredient that you should watch for as you choose your products. Used with abandon in nail polish, hardeners, and removers, formaldehyde is a carcinogen and has been found in studies to damage DNA. I'll go into detail about these and other chemicals in Chapter 13. Fortunately, there are non-toxic options available. Look for water-soluble products that don't require a remover when you want to change your look . (Removers strip your nail of necessary oil and water, leading to dry, peeling, and easily breakable nails.) As technology continues to catch up with demand, you should be able to find the quality, color, and shine in these products that you've come to expect from their conventional counterparts. As you switch to healthier and more fingernail-friendly products, make sure you allow enough time for damaged nails to grow out between polishings.

And once you've given the nails on your hands and feet some proper TLC, you might decide to show them off *au naturel* instead of coating them in color!

The All-Natural Pedicure

This recipe for comfort appeared in the chapter on treating your body's whole skin well (Chapter 8), but it's worth repeating here as a tonic for your toenails. Soak your feet in warm water for 10 minutes to soothe achy muscles and soften the skin on the bottoms of your feet. If you are doing an internal cleanse, adding Epsom salts to the water will help draw out toxins. For an invigorating soak, add peppermint or rosemary essential oil to the water, but for a relaxing end to your day, opt instead for lavender or rose oil. Use a nailbrush to clean under and around your nails, as well as the bottoms of your feet. Gently exfoliate with a pumice stone or foot scrub, taking care not to remove too much of the protective outer layer. Regular exfoliation should help remove painful corns and calluses.

When you've had your soak, thoroughly dry your feet and carefully push back your cuticle with an orange stick. Never cut your cuticle, as doing so can lead to infection. Using straight-edge clippers, trim your toenails to a length past the end of the nail fold without tapering corners to prevent the nail from growing painfully into the skin around your nail. Give yourself a well-deserved foot massage with coconut, olive, or avocado oil, and slip on a pair of cotton socks. Avoid wearing socks and shoes that are too tight. If ingrown toenails are a problem for you, you'll have to pass on pointy shoe trends and opt for a fashionable shoe with a wide toe area.

Pamper Your Fingernails

Constantly exposed to harsh elements, chemicals, and chores, give your fingernails the well-deserved treat of a 10-minute soak in olive oil. And if your nails are looking weak, soak them in warm water with horsetail or rosemary essential oil. Use evening primrose or calendula if you need to soften them, and myrrh will help to prevent breakage. Gently push back your cuticles with an orange stick, but never cut them. That could lead to infection. After drying your nails, replenish their moisture by massaging them with olive oil or a chamomile moisture cream. Buff to a shine with a buffer or soft cloth. Regularly moisturizing your nails and cuticles with lotions containing natural lactic, glycolic, or malic acid can help to keep the skin around them supple.

> ### Beauty Kit for Your Fingers and Toes
> Oil for soaking
> Pumice stone or Footscrub
> Toenail brush
> Toenail clippers
> Emery board
> Orange stick
> Buffer
> Moisturizer or massage oil
> and …
> A few minutes for you!

File your nails in one direction to the shape you prefer. If your cuticle is oval shaped, go with an oval-shaped nail tip. Squared cuticles look best with squared tips. Although nail length trends change with hemlines, remember that nails start to break easily when they are longer than a quarter-inch past the fingertip. Use a buffer to shine the tops of the nails on your fingers and toes. You might be amazed at the glow you can achieve without polish.

To protect your manicure, always wear gloves when doing chores. Moisturize your hands and nails morning and night to prevent them from drying out, and be sure to apply a sunscreen with at least SPF 15 to your hands whenever you're outside.

One last tip: don't think of beautiful nails as a sign of vanity. Healthy nails are an extension of healthy living.

Beauty Prescription for Healthy Nails

Take your *Living Beauty Essentials* daily, as described in Chapters 2 and 3. You will see that, for this prescription, some of those nutrients should be taken in the higher daily-total amounts shown below, along with any extra nutrients listed in this table.

Total Daily Amount

Vitamin A	10,000 IU	Helps your nails use protein
Vitamin B complex including biotin	100 mg	Strengthens brittle nails
Vitamin C with bioflavonoids	1,000 mg, 3 times per day or to bowel tolerance	Hangnails, inflammation, Helps treat infections
Zinc	50 mg daily. Do not exceed 100 mg from all sources.	Eliminate white spots
Iron (Ferrous fumerate)	Only on the advice of your health-care provider	To correct spoon-shaped nails
Dietary Silicon	3 mg choline – stabilized, concentrated orthosilicic acid once or twice per day	

Make sure that you drink plenty of pure, filtered water, and avoid refined sugars.

CHAPTER ELEVEN

A Healthy, Beautiful Smile

Beauty is power; a smile is its sword.
—*Charles Reade*

Ask anyone what feature they notice most when meeting someone for the first time, and they will likely answer: the eyes or
the smile. While the eyes are the windows of the soul, the
smile is the open door that invites you in. So it's really important to
have a smile that's friendly and warm.

Of course, this means having teeth and lips that are healthy and
attractive. But everyone has dental problems at some point, and in the
first part of this chapter, we'll look at a few of the key tooth and mouth
attackers. As you'll see, the majority of dental issues are caused by
improper oral care, but others come from some surprising sources.

Cavities

Cavities, or dental caries, represent tooth decay.
They start with dental plaque, a sticky film that
forms on and between the teeth, along the gum-
line, and in pits in the teeth. Plaque is made up of
a list of multisyllabic elements—micro-organisms, leukocytes, macrophages, and epithelial
cells—to name a few, and if it's not removed on a
regular basis, it will harden to become calculus,
or tartar, which can discolor teeth. Plaque can
also lead to inflammation of the gums (see
"Gingivitis," below). Meanwhile, when sugar
appears on the scene, the bacteria in plaque go to

Second-Hand Smoke and Tooth Decay

According to a study carried
out to determine the effect
of passive cigarette smoke
on the teeth of young children, second-hand smoke
inhalation is responsible for
27% of unfilled decayed
teeth and 14% of filled
teeth. More evidence that
smoking and health don't
mix—and that kids can be
caught in the crossfire.

work fermenting it, and this leads to the formation of acids that can destroy our pearly whites. If a cavity is not treated, decay will proceed through the surface enamel to the softer, second layer of the tooth called the dentin. At this stage, the cavity could start to cause pain, and if it's not treated, an abscess can form. The best way to avoid this situation is to prevent cavities from forming in the first place—through tooth brushing, daily flossing, and regular visits to the dentist for thorough cleanings. It's also a good idea to avoid constant snacking, as this provides a steady source of cavity-forming acid. If you can't brush your teeth after every meal, at least rinse your mouth with a glass of pure, unfiltered water.

Got a Cavity, Get a Filling, Right?

We've been brought up to think the solution to our tooth complaints is a handy filling. But it's actually not that simple. The problem lies in the fillings themselves. The common silver amalgams that many people have in their mouths contain 50% mercury, one of the most toxic heavy metals on earth. Why is it so poisonous? It loves taking up residence in the nervous system, with rather serious consequences. During the 19th century, in fact, English hat makers used mercury as a stiffener, and the chemical's effect on them gave rise to the expression "mad as a hatter."

Mercury in your mouth can also have damaging consequences. Vapors from mercury fillings combine with saliva to form methyl mercury, and this is absorbed into the bloodstream. From there, it travels throughout the body and accumulates in various tissues. Most of us would not think of our fillings when confused or depressed or when suffering from muscle spasms, tremors, poor coordination, weakness, high blood pressure, or pain in the back or face. But mercury poisoning

---

Try this delicious pesto recipe to help move metals out of your body.

Coriander Chelation Pesto

4 cloves garlic
1/3 cup Brazil nuts
1/3 cup sunflower seeds
1/3 cup pumpkin seeds
2 cups packed fresh coriander (cilantro, Chinese parsley)
2/3 cup flaxseed oil
4 tbsp lemon juice
2 tsp dulse powder
Sea salt to taste

Process the coriander and flaxseed oil in a blender until the coriander is chopped. Add the garlic, nuts, seeds, dulse, and lemon juice and blend into a paste. Add a pinch of sea salt to taste and blend again. Store in dark glass jars. Recipe freezes well. Take two teaspoons of this pesto daily for three weeks at least once a year. Try it on baked potatoes, pasta, and toast.

leads to these symptoms. *Candida*, dermatitis, and hair loss may also be linked to mercury in the body. This destructive chemical also causes kidney and liver damage, and it has been associated with Alzheimer's disease. Because mercury displaces iodine in the thyroid gland, this toxin may also be a factor in hypothyroid conditions.

If you have any of these symptoms or conditions, consider having your silver-amalgam fillings replaced. And if you are troubled by any other symptoms that simply won't go away, no matter what you do, you should also consider having your fillings replaced with a non-toxic material. Most people who do this experience almost immediate relief from symptoms they'd simply taken for granted as a part of aging. Vitamin E and antioxidant selenium are also useful for displacing (chelating) mercury, as is Aged Garlic Extract (AGE). At the same time, AGE protects red blood cells from damage due to heavy-metal poisoning.

Removing mercury fillings is not without complications. For instance, drilling out old fillings can release enormous amounts of mercury, so choose a dental professional who is experienced at this serious task. If you are a parent of young children, consider having their teeth sealed to protect against cavity formation.

Beauty Prescription for Mercury Fillings

Take your *Living Beauty Essentials* daily, as described in Chapters 2 and 3. You will see that, for this prescription, some of those nutrients should be taken in the higher daily-total amounts shown below, along with any extra nutrients listed in this table.

	Total Daily Amount
Vitamin A	20,000 IU for one month; then 5,000 IU
Vitamin B complex	100 mg
Vitamin C with bioflavonoids	4,000–8,000 mg or to bowel tolerance, in 2–3 equally divided doses
Vitamin E	400–800 IU
Selenium	200 mcg
Co-Enzyme Q10	50–60 mg, with food

Saliva

Saliva is a behind-the-scenes part of our body's cast of actors—that is, until we need to give a speech or are in some other stressful situation. That's when we really miss this helper, as our mouths go dry and we have a hard time swallowing. But on a day-to-day basis, saliva provides vital enzymes to help us break down our food—and it also acts to protect our teeth from cavities. People who suffer from an insufficient flow of saliva, known as xerostomia, also experience more cavities, plaque, and microbial overgrowth.

Saliva also contains the immunoglobulin A (IgA), which is the chief antibody in the gastrointestinal and respiratory tract, giving our bodies an early antibacterial and antiviral defense. A shortage of saliva necessarily means a shortage of this valuable defense mechanism. And research shows that a lower quantity of saliva and corresponding IgA were evident in patients diagnosed with oral carcinoma. We certainly feel parched when we haven't taken in enough water or when colds force us to turn into mouth-breathers. Although our mouths become less moist as we age, serious dryness is cause for medical attention. Xerostomia may be a symptom of systemic diseases like rheumatoid arthritis and Sjogren's syndrome. Sjogren's syndrome is an autoimmune condition in which the immune system attacks the salivary glands.

Diabetes, hypothyroidism, alcohol use, and some medications can also cause a parched palate. Left untreated, dry mouth leads to tooth decay and mouth infections such as thrush. Be sure to seek medical attention if your mouth is abnormally dry. To improve your moisture content, be sure to take in adequate water. Chew on healthy snacks like carrots and celery, and breathe through your nose.

The Best Antidote: A Good Friend

A recent study showed that having at least one close friend can reduce your risk of gum disease by as much as 30%. Friends typically help us deal with life's little stresses and often offer us opportunities for relaxing leisure activities. Call a friend. Among other things, it's good for your gums!

Gum Disease

Gingivitis

When sticky plaque builds up on teeth and starts to harden into tartar, the associated bacteria triggers inflammation of the gingiva, or gums. They become red and swollen and are prone to bleeding. Puberty and pregnancy can worsen the problem, as can the use of birth control pills. In cyclical fashion, swollen gums caused by medication, deficiency of vitamins C and niacin, or tobacco use make the removal of plaque more difficult, and this leads to more inflammation. Speak with your health-care provider if prescription medications have made your gums swell or bleed.

Probiotics will help maintain a healthy balance of bacteria in your system—and that includes your mouth. If you have no disease that affects your teeth and gums, you can stay that way by following the advice you learned when you were a child: brush your teeth at least twice a day and floss daily. We're all tempted to leave flossing off the agenda. It seems such a bother to wind those threads between every pair of teeth, especially when we're tired. But skipping the routine can lead to bleeding gums and gum disease. Besides, flossing feels good when you get used to it. It's a tingly and invigorating gum massage. Once you're proficient at the process, you'll likely find you're not in the dentist's chair quite as long at cleaning time!

> ## Green Tea for a Perfect Smile
>
> Research shows that drinking green tea on a daily basis helps kill the bacteria that lead to gingivitis and periodontal disease.

Periodontitis

Periodontal disease occurs when gingivitis is not treated and invading bacteria spread through the gums to the underlying bone. Symptoms include red, swollen gums that may be bleeding and shrinking away from the tooth—not to mention bad breath. Eventually, if left untreated, the foundation of the tooth is weakened, becomes loose, and falls out. An abscess can also develop, causing extreme pain. Medical conditions such as diabetes mellitus, Crohn's disease, and AIDS increase susceptibility to periodontal disease—a condition that requires professional medical attention.

Beauty Prescription for Gum Disease

Take your *Living Beauty Essentials* daily, as described in Chapters 2 and 3. You will see that, for this prescription, some of those nutrients should be taken in the higher daily-total amounts shown below, along with any extra nutrients listed in this table.

Total Daily Amount

Vitamin A	20,000 IU for one month; then 5,000 IU
Vitamin B complex	100 mg
Vitamin C with bioflavonoids	3,000–8,000 mg or to bowel tolerance, in 2–3 equally divided doses
Vitamin E	400–800 IU
Zinc lozenges	100 mg. Do not exceed 100 mg daily from all sources.
Co-Enzyme Q10	50–60 mg, with food
Cranberry	Simmer 2 tbsp dried cranberries with 8 oz. water for 10 minutes; strain. Drink 2–3 cups per day to kill bacteria.

How to Brush Your Teeth

Many of us have been brushing our teeth for decades, but dentists know that we don't always do it the right way! Here's how you can brush up on your brushing. Make sure your toothbrush isn't too big or too small and choose one that's in a good shape for your mouth. The brush should let you reach every nook and cranny of your mouth, and its bristles should be soft. Replace your toothbrush every three months or after a cold, flu, mouth infection, or cold sore.

Now here's the skinny on your morning, evening, and after-meals tooth-care routine. Place the side of your brush along your bottom gum-line at a 45-degree angle. Then, using a gentle side-to-side motion, move the brush upwards, away from the gum-line to the top of the tooth. Your brush should be in contact with two or three teeth at a time. When you've done the first batch, lift your brush and move on to the next group of teeth. For your top teeth, start the brush at the gum-line and move downward. Then move on to the chewing surfaces. Gently clean them with a back-and-forth motion and hold the brush vertically to get behind your back teeth. But when doing any of these tooth routines, don't scrub too hard! That can cause gum irritation and recession, and it can damage the structure of the tooth. Last but not least, give your tongue a scrub to remove bacteria.

Even if we use the right brushing techniques, we often just do a going-through-the-motions, lick-and-a-promise type of tooth-cleaning operation. While you're at it, you might as well do it the right way and take at least three minutes before rushing away.

How to Floss

And here are the facts of floss. Start with about 18 inches of floss, and wrap one end around the middle finger of one hand. Leaving about 2 inches to work with, keep the remaining floss in your other hand. Using the thumb and forefinger of each hand, grasp the floss and ease it between your teeth, reaching the gum-line. Create a C-shape with the floss around your tooth, covering as much of the surface of the tooth as possible. Gently move the floss up and down and back and forth to remove plaque from the side of the tooth. Move on to the other side of the tooth, releasing clean floss from your inventory as you go.

Be gentle, as aggressive flossing can cause damage to the gums. Don't be surprised if your gums bleed the first few times you floss. As flossing becomes part of your daily routine, you'll wonder how you lived without the incredible feeling of clean teeth and gums.

The Health Connection

It's a good idea to take care of your teeth and gums for the sake of your appearance, but serious health matters may be at stake, as well. Recent studies indicate that gum disease is associated with diabetes, respiratory disease, cardiovascular disease (including stroke and heart disease), and even premature babies. In fact, many studies have linked gum disease with infective endocarditis, an infection that targets the endocardium (the lining) and the valves of the heart. This disease takes hold when bacteria enter the bloodstream and travel to the heart, where they lodge in the valves. Bacterial entry is simplified when the gums are injured by disease. People with damaged heart valves are most at risk, but aggressive bacteria can harm normal heart valves too.

Bacteria in the bloodstream is a condition called bacteremia, and if left untreated, it may also turn into the severe blood infection known as septicemia, whose symptoms include chills and shaking, along with elevated fever and low blood pressure. People who develop septicemia are at high risk of developing infective endocarditis. With this heart infection, clots and accumulations of bacteria called vegetations can break away and travel through the bloodstream to other locations, where they can block arteries. These blockages can lead to heart attack and stroke, as well as causing infection and damage to nearby organs. Acute infective endocarditis can come on suddenly or it can develop slowly over a period of several months, but whatever its speed, infective endocarditis is a life-threatening condition.

You may remember from the introduction to this book that my son was born with a minor heart imperfection. Instead of having three leaflets on his aortic valve, he has only two. About 1% of girls and 2% of boys are born with a bicuspid aortic valve, which causes leakage of blood from the valve every time the valve relaxes. The effect is commonly known as a heart murmur. Although my son and others who have this condition can lead healthy, active lives, they are at higher-than-average risk of developing infective endocarditis. And anyone with a heart concern needs to be especially attentive to good oral care, to make sure that bacteria have no point of entry through the gum. They also need to tell their dentists about their condition before any invasive procedure, as cut gums could allow bacteria to enter the bloodstream. Typically, a round of antibiotics is used as a preventive measure for dental and surgical procedures.

As a final caution, I urge you to have your doctor check your heart for a heart murmur. A close friend of mine lived 37 years of her life unaware that she, too, had a bicuspid aortic valve and mild murmur! After a visit to the dentist for a minor procedure, she developed a high fever, with chills and shaking. She was eventually diagnosed with septicemia, and only then did a heart examination uncover the valve imperfection. Fortunately, she did not develop infective endocarditis, but her recovery was painstaking and slow. Mild heart murmurs are more apparent when fever is present, so ask your physician to have a listen to your heart the next time you are feeling under the weather.

And be sure to enjoy a full regime of brushing and flossing.

Tooth Discoloration

Everybody wants pearly whites, but many factors determine the color of our teeth: heredity, metabolism, reactions to chemicals, and infections. Thickness of enamel, as well as the protein and calcium content of teeth, can also have an impact on their color. Drugs such as tetracycline can discolor a child's teeth and affect the hardness of the enamel if it is taken by the mother during pregnancy or by the child when teeth are being formed. Drinking coffee, tea, and red wine can also temporarily stain teeth. Talk to your dentist about how to improve the appearance of your choppers and how to prevent problems for your children.

> **Although mottling may seem more like an issue of vanity than one of health, excess fluoride has been linked to pitted, brittle teeth and an increase in cavity formation.**

And then there's your drinking water. Yes, you read that correctly. If your water is fluoridated, the fluoride can accumulate in your teeth in a condition called dental fluorosis. Fluorosis causes chalky white patches to appear on the surface of teeth, and these may eventually turn brown or yellow. Although mottling may seem more like an issue of vanity than one of health, excess fluoride has been linked to pitted, brittle teeth and an increase in cavity formation. Moving beyond the mouth, fluorosis can also affect the health of bones, and it's associated with the development of osteoporosis and osteofluorosis. A condition that doesn't get as much press as osteoporosis, osteofluorosis is the abnormal hardening of bone caused by prolonged overdose of fluoride. You might be surprised to learn what research has proven about the fluoride that may be in your drinking water.

The Fluoridation Debate

Between the years 1908 and 1925, Dr. Frederick McKay of Colorado observed that the same element in drinking water that caused brown staining and mottling of teeth also seemed to prevent cavities. By 1942, Dr. H. Tredley Dean had determined that optimal fluoride levels of 1 part per million in drinking water could prevent cavities without promoting the mottling associated with fluorosis. After fluoride was duly added to drinking water in many North American communities, studies in both Canada and the United States saw a decline in numbers of cavities. As a result, today, about 56% of the U.S. population regularly drinks fluoridated water.

Health problems related to fluoride have arisen because levels determined to be fluorosis-preventive for teeth were not tested for their effect on the entire body before fluoride was added to the water supply. Although 1 part per million in drinking water is arguably optimal for dental health, we are now overexposed to fluoride. This trace element—which in high concentrations is toxic—is now added to toothpaste, mouthwash, and chewing gum, and when it is in the relevant water supplies, it is also present in our fruits and vegetables.

Because fluorine is actually a trace element in the earth, it also finds its way naturally into our food supply, thus increasing our exposure even more. A 2004 study, for example, showed that teas made with *Camellia sinensis,* including Oolong and black tea (the kind that most people drink most of the time) contain significant amounts of fluoride—high enough levels that drinking them may increase the risk of developing dental fluorosis.

Young children are also at risk. Infant beverages, especially baby formulas prepared with fluoridated water, can increase the chances of fluorosis appearing in primary teeth. In the past, it was believed that fluoride was necessary during tooth development, but recent studies have concluded that the caries-preventive effect of fluoride occurs almost entirely *after* teeth have appeared.

With all the fluoride exposure, it's no wonder that more problems are beginning to surface. Excess fluoride has also been linked with thyroid imbalances, particularly hypothyroid. So if you are concerned about underactive thyroid, you might be wise to stay away from fluoride. (See Chapter 6 for more information about thyroid conditions.) Although initially touted as a bone builder, fluoride is actually detrimental to bones. In July 2002, the government of Belgium banned supplemental fluoride tablets, drops, and chewing gum, basing their decision on research that linked fluoride with joint problems, skeletal deformities, bone cancer, osteoporosis, and problems with the central nervous system. Austria, Denmark, Germany, Japan, and Sweden have also ended water fluoridation, many of them citing the link to an increased risk of bone cancer.

Studies also show that we don't need to add fluoride to our water supplies in order to protect our teeth. Recent research in areas stretching from British Columbia and Cuba to the former East Germany indicate that the rate of cavity development does not increase in localities that remove fluoride from the water supply. Although explanations for this finding vary in each study, it's possible that in many cases, people are simply taking better care of their teeth. It's also likely that fluoride in toothpaste is helping prevent cavities. And since most toothpaste is not swallowed, it doesn't enter our bloodstream, where it would be a greater threat to our health. It's a bit ironic that communities add fluoride to drinking water, while instructions printed on toothpaste tubes indicate that we should avoid swallowing their product. Talk about a mixed message!

I urge you to do your own research about fluoride use in your community. That way, you can make an informed decision about whether fluoride will likely do you more harm than good. And if you opt to go the route of bottled water, don't assume that it is fluoride free. Let the buyer beware!

If you are concerned about the amount of fluoride that you may be taking in, supplementing with calcium and magnesium might help to offset fluoride toxicity.

Canker Sore

A canker sore is a small white spot that appears on the lips, gums, soft palate, and inside of the cheeks—and even the throat. The scientific name, *aphthous ulcer,* seems to more accurately suggest the amount of pain caused by these small lesions. Women are more inclined to experience cankers, and not surprisingly, stress appears to be a trigger. Food allergies, hormonal imbalances, poor dental health, and Crohn's disease have also been associated with canker development, the link with Crohn's suggesting a digestive system connection. Nutritional deficiencies of vitamin B12 and folic acid, iron, and the amino acid lysine may also be factors in the development of canker sores. You will find iron in green vegetables, blackstrap

> Women are more inclined to experience cankers, and not surprisingly, stress appears to be a trigger. Food allergies, hormonal imbalances, poor dental health, and Crohn's disease have also been associated with cankers.

molasses, nuts and seeds, fish, millet, and parsley. When you eat foods containing iron, be sure also to take in a source of vitamin C to enhance absorption—and never take iron supplements without the advice of a medical professional.

A diet focused on fresh fruits, vegetables, legumes, nuts and seeds, and whole grains will also tend to keep canker sores at bay. But if you do experience an episode of these sores, cut down on meat products, as these trigger acidity in the body, thus delaying healing. Of course, continue with your probiotics supplementation, and eat plenty of yoghurt, sauerkraut, kefir, and other natural food sources of beneficial bacteria. Identify sensitivities to products that you use in your mouth, such as toothpaste and mouthwash. Opt for natural products that do not contain alcohol, and instead of using mouthwash, rinse your mouth with tea tree oil. But be sure not to swallow. Tea tree oil is a powerful disinfectant!

Beauty Prescription for Canker Sores

Take your *Living Beauty Essentials* daily, as described in Chapters 2 and 3. You will see that, for this prescription, some of those nutrients should be taken in the higher daily-total amounts shown below, along with any extra nutrients listed in this table.

Total Daily Amount

Vitamin A	20,000 IU for one month; then 5,000 IU
Beta carotene	25,000 IU
Vitamin B complex	50 mg, 2 times per day (max 100 mg daily)
Vitamin C with bioflavonoids	3,000–8,000 mg or to bowel tolerance, in 2–3 equally divided doses
Vitamin E	400–800 IU
Zinc lozenges	Do not exceed 100 mg daily from all sources
L-Lysine	500 mg, twice per day, on an empty stomach (max, 1,000 mg daily)
Chamomile	Rinse with cooled tea made from 2–3 tsp of dried chamomile in 8 oz. of water

Cold Sores

Unlike canker sores, cold sores are caused by a viral infection. Herpes Simplex 1 (HS1) is a highly contagious virus, spread via skin-to-skin contact, including kissing and sexual contact. It is similar to, but not the same as, the virus that causes genital herpes.

People are often exposed to HS1 in childhood, when small blisters form in the mouth, accompanied by fever and general discomfort. Caregivers often think the symptoms result from teething. After primary exposure, the virus hides in the nervous system near the mouth, waiting to be awakened by a cold, fever, food sensitivity, sunlight on the lips, or stress. Cold sores then start to appear on the outer lips or on the palate inside the mouth. These bothersome sores start with a tingling or itchy sensation in one spot, in what is known as the prodome stage. The spot then erupts with a painful open sore that scabs over and then finally heals without a scar in about 10 days. High doses of vitamin C taken at the prodome stage may help to speed this process, so the cold sore doesn't stay around too long.

The herpes virus depends on the amino acid arginine for replication, so avoid food sources of arginine, including dairy products, chocolate, coconut, meats, soybeans, white flour, walnuts, and wheat germ. The essential amino acid lysine actually displaces arginine and is proven to prevent and speed recovery from herpes outbreaks. Look for lysine in eggs, fish, lima beans, and potatoes. Supplemental lysine is also available for those who suffer from cold sores.

Beauty Prescription for Cold Sores

Take your *Living Beauty Essentials* daily, as described in Chapters 2 and 3. You will see that, for this prescription, some of those nutrients should be taken in the higher daily-total amounts shown below, along with any extra nutrients listed in this table.

Total Daily Amount

Vitamin A	20,000 IU for one month; then 5,000 IU
Vitamin B complex	100 mg
Vitamin C with bioflavonoids	3,000–8,000 mg or to bowel tolerance, in 2–3 equally divided doses

	Total Daily Amount
Vitamin E	400–800 IU
Zinc lozenges	Do not exceed 100 mg daily from all sources
L-Lysine	500 mg, twice per day, on an empty stomach (max. 1,000 mg daily)

Bruxism

Even the word sounds painful. Bruxism refers to the clenching and grinding of teeth that can occur during the day but seems to cause most damage at night. People who grind their teeth are usually asleep during an episode, so they are often unaware that bruxism is a problem until daytime symptoms appear. Grinding leads to earache and neck and jaw pain—as well as possible marital problems if the noise is loud enough to wake up a sleeping partner!

When teeth are ground, their enamel wears down, so they become more sensitive to heat and cold. The pressure from grinding can also actually crack teeth and damage dental work. Pain from bruxism can lead to insomnia, depression, and eating disorders. Stress is usually a trigger for bruxism, while alcohol and allergies seem to make it worse. If you suspect (or someone has told you!) that you are a nighttime grinder, talk to your dentist about your options. Sometimes a dental guard can be worn during the night to prevent further tooth damage. Make a habit of regularly relaxing your face and jaw muscles during the day, and find ways to reduce stress in your life. Go for a walk, take up yoga, relax in a warm bath!

Halitosis

Bad breath is often caused by food stuck between teeth, poor oral hygiene, or gum disease. To help prevent this unwanted consequence, follow the cleaning protocols described earlier in this chapter under "How to Brush Your Teeth" and "How to Floss." Certain foods like onions and garlic contain volatile oils that travel through the bloodstream to the lungs from where they are eventually exhaled. And that exhalation causes the knock-'em-dead breath associated with these otherwise desirable veggies. Dieting can also cause bad breath as the body breaks down fat stores and protein to be used as fuel, and incomplete protein digestion can also cause a foul odor. To determine whether you have underactive digestion, try the hydrochloric acid self-test described in Chapter 3 and follow the recommendations given.

Infection of the respiratory tract, postnasal drip, or an imbalance of bacteria in the colon can also cause malodorous breath. Read Chapter 5 if you think that *Candida* overgrowth might be a factor contributing to your breath troubles. An overload of toxins is another possible explanation for halitosis, so you might consider doing a cleanse to clear the air. Halitosis can also be a symptom of serious health conditions such as diabetes and liver or kidney problems. Kidney failure can cause a urine-like aroma, while the smell of nail-polish remover (acetone) is associated with uncontrolled diabetes. Talk to your health-care provider if you can't get rid of your bad breath on your own.

> Chlorophyll is a powerful blood cleaner that's commonly found in green health drinks. In fact, rather than using an alcohol-based mouthwash, find one that's formulated with chlorophyll.

Chlorophyll is a powerful blood cleaner that's commonly found in green health drinks. In fact, rather than using an alcohol-based mouthwash, find one that's formulated with chlorophyll. After a delicious garlic-and-onion-filled meal, you can also chomp on the parsley that often decorates your plate at a restaurant. Parsley is full of breath-freshening chlorophyll.

As part of your twice-daily cleansing ritual, don't forget to brush your tongue, especially toward the back. And drink plenty of water to help disperse the bacteria that always accumulate in your mouth.

Beauty Prescription for Halitosis

Take your *Living Beauty Essentials* daily, as described in Chapters 2 and 3. You will see that, for this prescription, some of those nutrients should be taken in the higher daily-total amounts shown below, along with any extra nutrients listed in this table.

	Total Daily Amount
Vitamin A	10,000 IU
Vitamin B complex	100 mg
Vitamin C with bioflavonoids	3,000–5,000 mg or to bowel tolerance, in 2–3 equally divided doses

	Total Daily Amount
Vitamin E	400–800 IU
Zinc	50–100 mg. Do not exceed 100 mg daily from all sources
Chlorophyll	From alfalfa, wheatgrass, barley, etc. Available in green drinks or as liquid supplement. Follow label directions

Oral Cancers

Benign and malignant growths can develop anywhere in the mouth, including the tongue, the lining of the cheek, the gums, and the salivary glands. They can also appear on the floor of the mouth or on the soft palate (the back part of the roof of the mouth). If you notice changes in your mouth such as a variation in pigmentation (red spots, white spots, or dark areas) report them to your doctor. Textural changes including rough spots, growths, or the development of wart-like bumps should also be discussed with your doctor. Be sure that your health-care provider includes an oral checkup as part of your regular health exam. When detected early, oral cancers are highly curable. Unfortunately, since many oral cancers aren't found until the lymph nodes are involved, 25% of oral cancers are fatal. That's why you must see your doctor immediately if you notice any of the changes described here.

Luscious Lips

Soft, luscious, and plump lips symbolize youth and beauty, so your lips deserve some attention. Sun damage can lead to dryness, hardness, and cracking, so be sure to wear a lip balm that will offer some sun protection when you're outside. For a natural alternative to chemical sunscreens, look for a product containing coconut oil. A wide-brimmed hat will help shade your pucker from the sun, possibly preventing an outbreak of cold sores and sunburned lips, while at the same time shielding your skin. Freckles on lips are safe, but brownish-black spots may indicate the inherited stomach and intestinal disease called Peutz-Jeghers syndrome. Red lip spots may indicate an increased risk of cancer. Report these possibly dangerous changes to your doctor. Inflamed lips caused by trauma, allergic reactions to sunburn, or the inherited swelling condition called angioedema can lead to irritation in the corners of the mouth. This can lead to cracks, which create an open invitation for the fungus thrush to develop.

Deficiencies in vitamin B2 can cause dry skin around the lips, as well as cracks in the corners of your mouth. Lips tend to become thinner as we age, partly due to the constant pull of gravity. So if you'd like to keep your lip-line without resorting to injections of foreign substances, try using gravity to your advantage by turning upside down every so often. (See "Going in Another Direction" at the end of Chapter 7 for more information.) And you can always cheat a little with some properly applied make-up. (See Chapter 14 for details.)

> ## Geranium and Olive Lip Balm
> Recipe for healing cracked lips: Add a few drops of geranium essential oil to some olive oil and lather it on your lips to soothe and speed healing.

Watch Your Tongue!

Your tongue can tell you a lot about what's going on in your body, so pay attention to what it has to say. A healthy tongue is pink. If your tongue is red, pernicious anemia or a deficiency in folic acid may be the cause. (I discuss pernicious anemia in Chapter 9, in the section "The Colors of Your Life.") A pale, smooth tongue might also indicate an iron shortage, so eat more asparagus, nuts and seeds, whole grains, beef, fish, legumes, and eggs if things are looking that way. Always take your iron food with a source of vitamin C to increase absorption, and never supplement iron without the advice of a physician. Avoid caffeine and chocolate, as these interfere with iron absorption. If your tongue is smooth and red and your mouth is painful, you might be experiencing a deficiency of niacin. Signs of cancer include painless bumps or patches of red or white on either side of the tongue. Be sure to see your doctor if you notice these changes.

And the most important beauty tip of all? Keep smiling!

CHAPTER TWELVE

Looking Good: The Eyes Have It

Tell them dear, that if eyes were made for seeing,
Then beauty is its own excuse for being.
—**Ralph Waldo Emerson**

When my six-year-old son jumps off the couch, in some sword-swinging, monster-slaying, acrobatic maneuver, he usually gets a lecture that goes something like this: our eyes are a precious gift, and we only get two of them. We can't just go to the store and buy a working replacement if we damage or lose an eyeball! Mothers throughout the ages have no doubt made similar pronouncements, but these words of wisdom also apply to you, gentle reader. We all need to treat our eyes with respect.

If beauty is your main motivation, taking care of your eyes will help prevent crow's feet, those wrinkles around your eyes that form after years of squinting to read food labels in the grocery store. And if you think that your good looks are hampered by a set of bifocals or if, like me, the thought of poking a contact lens into your eye makes you squeamish, you might be able to defer the purchase of seeing aids with proper eye health maintenance. (Of course, if you like the way you look in spectacles, you can indulge your sense of style with an awesome pair of fashion glasses or sun shades!) After a certain age, we don't need to worry about slaying monsters anymore, but we all make daily choices that can affect our eye health.

Starting at the Finish Line

In order to understand how to protect eye health, it's easiest to start backwards and discuss eye problems. Several of the most common degenerative eye conditions have been associated with lifestyle and nutritional factors. Addressing these concerns now could protect your sight from these conditions later—whether you are a college student or a retiree.

Age-Related Macular Degeneration

The most common cause of irreversible vision loss for people over the age of 60, Age-Related Macular Degeneration (AMD) can also affect people in their 40s and 50s. According to the World Health Organization (WHO), 25% of those over the age of 80 are affected. In 2001, the United Nations predicted that the number of people over the age of 60 would more than triple from 606 million in that year to nearly 2 billion by the year 2050 and that the number of people over the age of 80 would increase more than five times from 2001 to an astounding 379 million in 2050. Suffice it to say that AMD could reach epidemic proportions over the next several decades.

The macula is the central and most sensitive portion of the retina—a nerve-rich area at the back of the eye. As we age, the macula breaks down, causing deterioration of central vision and fine-detail perception. Some scientists have suggested an association between macular degeneration and diets that are high in saturated fat and low in carotenoid pigments. Cigarette smoking, sun exposure, high blood pressure, and high cholesterol are also significant factors, because these conditions all generate free radicals, which are responsible for the retinal damage. Unfortunately, deterioration begins long before a person is aware of it.

Cataracts

Cataracts, another condition associated with aging, involve the clouding of the normally transparent lens of the eye, which impedes light from entering. The cataract is not a tumor or a new growth of tissue over the eye but a fogging of the lens itself. Depending on the size and location of the cataract, impairment would range from negligible to complete loss of sight. Vision is often restored by the surgical removal of the cataract. The most common cataracts are age related, but they can also occur in people as young as age 40. Along with aging, most cataracts are the result of birth defects or heredity, but eye injury (including sun damage) can also cause this condition, even in the very young. Secondary cataracts can also form as a result of infections or diseases such as diabetes. As with AMD, free radicals appear to be responsible for much of the damage.

Computers: The New Threat to Eye Health

Unfortunately, a new type of eye problem has appeared in recent years, and this one affects people long before retirement. Symptoms of Computer Vision Syndrome include eyestrain, headaches, blurred vision, and fatigue. If your occupation involves staring at a computer screen, you may notice itchy, sore, or heavy eyes and blurred or double vision during or immediately after work. If these symptoms occur three or more times a week, you may be putting too much stress on your eyes. Be sure to take regular breaks from the glare of the screen to give your eyes a change of focus. And blink regularly to keep your eyes moist.

> ### Rest Those Tired Eyes!
>
> When you've been focusing on a task for a while, try this exercise to give your eyes a break. Close your eyes, then slowly roll them up and down, then side to side. It's good for your eye muscles, which tend to stay in one position when you've been staring at a computer screen—or a hobby like needlework—for too long.

Back to the Beginning

Now that you know what might be ahead of you sooner than later if you don't take care of your eyes, let's talk about ways to preserve your eye health. By now you must be more than familiar with the destructive potential of free radicals, so you would probably not be surprised to learn that they're a factor in several degenerative eye conditions. Even cataracts and AMD might be delayed by enhancing the antioxidant status of your eye. Studies show that a diet high in serum carotenoids, especially the lutein and zeaxanthin found in leafy green vegetables like spinach, kale, parsley, and collard greens, protects the retina from the effects of the highly reactive radicals generated by exposure to sunlight. Carotenoid pigments have also been proven to form macular pigment, which scavenges hazardous free radicals in the macula. Antioxidant vitamins may also have positive effects. Retinol, better known as vitamin A, is essential for the production of one of the photopigments responsible for night vision. A diet deficient in vitamin A will lead to a condition called "night blindness." Vitamin B2, or riboflavin, is also important for eye health, and sensitivity to light is one symptom of riboflavin deficiency. Meanwhile, vitamin C is known to absorb UV light, and it also neutralizes free radicals. Researchers have found that vitamin C may help prevent cataracts by stopping photo-oxidation of the lens. Vitamin E is also responsible for the proper functioning of the immune system and for maintaining healthy eyes and skin. Research suggests that supplementing with vitamin E may also help. People with Type 1 diabetes can also reduce the risk of developing some retinal abnormalities.

Bioflavonoids, (antioxidants found in bilberries), help promote circulation and improve the strength of blood vessels throughout the body—especially small capillaries like the ones that supply nutrients to the eyes. Gingko biloba also improves circulation to the eyes and should be considered by those who are locked in front of a computer screen every day.

Along with antioxidants, zinc is a trace mineral that is highly concentrated in the retina and surrounding tissues, and it's required for chemical reactions in the retina. Zinc deficiency can cause the optic nerve to become swollen, it can damage color vision, and it's one factor that causes the formation of cataracts. Zinc is also an important component of the immune system. Since meats are the best sources of zinc, strict vegetarians and vegans are among the groups most likely to be deficient in this nutrient. Look for zinc in pumpkin seeds, brazil nuts, fish, meat, shellfish, whole grains, and brewer's yeast.

Wear Your Shades

While 79% of Americans realize that too much time basking in the sun can cause skin cancer, only 6% realize that the sun causes eye damage This might explain why the number of cases of conjunctival melanoma, a form of eye cancer, has tripled in white males over the age of 40 since 1973. Researchers speculate that this may be because males are less likely than females to wear eye protection and sun hats. To protect your eyes, wear your shades, whether you're in the shade or not.

Glaring Problems

Remember that the dangers of too much sun can also extend to your eyeballs. Be sure to wear sunglasses that offer both UVA and UVB protection. You should also take care when using a computer or watching television that you don't stare too long at the screen without looking away. Take regular breaks. At the risk of sounding like your mother, you should also make sure that you have enough light when you're reading. It makes no sense to strain your eyes intentionally.

Your Eyes Speak Volumes

As we work to preserve our sight, it's important to realize that while eyes provide a window to the soul, they also offer some vital clues about our internal health.

Blepharitis

Inflammation of the eyelid can cause burning, itching, and redness in a condition called blepharitis. Swollen lids, tearing, light sensitivity, and feeling as if there's an irritant in the eye are common symptoms. Nighttime secretions can make the lids sticky in the morning, and lashes may also fall out. Blepharitis is typically caused by an infection, and it's associated with inadequate sleep, improper cleaning of the eye area, nutritional deficiencies, or an underlying immune-system weakness. There are three major types of blepharitis.

With infectious blepharitis, glands along the eyelid become infected by bacteria. In the second form, an allergy is caused by something that's come into contact with the eyelids, like make-up. This can lead to a localized inflammation known as contact dermatitis blepharitis. Finally, an improperly functioning oil gland can cause skin cells to shed too rapidly, resulting in seborrheic blepharitis. The excess skin cells and oil encourage bacterial growth. Seborrea of the scalp or face may also be present. Blepharitis tends to recur, and treatment typically involves making sure that the eye area is clean. If you develop this condition, support your immune system with a diet high in antioxidant fruits and vegetables and avoid refined foods and sugar. Use appropriate supplements to strengthen your immune system, and remember that adequate vitamin A is essential as a remedy for all eye conditions. Get enough restorative sleep and don't stress your eyes with too much time in front of the computer. Whatever you do, keep dirty fingers away from your eyes and discard make-up that you were using when the infection began.

Beauty Prescription for Blepharitis

Take your *Living Beauty Essentials* daily, as described in Chapters 2 and 3. You will see that, for this prescription, some of those nutrients should be taken in the higher daily-total amounts shown below, along with any extra nutrients listed in this table.

Total Daily Amount

Vitamin A	20,000 IU
Beta carotene	25,000 IU
Vitamin B complex	100 mg
Vitamin C	3,000 mg, in 2–3 equally divided doses
Vitamin E	800 IU
Selenium	400 mcg
Zinc	50–100 mg. Do not exceed 100 mg daily from all sources

Stye

Known in medical terms as a hordeolum, a stye is a small boil or infection that occurs at the base of your eyelash. Bacteria cause the gland located inside the lash follicle to become inflamed, causing redness and pain. Staphylococcus bacteria are usually responsible. Styes are also associated with blepharitis. A stye will normally develop over several days, eventually forming ahead, which soon ruptures, releasing pus. When a stye is present, eyes tend to water and become sensitive to light. You may also feel as if you have sand or some other irritant in the eye.

To prevent styes from developing, be sure to clean your eyes daily, removing all traces of make-up and oil. Avoid touching your eyes with unwashed hands. Keep your immune system strong to prevent or quickly extinguish an infection and work to reduce cholesterol and blood lipid levels.

Styes will heal on their own, and they should never be squeezed or poked. Although antibiotics are sometimes used, they are frequently ineffective. To speed healing, bathe your eyes several times per day with a warm, wet face cloth. The heat will help destroy bacteria. A stye that develops deeper within the gland is known as an internal hordeolum. This type is usually more painful and rarely ruptures on its own, but a doctor can open and drain it. A stye is not dangerous, but if left too long, it can lead to the development of a chalazion, described in the next section.

To prevent styes from developing, be sure to clean your eyes daily, removing all traces of make-up and oil. Avoid touching your eyes with unwashed hands. Keep your immune system strong to prevent or quickly extinguish an infection and work to reduce cholesterol and blood lipid levels. (Blood lipids may encourage blockage of oil glands.) Drinking eyebright herbal tea may be helpful during an episode with a stye.

Beauty Prescription for Stye

Take your *Living Beauty Essentials* daily, as described in Chapters 2 and 3. You will see that, for this prescription, some of those nutrients should be taken in the higher daily-total amounts shown below, along with any extra nutrients listed in this table.

	Total Daily Amount
Vitamin A	20,000 IU
Beta carotene	25,000 IU
Vitamin B complex	100 mg
Vitamin C	3,000 mg, in 2–3 equally divided doses
Vitamin E	800 IU
Selenium	400 mcg
Zinc	50–100 mg. Do not exceed 100 mg daily from all sources.
Grapeseed extract	50–200 mg, 3 times daily

Chalazion

The meibomian gland produces an oily substance that lubricates the front of the eye and the margins of the eyelid. A blockage in the duct leading from this gland to the eyelid is known as a meibomian cyst or chalazion (pronounced sha-lazy-on.) The blockage causes the meibomian secretion to harden, forming a cyst. As the blockage is typically caused by inflammation of the eyelid, a chalazion often follows the formation of a stye. The chalazion can be as small as a grain of sand or it can grow to seven or eight millimeters in diameter (about the size of a pea). Chalazia are known to become red and swollen due to infection, and a red or gray area may develop underneath the eyelid. Although not painful, a large chalazion can exert pressure on the eyelid, causing blurred vision. People who experience rosacea and chronic blepharitis are prone to develop these.

Home care for a chalazion involves bathing the eye in warm water for 15 minutes, several times per day. (See below for instructions.) The chalazion should disappear on its own, but if it continues to grow, you should seek medical attention, as surgical removal may be necessary. Whenever a lump on your eyelid does not clear up within a few days of committed eye bathing, it is wise to seek the advice of a qualified eye professional. A report from McGill University in Montreal, Canada, concluded that several pre-malignant and malignant conditions (including sebaceous cell carcinoma) often look like chalazia. Recurrent chalazia may also be problematic and should be reported to your eye doctor. To avoid infection that can lead to the development of a chalazion, always wash your hands before touching your eye area. It's also a good idea to avoid eye make-up when you're dealing with a chalazion. If you are prone to developing styes and chalazia, avoid using oily make-up removers and eye products too close to the lash-line. If you've ever experienced surgical removal of a chalazion, you've probably decided that prevention of recurrence is a very good idea. Use the following technique daily to be sure that your eye area is thoroughly cleaned, morning and night.

Eye Bathing

Use very warm water (not hot!) and a clean face cloth, twice per day. Starting at the outside corner of your eye, use your fingertips to apply gentle pressure through the face cloth against the eyelid, moving slowly toward your nose. This massages the glands and releases any trapped secretions. Do this on the top and bottom lids, continually refreshing your face cloth in warm water. After you have done both eyes, rinse out your face cloth in very warm water. Then use the face cloth to apply heat to the lids to kill any bacteria.

Beauty Prescription for Chalazion

Take your *Living Beauty Essentials* daily, as described in Chapters 2 and 3. You will see that, for this prescription, some of those nutrients should be taken in the higher daily-total amounts shown below, along with any extra nutrients listed in this table.

Total Daily Amount

Vitamin A	20,000 IU
Beta carotene	25,000 IU
Vitamin B complex	100 mg
Vitamin C with bioflavonoids	3,000–6,000 mg or to bowel tolerance, in 2–3 equally divided doses
Vitamin E	800 IU
Selenium	400 mcg
Zinc	50–100 mg. Do not exceed 100 mg daily from all sources

No More Tears

Our tears are the unsung heroes of our eye health, and we don't seem to appreciate them until they are gone. Tears are composed of three distinct layers. The inner mucin layer is made up of mucus that allows tears to adhere to the surface of the eye; the watery middle lacrimal layer cleanses the eye and washes away irritants; and the oily outer lipid layer prevents tears from evaporating. Tears also contain the antibacterial lysozyme, which helps prevent infections. Blinking helps bathe our eyes in tears.

Dry eyes lead to burning, stinging, and redness, and if left untreated, they could progress to infection and corneal scarring. A lack of tears could be caused by outdoor or indoor environmental factors like sun, wind, dust, smoke, air conditioning, or heating. As we age, our eyes become drier because tear production slows down. This is particularly true for women after menopause. Medications for blood pressure, allergies, depression, and Parkinson's disease can all lead to eye dryness, as can a deficiency in vitamin A and Essential Fatty Acids. Systemic diseases such as lupus, rosacea, and rheumatoid arthritis also involve dry eyes.

Perhaps not surprisingly, contact lens wearers are also susceptible to eye dryness. If you wear lenses, be sure that they're properly fitted, and take regular breaks from them if dry eyes are a problem for you. People who work in front of a computer must be sure to blink regularly and to rest their eyes for several minutes every hour.

Beauty Prescription for Dry Eyes

Take your *Living Beauty Essentials* daily, as described in Chapters 2 and 3. You will see that, for this prescription, some of those nutrients should be taken in the higher daily-total amounts shown below, along with any extra nutrients listed in this table.

	Total Daily Amount
Vitamin A	20,000 IU
Borage oil	1,000–3,000 mg

Thinning Lashes

Besides making your eyes look attractive, your lashes serve a useful pur-pose by providing a barrier against foreign particles. Glands at the base of the lash follicle also supply an oily lipid substance that prevents tears from evaporating. Eyelashes may be lost as a result of allergic reactions to skin products and make-up, as a side effect of certain drugs, or because of blepharitis or a chalazion. Thinning lashes may also be con-nected to total body hair loss caused by an underlying medical condi-tion. (See the description of alopecia toward the end of Chapter 9.) Lash loss, for example, can be a symptom of hypothyroidism. Nutritional deficiencies can also be a factor. If your lashes are thinning or falling out, first treat any infection, stye, or chalazion that you might have. Avoid rubbing or irritating the lash area. Do not use waterproof mas-cara, as it's much harder to remove than the regular version, and it causes too much tugging at the lids. If lashes are lost, steer clear of eye make-up until the lash-line is restored—and follow the *Beauty Prescription for Thinning Lashes*.

Beauty Prescription for Thinning Lashes

Take your *Living Beauty Essentials* daily, as described in Chapters 2 and 3. You will see that, for this prescription, some of those nutrients should be taken in the higher daily-total amounts shown below, along with any extra nutrients listed in this table.

Total Daily Amount

Vitamin A	20,000 IU
Vitamin B complex	100 mg
Vitamin C with bioflavonoids	3,000–6,000 mg or to bowel tolerance, in 2–3 equally divided doses
Vitamin E	800 IU
Selenium	400 mcg
Zinc	50–100 mg. Do not exceed 100 mg daily from all sources
Dietary silicon	3 mg choline-stabilized, concentrated orthosilicic acid, once or twice per day (max 6 mg daily)

Undereye Bags

Puffiness, bags, and dark circles under the eyes make us look tired. Not surprisingly, they appear when we *are* tired, as most eye baggage is caused by a lack of sleep. Our bodies need restorative sleep to repair daily damage, and when we don't get it, the evidence appears on our faces. Age is another factor, as eyelid muscles lose strength and skin starts to sag over time. Exhausted adrenal glands from too many late nights, followed by rounds of coffee for a pick-me-up and alcohol for a relaxant also trigger tell-tale facial puffiness and bags. (See "Symptoms of Adrenal Exhaustion" near the beginning of Chapter 6 to determine whether you are experiencing exhausted adrenal glands.)

> Our eyes betray much of the stress that comes our way, but we can make them look and feel better by improving our nutrition and circulation and giving our baby blues some time to relax.

Allergies can cause puffy eyes, as can having too much salt in the diet. If you're a smoker, getting rid of undereye circles and bags is another great reason to quit—and second-hand smoke should be avoided too. Our eyes betray much of the stress that comes our way, but we can make them look and feel better by improving our nutrition and circulation, and giving our peepers some time to relax. To reduce eye-area issues, avoid caffeine, soft drinks, salt, and monosodium glutamate and focus on a diet of fresh fruits, vegetables, whole grains, and lean protein. Also be sure to drink at least eight glasses of pure, filtered water daily. To reduce early morning swelling, apply a cold compress or cold cucumber slices to the eye area.

Beauty Prescription for Undereye Bags

Take your *Living Beauty Essentials* daily, as described in Chapters 2 and 3. You will see that, for this prescription, some of those nutrients should be taken in the higher daily-total amounts shown below, along with any extra nutrients listed in this table.

	Total Daily Amount
Vitamin B complex	100 mg
Vitamin C with bioflavonoids	3,000–6,000 mg or to bowel tolerance in 2–3 equally divided doses
Vitamin E	800 IU
Zinc	50–100 mg. Do not exceed 100 mg from all sources.
Milk thistle (as silymarin)	900 mg, in 3 equally divided doses (max. 900 mg daily)

Yellow Eyes

If the whites of your eyes turn yellow, it's time to visit the doctor. Yellow eyes are a symptom of jaundice, a discoloration of the skin and eyes that results from excess bilirubin in the blood. Bilirubin is a yellow-brown pigment that's left over after damaged red blood cells are removed from circulation. Most of the red-blood-cell cleanup is done in the spleen, but the hemoglobin, (the oxygen-carrying part), is broken down into bilirubin and sent to the liver before going to the intestine, where it becomes a component of the bile that helps digestion. Bilirubin in the bloodstream could indicate one of a number of medical problems. Gallstones or a tumor may be blocking the bile duct or the liver may be inflamed or diseased.

Jaundice is also common in cases of cirrhosis of the liver, pernicious anemia, and hepatitis. It also appears in newborns because bilirubin production increases in the few days after birth, but newborn jaundice normally corrects itself. However, adults with jaundice must consult with their health-care providers to determine and treat the underlying cause of the condition. At-home treatment must focus on supporting the liver, but do not do a liver cleanse without talking to your doctor.

Beauty Prescription for Yellow Eyes

Take your *Living Beauty Essentials* daily, as described in Chapters 2 and 3. You will see that, for this prescription, some of those nutrients should be taken in the higher daily-total amounts shown below, along with any extra nutrients listed in this table.

	Total Daily Amount
Vitamin A	5,000 IU
Vitamin B complex	100 mg
Vitamin C with bioflavonoids	3,000–6,000 mg or to bowel tolerance in 2–3 equally divided doses
Vitamin E	800 IU

You're looking better already!

CHAPTER THIRTEEN

If Looks Could Kill

There is no beautifier of complexion, or form, or behavior,
like the wish to scatter joy and not pain around us.
—*Ralph Waldo Emerson*

S o, you've done everything I've asked, right? You've taken steps to improve your digestion, your immune system is strong, and you're now giving your body the nutrients it needs for you to feel energetic, alive, and beautiful. You skin is soft, supple, and healthy. Your hair shines, and your fingernails inspire awe and admiration from men and women alike. You're doing all that you can to fulfill your beauty potential from the inside, and yet you and I both know that there's more to the equation than that.

Living in the real world as we do, we're sometimes expected to leave the safe cocoon of our homes and venture out into public— where people can actually see us! And, frankly, not all of us were blessed with pillow lips and a glorious mane of hair. And, frankly, not all of us look like movie stars and fashion models, not even most of the time. Most of us prefer to help Mother Nature a little. We like to add a splash of color to our hair or pink to our cheeks, and we like to create some mystery with our eyes. We also prefer not to smell as if we just came from the gym. We like hair products and make-up and perfume. And there's nothing wrong with that.

Unfortunately, however, there may be something wrong with the products we're using. In fact, in many ways, the chemicals in our favorite products may contribute to our health problems, from lung and liver disease to various forms of cancer. It would be rather ironic to go to great lengths to radiate health and beauty and then coat ourselves in chemicals that can lead to skin problems and disease. In the next few pages, I'll be highlighting some of the major concerns about chemicals used in our personal-care products, and I'll offer some suggestions for alternatives.

Before I do so, however, I would like to make a few things clear: first, I am not a chemist. I'm a consumer, like you, who is concerned about the potential dangers of products that I use on my body and on my children's bodies—not to mention how they might affect the health of our environment. Second, I certainly understand the law of supply and demand, particularly as it relates to creating products that work safely, are priced well, and have a reasonable shelf life. I realize that some chemicals are less expensive than others, and I also understand that the use of some ingredients, at this point, could be cost-prohibitive. Actually, I have such faith in economics and the power of the almighty dollar, that I know consumers have the power to force manufacturers to stop producing products that could endanger our health—simply by refusing to buy them.

Finally, as anyone who knows me or has seen a picture of me already knows, I'm not what anyone would call a natural beauty— unless a natural beauty has a penchant for eye make-up reminiscent of Audrey Hepburn in *Breakfast at Tiffany's* and absolutely no fear of bright red lips. Yes, it takes a drawerful of creams, powders, and colors to keep this girl happy. I even have a favorite perfume that I wear on special occasions. So I'm not a "go-natural, no make-up" type. I just want to make sure I'm not spreading toxic substances on my body. Like you, I have no intention of throwing out the baby with the bathwater. Rather than giving up my love of beauty products, I choose to buy products that will give me the look I want without endangering my health. It would be a good idea for you to do your own risk-reward analysis, to determine what you can comfortably accept in your products and what you must change. My suggestion is that, whenever possible, make choices that minimize your risk of harm from the products you use on a regular basis.

Who's in Charge?

Although you'd think the government would control the ingredients that are poured into beauty products, you might be surprised to learn that, in the United States, body-care products are not regulated by any government agency. In fact, the Food and Drug Administration (FDA) is not authorized to require companies to safety-test their cosmetic products before marketing them; it's allowed to regulate cosmetics only after they're released to the marketplace. According to the FDA, a cosmetics manufacturer may use almost any raw material except color additives and a few prohibited ingredients. The FDA does not have the authority to require manufacturers to file data on ingredients or report cosmetics-related injuries, and it is also not allowed to order recalls of cosmetics that have or might cause an unwanted reaction if those products don't contain any of the few prohibited ingredients. The only thing they can do, it seems, is to look for products in the marketplace that contain prohibited ingredients.

That would be more reassuring if the list of restricted ingredients was not so short. Another agency—the Cosmetic Ingredient Review (CIR)—has been set up to determine the safety of ingredients used by American cosmetics manufacturers, but it's a self-regulating organization of the cosmetics industry. According to their website, the CIR was established in 1976 by the Cosmetic, Toiletry, and Fragrance Association (CTFA), with the support of the U.S. Food and Drug Administration and the Consumer Federation of America. The CIR states that although it is funded by the CTFA, it is independent from that association and the cosmetics industry. The CIR also asserts that it reviews and assesses the "safety of ingredients used in cosmetics in an open, unbiased, and expert manner, and publishes the results in the open, peer-reviewed scientific literature." Unfortunately, a report containing full results of their analysis of tested cosmetic products will set you back $350. According to the website of the U.S.-based Environmental Working Group (a health and environmental watchdog), in nearly 30 years, the CIR has assessed only about 11% of the 10,500 ingredients found by the FDA to be used in cosmetics manufactured in the U.S.A. And of the 1,175 ingredients studied by the CIR, only nine have been deemed unsafe. Wow. By comparison, in this small chapter, I've written about more than nine ingredients, and none of them appear on the FDA Restricted List.

In an approximate parallel to the American situation, companies in Canada are not required to present Health Canada with ingredient listings before cosmetics products are introduced to the market. Ten days after the first sale of a product, however, companies must forward ingredient information to this government department. Health Canada then checks to make sure that no restricted ingredients are included in the formulation and that labeling requirements have been met. The list of restricted ingredients in Canada is in the hundreds, though some are on the hotlist because they are used as prescription drugs. It is likely that some of them may not have a purpose in cosmetics anyway.

The descriptions in the rest of this chapter merely represent a survey of various chemicals that are used today. According to the National Toxicology Program, an interagency program that researches the toxicology of chemicals, there are over 80,000 chemicals registered for use in the United States, and 2,000 new ones enter the market each year. Of course, many of these chemicals are also used for manufacturing in Canada. According to an Environmental Working Group Survey of 2,300 people, the average adult uses nine personal-care products each day and is therefore being exposed to 126 chemical ingredients on a daily basis. Over a six-month period, the EWG studied 10,000 products found in beauty and body-care products and discovered 356 synthetic ingredients that have absolutely no safety research to support their use.

Using synthetic chemicals wouldn't necessarily be a bad thing if we knew for sure that our bodies were able to break them down. Taking the argument a bit further, it would also be great to know that our earth has the ability to break them down. Although some natural chemicals can also be dangerous or deadly to our bodies, we can at least argue that the earth knows what to do with them when they eventually return there.

> According to an Environmental Working Group Survey of 2,300 people, the average adult uses nine personal-care products each day and is therefore being exposed to 126 chemical ingredients on a daily basis. Over a six-month period, the EWG studied 10,000 products found in beauty and body-care products and discovered 356 ingredients that have absolutely no safety research to support their use.

The term used for "things that aren't in the body naturally" is xenobiotics. "Xeno" (pronounced "zeeno") means foreign, so the word can be literally translated as "foreign to the body." More recently, however, the term has come to be associated with the hormone-disrupting chemicals such as petrochemical compounds found in adhesives, herbicides, pesticides, plastics, solvents, and personal-care products. Anything that the body can't assimilate or break down into a form that it understands is considered foreign, and the body will either find a way to use the foreign substances, try to get rid of them, or store them. In the process, strange things can happen. Xenoestrogens fall into this category.

Starting with Hormones

Trust me, a discussion of hormones is relevant to your choice of beauty products. Just be patient. You will recall from our earlier discussion that hormones are substances released from a gland or organ into the bloodstream. They can be composed of amino acid chains, steroids, or fatty substances derived from cholesterol. Tiny quantities of a hormone can cause huge changes in the body, and they operate through altering cellular function by binding to a cell at the hormone-receptor site. Xenoestrogens, which you will recall are false estrogens, bind with the estrogen-receptor sites on our cells. When this occurs, cellular functions can change, and hormonal balance shifts in favor of estrogen. (See Chapter 6 for details about the consequences of estrogen dominance.)

Xenobiotics: The Insidious Invaders

Xenobiotics enter our food supply from the chemical fertilizers and pesticides used on so many of our crops. We also voluntarily expose ourselves to xenobiotics in our body-care products, and these items don't undergo the same government scrutiny as our food supply does. Although these foreign substances can enter our systems in many ways, one of the largest ports of entry is our skin. Remember that the skin, as the largest organ, is permeable. Since the 1960s, scientists have known that all chemicals penetrate the skin to some degree. Think about medicinal patches used for nausea or hormone therapy, and you'll realize how modern medicine has taken full advantage of this knowledge. Unfortunately, however, the skin cannot discriminate between beneficial substances and toxic ones and welcomes them all with open pores.

Ingredients for Disaster

Unless you read health magazines, it's quite likely that you've never heard of phthalates, let alone what research is now revealing about them. Phthalates (pronounced "thay-lates") are used in some hairspray, deodorant, nail polish, and cologne formulations. They can be inhaled or absorbed through the skin and are known to damage the liver, lungs, and reproductive system.

Mono-(2-ethylhexyl)phthalate (MEHP), a metabolite of Di-(2-ethyl-hexyl)phthalate (DEHP), has been proven to be a contributing factor in female infertility by suppressing the production of estradiol, a hormone essential for the release of an egg from the ovary. In animal studies, MEHP has also been implicated as a cause of decreased levels of the natural estrogen estradiol in the blood, prolonged estrous cycles, and lack of ovulation. All of you mothers, grandmothers, and potential mothers out there should be alarmed to learn that phthalates have also been found in breast milk. (Please note, however, that the benefits of breast feeding babies still far outweigh the risks from toxicants.)

The Male Perspective

It isn't all about women. Just as some xenobiotics act like estrogens, others act like anti-androgens, interfering with the action of androgen in males. Although no definitive studies have been performed concerning the connection between phthalates and cancer, testicular cancer has increased in Caucasian men worldwide. Despite the initial test results of phthalates that showed no serious effect on males, it is now evident that these compounds drastically affect the genital development of male fetuses. One study done at a hospital in Italy showed that either DEHP or MEHP or both were found in 88.1% of umbilical cords of babies, born to mothers with average exposure to phthalates.

Phthalates have also been associated with undescended testes, which occurs when a testis remains in the abdomen for more than a year after the birth of a male baby. To prevent infertility and painful twisting of the testis and to reduce the risk of testicular cancer, the condition must be surgically corrected before the child reaches the age of five. Various compounds, including monobutyl phthalate, monobenzyl phthalate, and monoethyl phthalate (MEP), have been shown to affect the quantity and quality of semen and the motility of sperm. Estrogenic DEHP has also been demonstrated to trigger the loss of spermatogenic (sperm-producing) cells. Most alarmingly, a recent Harvard study has determined that phthalates damage the DNA of sperm in adult males. Scary stuff.

Studies also show that phthalates increase free radical production in the liver—and we can't forget how those free radicals attack our cells, leading to aging and disease.

Diethyl phthalate (DEP) is found in many soaps, lotions, perfumes, and fragrances used in Canada and the United States. Think about the number of products in your home that contain fragrance: candles, room deodorizers, dish detergent, laundry soap, feminine products, garbage bags, carpet freshener, and furniture polish are just a few examples. Now think of how many products you use directly on your body that have a fragrance: shampoo, conditioner, gel, mousse, spray, shaving gel or cream, soap, body lotion, facial cleanser, moisturizer, make-up, lipstick, deodorant, and of course, perfume. It doesn't take a mathematician to add up our exposures to synthetic fragrance.

Although DEHP and DEP were banned from Europe in late 2002, at the time of writing, no such restriction exists in Canada or the United States. So I'd recommend that you go through your cupboards, isolate the products that contain phthalates, and be sure never to buy them again. Opt for products that are fragrance free or that use natural essential oils. Note that some products are labeled "unscented" because they have no aroma, but a synthetic fragrance could still have been used to mask a possibly unpleasant odor. Unfortunately, there is no law against the use of phthalates in personal-care products, and they are often included in the umbrella term "perfume" in Canada and the United States. So do your best to decipher ingredients, but contact the manufacturer if you are uncertain.

You might also like to know that when professionals use products made for exclusive use in salons, the ingredients in those products do not, by law, have to be declared on the product. But they are still absorbed into your skin as you are sitting in the chair—whether they are listed on the label or not. And what if you are the professional working in the salon? As early as 1982, a population-based cancer registry showed that cosmetologists, hairdressers, and manicurists had above-average rates of multiple myeloma, a type of cancer affecting plasma cells that produce antibodies. As yet, the exact cause of multiple myeloma has not been established.

Preserving Your Looks?

The parabens are a bunch of chemicals distinguished by their first names, the most common being *butyl, ethyl, methyl,* and *propyl.* Parabens are used extensively as preservatives in everything from shampoos to moisturizers. They are readily absorbed into our bodies from the skin and the intestinal tract and typically do not cause skin sensitivities or allergic reactions. In fact, it is their non-irritating quality that makes parabens so popular—and ultimately why they are a cause for concern, because we are constantly exposed to them. Although generally regarded as safe, multiple studies show that parabens exert a weak estrogenic activity that affects both men and women.

Studies show that all four parabens listed above, along with isopropylparaben and isobutylparaben, stimulate the growth of the breast-cancer-causing MCF-7 cells. Of these, butylparaben is the most potent, and these parabens have also been found intact in the human breast. This isn't information that we can ignore. Breast cancer rates have increased dramatically in the last 40 years in North America. Since 1960, the odds of developing breast cancer have increased from 1 in 20 to 1 in 7 in the United States. Is it merely coincidental that cancer rates have increased along with the use of parabens and other xenoestrogens?

And, of course, I can't leave out the men. Studies show that parabens adversely affect testosterone and the proper functioning of the male reproductive system. Japanese researchers learned that propylparaben decreased the quantity and quality of daily sperm production in the testes. Interestingly, blood testosterone levels also decreased as paraben levels decreased in male study participants. These effects were obvious at levels considered to be at the upper limit of daily exposure in Japan and the European Community. Tests to determine the impact of butylparaben on males found that the presence of butylparaben resulted in a 1% drop in blood testosterone levels and damage to the final stages of sperm production. The amounts of butylparaben used in this study were well below Japan's accepted daily intake. The bottom line is that we don't know enough.

Preservation without Reservation

Plant essential oils and antioxidants like vitamin E have been clinically proven to have anti-fungal, anti-microbial, and antiseptic properties, making them safe and effective options as preservatives for beauty-care products. A combination of different oils, including those from tea tree, oregano, rosemary, cinnamon, and vanillin, are more effective as preservatives than one essential oil used alone.

So it would make sense for us all to be interested in more research. Studies need to determine the extent to which parabens will accumulate in our tissues, and the long-term impact of their use should be reviewed.

Propylene Glycol

According to the 10th edition of the *Report on Carcinogens* (2002) available on the Environmental Health Perspectives website, propylene oxide is now suspected of being a human carcinogen. Propylene oxide is used as an intermediate in the production of propylene glycols (20–25%) and glycol ethers (3–5%).

You will find propylene glycols in antifreezes, drugs, emollients in food, heat transfer and hydraulic fluids, plasticizers, solvents, and, yes, as a delivery agent in nearly every category of cosmetic product manufactured in North America.

Mineral Oils

Ah, finally, I hear you sigh, an ingredient I've heard of and can pronounce. Unfortunately, its popularity doesn't mean it's good for you. Mineral oil is known to cause skin irritation. According to the website of the Occupational Safety and Health Administration, a division of the U.S. Department of Labor, people who work with this chemical are cautioned that If the mineral oil comes into contact with their skin, they should immediately wash the affected areas with large amounts of soap and water.

Mineral oil is a stable lubricant and emollient oil derived from crude oil, and it's used because it's cheap and plentiful. You may also be surprised to learn that, according to the 10th edition of the *Report on Carcinogens* (2002), it has been classified as a carcinogen. As a petrochemical product, mineral oil may contain xenoestrogenic polycyclic aromatic hydrocarbons (PAH). According to the Agency for Toxic Substances and Disease Registry (part of the U.S. Department of Health and Human Services), PAHs are byproducts of charbroiled meat, as well as of the incomplete burning of coal, gas, oil, garbage, wood, and tobacco. PAHs also occur naturally. Some are used in the making of dyes, medicines, pesticides, and plastics. Studies also show that PAHs cause tumors in laboratory animals through inhalation, via food, or through prolonged contact with skin. Some PAHs are known to activate estrogen receptors, and a 2004 study found that PAHs stimulated the proliferation of MCF-7 breast cancer cells.

Dioxins

Dioxins are environmental pollutants created as a byproduct of commercial or municipal waste incineration and the burning of fuels. Forest fires, trash burning, and cigarette smoke all contribute to dioxin production. Between 90% and 95% of human exposure comes via the diet, particular through animal fats. The reason I'm including dioxins in our beauty products section is that chlorinated dioxins are often formed through the bleaching of pulp and paper, and this is used in many types of cotton balls, facial tissue, toilet tissue, sanitary pads, and tampons. Some of these products are used in our beauty routines, and all of them have rather intimate contact with our bodies.

> ### Jojoba, Olive, and Almond!
> Instead of using carcinogenic mineral oils, opt for organic jojoba oil, olive oil, or almond oil. These can all be used for removing makeup, as skin moisturizers, and for your baby!

Studies have shown that exposure to dioxins may cause a number of serious health consequences. People who are exposed to large amounts of this substance can experience chloracne, a serious skin disease involving acne-like lesions on the upper body and face. High levels of dioxins in the workplace also seem to increase the risk of cancer in workers. Other research shows that long-term, low-level exposure might result in weight loss, liver damage, and developmental or reproductive damage. Disruption of the hormonal system, birth defects, and miscarriage are also linked to dioxins. Several studies have highlighted a connection between dioxins and endometriosis, and they've been associated with an increase in cancer-causing metabolites in breast cancer cells.

Another Reason to Stay in the Shade

If your love affair with the sun isn't experiencing enough turbulence, this will send you running for cover! In a study of common sunscreen ingredients, including benzophenone-3 (Bp-3), homosalate (HMS), 4-methylbenzylidene camphor (4-MBC), octyl-methoxycinnamate (OMC), and octyl-dimethyl-PABA (OD-PABA), animals exposed to these ingredients experienced an increased proliferation of MCF-7 breast cancer cells. Use of 4-MBC, OMC, and Bp-3 also resulted in an increase in the weight of the uterus, showing that these chemicals affect other reproductive organs, as well. Only one chemical, butyl-methoxydibenzoylmethane (B-MDM), did not result in estrogenic activity. So as you're adding up your exposure to xenoestrogens, don't forget to consider your sunscreen.

> ### The No-Bleach Zone
> When choosing your toiletries and feminine products, you can decrease your exposure to dioxins by avoiding bleached varieties.

No Safety in Numbers

While it's true that xenobiotics appear in very small quantities in our personal-care products, give some thought to how many and what variety of products you use on a regular basis. Although many xenoestrogens are used at levels that cause no observable effect (affectionately known as NOE), studies show that combining xenoestrogens has an additive effect. In fact, research indicates that combining a variety of xenoestrogens below NOE produces an estrogen-mimic effect. More simply, this means that your daily bathroom and beauty routine, complete with tiny amounts of harmful chemicals in each bottle or jar that you use, may add up to a good dose of xenoestrogens before you leave the house. You need to keep this in mind when reading findings of the CIR and manufacturers who state that cosmetic products don't contain these chemicals in the same quantities that produced disastrous results in experiments.

Limiting the Effects of Xenobiotics

In this brief survey, I have not by any stretch of the imagination discussed every possible way that we are exposed to xenobiotics. And I have not dis-

> ### Do-It-Yourself Sunscreen
> Mix together 2 oz. (60 mL) each of jojoba oil, sesame oil, and coconut oil, and add 10 drops of carrot seed oil. Add 8 drops each of lavender and geranium essential oils. Then add 1 tsp (5 mL) vitamin E. Store in a tightly capped amber bottle in a cool, dry place. Yields about 6 oz. (150 mL).
>
> As with any sunscreen, this formula does not replace common sense! Stay out of the sun's direct rays between the hours of 10 AM and 4 PM, and wear long-sleeved cotton tops and long pants when you are under the strongest rays.

cussed every potential chemical that has hormone-disrupting ability. Research into the effects of xenoestrogens is actually a relatively new area of study, and I'm sure that we will continue to read about new discoveries. I urge you to stay informed.

Avoiding xenobiotics is both the simplest and the most difficult means of reducing your exposure to foreign chemicals—because they can potentially be found in our foods, drinks, medications, and beauty products.

So how can we avoid this hidden threat? Buy organic food whenever possible. Organic crops are grown using traditional farming methods that honor the soil through crop rotation and the use of only natural fertilizers and pesticides. Organically raised meats are often taken from free-range animals, who are not injected with either hormones or antibiotics. Due to their respectful and not overcrowded living environments, these animals have less need for antibiotics and other medications to stave off disease. If you drink dairy milk, buy organic, again to limit your exposure to hormones and drugs.

Better a thousand times careful than once dead.
—*Proverb*

Due to production costs, organic foods can be more expensive than other options, but as a result of growing demand, prices are starting to level out. You have to decide what price to put on your health. Or, as I often say, you can pay a bit more for your foods now to protect your health or you can pay for medications and treatments in the future when your body finally reaches its toxic limit. It's your call.

Eat a diet that is high in antioxidant vitamins to help your immune system stay strong. Do not heat foods in the microwave using plastic bowls or wrap, as xenoestrogens will leach from the plastic into your food. Opt for glass containers if you must use the microwave. Buy only unbleached bathroom tissue, feminine products, and other paper goods to reduce exposure to dioxins. For birth control, use condoms without spermicide rather than taking the pill, and talk to your healthcare provider about natural alternatives to hormone replacement therapy (HRT) to treat the symptoms of menopause. Limit your use of alcohol and non-essential drugs, keep your stress levels under control, and make sure to get at least 15 minutes of exercise each day. These lifestyle choices will limit the impact of xenoestrogens on your body.

Before you buy any more shampoo, soap, skin cream, make-up, or other body-care item, read the product labels. Avoid the xenoestrogens mentioned in this chapter whenever you can. It will be a challenge, but it will be well worth the effort.

On to the Noxious Substances

The chemicals I'm about to cover in this section are just as foreign to the body as the ones discussed above, but there is no evidence that they disrupt our hormone function. What they have in common is that they are linked to cancer.

Nitrosamines

Products that contain amines or amino derivatives may form nitrosamines if they also contain a nitrosating agent such as the alkanoamides diethanolamine (DEA), triethanolamine (TEA), or monoethanolamine (MEA). Many nitrosamines (the result of combining an amine or amino derivative with a nitrosating agent) have been found to cause cancer in laboratory animals.

Unfortunately, chemical nitrosating agents not listed on the label could appear in a cosmetics formulation, turning the product into a potentially deadly concoction. Contamination could occur because nitrosating agents could be present in raw materials or perhaps because, between batches, the vats were cleaned with a product that contained a nitrosating agent. As a result, the U.S. Food and Drug Administration has urged cosmetics manufacturers to remove any ingredient that could form with others to create nitrosamines. It's important to note that the nitrosation may occur while the product is being stored, as well as during manufacture. To protect yourself, you might want to consider avoiding products containing chemicals that begin with DEA, TEA, and MEA.

> ### Youthful Skin
>
> Try these natural options for supple, youthful, healthy skin:
>
> **Biotin:** an important B-vitamin that helps the skin make use of protein
>
> **Chamomile:** a soothing moisturizer that nourishes and softens fine lines
>
> **Cocoa butter:** an ultra-rich emollient for dry body skin
>
> **Coconut oil:** a skin-softening sunscreen, and it has a wonderful aroma
>
> **Dietary silicon:** to soften the skin, speed healing, and promote elasticity
>
> **Green tea:** to offer clinically proven protection from sun damage. Drink up!
>
> **Jojoba oil:** to soften and hold in moisture without clogging pores
>
> **Panthenol:** a vitamin B derivative that retains moisture and softens fine lines
>
> **Rosehip oil:** to replenish lipids and reduce fine lines

Formaldehyde

You are likely familiar with the term formaldehyde because of its use as embalming fluid. Because it's an effective preservative, it is also used in many beauty products—such as some nail-care items. However, one Occupational Safety and Health Administra-tion report states that long-term exposure to formaldehyde is associated with an increased risk of nose and lung cancer in humans. Evidence of the cancer-causing potential of formaldehyde includes DNA binding, genotoxicity, and cell changes. Irritation of the skin and contact dermatitis can also result from exposure to formaldehyde solutions. Widely used preservatives such as 2-bromo2-nitropropane-1, 3-diol, Diazolidinyl urea, DMDM hydantoin, Imidazolidinyl urea, Quaternium 15, or Bronopol also break down to release formaldehyde. Avoid any formulation that combines these preservatives with DEA, TEA, or MEA due to the potential for nitrosation.

> ### Nitrosamine Blockers in Your Food
>
> Nitrosamines can also form in response to the foods we eat. For instance, they can result from taking in nitrates, the chemicals added to cold meats and bacon to prevent spoilage. Look for nitrate-free meat products to limit your consumption of these potentially dangerous chemicals.
>
> The good news is that certain foods can help block the process of nitrosamine formation! Carrots, green peppers, pineapples, strawberries, and tomatoes are all proven to inhibit nitrosation. Scientists have also hypothesized that other fruits and vegetables have the same power, but sufficient study hasn't been done. One remedy is this: the next time you order a deli sandwich with nitrate-preserved meat, make sure you load it with tomatoes and green peppers! Aged Garlic Extract is also known to inhibit the formation of dangerous nitrosa-mines. Because nitrosamines may also form in your beauty-care products, be sure that you eat some of the proven nitrasamine blockers every day.

Changing Your Locks

Let's face it, we all like to play with our hair. Whether it's to find out if blondes do indeed have more fun, to test-drive the passion of red, or (gasp!) to camouflage gray hairs, 40% of us color our tresses. But is our quest for color causing us harm? In a word, possibly.

In 2001, researchers at the University of California discovered that women and men who used permanent dyes once a month for a year or more had twice the risk of developing bladder cancer. Hairdressers and barbers who came into contact with hair dyes had five times the risk. A 1994 American Cancer Society study found that prolonged use of permanent dark-hair colors made of coal-tar dye may result in an increased risk of fatal non-Hodgkin's lymphoma and multiple myeloma. Another study concluded that women who used hair dyes five or more times per year were at greater risk of developing ovarian cancer than those who did not dye their hair. In fact, many obstetricians and gynecologists now advise pregnant and nursing women not to use synthetic chemical hair dyes, to avoid the possibility of transferring harmful chemicals to infants.

I mentioned earlier that the FDA has very little power in the beauty business, except in one area—color. According to the FDA website, several coal-tar hair-dye ingredients have been found to cause cancer in at least one animal species in lifetime feeding studies: 4-methoxy-m-phenylenediamine, 4-chloro-m-phenylenediamine, 2,4-toluene-diamine, 2-nitro-p-phenyle-nediamine and 4-amino-2-nitrophenol. Do not take lightly the warnings on home hair-color products that instruct you not to let the product touch your skin. The warning is there because the ingredients in the box are readily absorbed.

And Speaking of Color

In the United States, synthetic colors are placed in two categories: certifiable colors and natural colors. (Canadians also use the U.S. system.) Certifiable colors are those known as coal-tar colors, and they're often labeled with an FDC number. Each batch of these colors must be tested for safety and

Au Naturel

When it comes to hair, going natural doesn't have to mean letting the gray hairs take over or being stuck with one color. Natural hair colors (both permanent and semi-permanent) are smart choices if you'd like a subtle enhancement of your natural color or if you want to disguise a modest amount of gray. They typically use less hydrogen peroxide or ammonia to penetrate the hair shaft, but be sure to read and compare labels.

Products like henna are great for intensifying reds, but beware: a henna product that comes in a color other than the naturally occurring red has been chemically altered. If, on the other hand, you truly believe that blondes have more fun, foil highlighting allows your hairdresser to apply the bleaching chemicals without letting the product touch your scalp. This way, you can achieve a lighter look with fewer potentially damaging chemicals.

Or you can try these pantry solutions for your color needs:

Dark hair. Steep a pot of strong black tea from the tea leaves. After the solution has cooled, use it as a rinse after shampooing. Brunettes will also get shine from a diluted apple-cider vinegar rinse.

Blonde hair. Steep a pot of chamomile tea, allow it to cool, and use it as a rinse after shampooing. Lemon juice is also a good rinse for blondes.

approved by the FDA. Different colors have been banned since the 1950s because they've been proven to cause adverse reactions or tumors. Exempt from individual batch testing are those colors historically derived from animal, mineral, or plant sources, as they are considered "natural." Nowadays, however, components of natural colors, such as beta carotene, can also be produced synthetically. So if you see these names on a product, it does not necessarily mean its color is natural. If you would like to know whether an ingredient is natural or synthetic, call the manufacturer.

The FDA has the authority to prohibit the use of any color additive that is proven to cause cancer in animals or humans. Whether or not they are proven carcinogens, however, some colorants may cause adverse reactions. Tartrazine (FDC Yellow No. 5), for example, is used to color everything from soup to soap and has reportedly caused hives, swollen eyelids, behavioral problems like ADD and ADHD, and headaches. A 2002 animal study showed that ingesting tartrazine at a low dose (10–100 mg/kg) induced dose-related DNA damage in the stomach, colon, and urinary bladder, and in the gastrointestinal organs. More study of tartrazine and other colorants is definitely needed.

Color Dictionary

Coal-tar dyes	Originally derived from coal sources, these colorants are now petroleum based
Lakes	Water-soluble colors created by precipitating dye into an absorbent material
Provisional listing	Colors whose use is permitted provisionally until sufficient safety data is available to prohibit or allow their use on a permanent basis
Permanent listing	Colors determined to be safe for human consumption
FD&C Colorants	Certifiable for coloring food, drugs, and cosmetics
D&C Colorants	Considered safe for use in drugs and cosmetics that can be ingested or that have direct contact with mucous membranes

Ext. D&C Colorants	Not certifiable for products intended to be ingested (due to oral toxicity), but considered safe for products applied to the skin. Remember that the skin is permeable. I recommend not using any colorant that is not approved as a food colorant.
Allura Red AC	Uncertified FD&C Red No. 40
Indignotine	FD&C Blue No. 2
Erythrosine	FD&C Red No. 3
Tartrazine	FD&C Yellow No. 5

It's important to remember that natural chemicals are still chemicals! And although an ingredient may be natural, it may still cause harm in the body. Furthermore, natural ingredients taken from our polluted environment are possibly contaminated. One could argue that, in some cases, certified colors (FD&C Colors) might be safer for consumers because they are so strictly monitored. If you choose products that are colored with natural ingredients like chamomile, annatto, or beet, for example, you should obtain backup information to prove that the manufacturer has acted with due diligence and has sourced contaminant-free ingredients.

Just Plain Irritating

Oddly enough, I firmly believe that when a product gives you some sort of adverse reaction—such as a rash, hives, or acne—it's actually a blessing in disguise. This way, you know immediately that the product contains an ingredient that is harmful to you, and you can stop using it. Through trial and error you can even isolate the offending ingredient and put it on your own personal restricted list. This is much better than using a product for years that gives no outward indication of the harm it's doing inside your body. In the next few pages, I'll discuss some products that are known to be irritants for some people. Perhaps these examples can help you solve a few of your own skin problems.

Sodium Laurel Sulfate

Nothing seems to spark so much debate as this ingredient. Some sources claim that it causes cancer, although there is as yet no clear indication that it does. It can, however, combine with other ingredients to form nitrosamines, and it may contain dioxins. Sodium laurel sulfate (SLS) is used in shampoos and cleansers because of its excellent foaming properties, although it can be a skin irritant for many. One study showed that SLS encouraged water loss from the skin, a consequence of particular concern for those with eczema. Consecutive applications of SLS led to a pronounced increase in water loss.

According to the Cosmetic Ingredient Review (CIR) website, SLS is safe in formulations designed for discontinuous and brief use, but it should be thoroughly rinsed from the skin. It's probably wise to avoid products containing this chemical, particularly if you have sensitive skin.

Sodium Laureth Sulfate

This is the alcohol form of SLS, and although it's gentler on the skin, it comes with all the same concerns.

Talc

Yes, I'm referring to the soft, white powder that you apply to your baby's bottom to help keep the little dear dry. Unfortunately, some studies link lung conditions with inhaled talc and an increased risk of ovarian cancer in women with the use of talc products in the genital region. The problem lies in determining whether talc is the problem or whether asbestos or other possible contaminants in talc could be the carcinogens. At this point, the evidence is inconclusive, and the National Toxicology Program deferred consideration of the listing of talc on the *Report on Carcinogens* until more information becomes available. In the meantime, I would suggest using corn starch on your baby's skin. It would also be a good idea to carefully investigate the source of talc in products that you use. Call up the manufacturer. They'll be glad to hear from you.

> ### Corn, Rice, and Your Baby's Skin
>
> Rather than taking a chance with talc, use cornstarch or rice powder for your baby's bottom or to absorb excess moisture. Be cautious of corn allergies if using cornstarch.

A Little Bit Sensitive?

I know I haven't written about every product out there, and I possibly haven't addressed the one that you know irritates you. There are hundreds of chemicals that we could be exposed to in our beauty products and more people who react to them. A 1988 study of the causes of allergic contact dermatitis from cosmetics showed that 56.3% of reactions were caused by skincare products. Nail products (13.4%), perfumes (8.4%), and hair products (5.9%) rounded out the results. Researchers determined that preservatives caused most of the problems (32%) and fragrances ran a close second (26.5%). Emulsifiers finished third, causing 14.3% of the problems. The preservative Kathon CG was most annoying, bothering 27.7% of the study group, and formaldehyde irritated 12.6% of the participants. The numbers add up to more than 100, because some people reacted to more than one product.

It should go without saying that if a product bothers you, you should stop using it. You should also contact the manufacturer to report your reaction. A responsible company will record and follow up on your complaint. Finally, don't underestimate the power of reporting an adverse reaction to the FDA or Health Canada. These governing bodies can't address a problem if they don't know it exists.

CHAPTER FOURTEEN

Making Up

Beauty is an ecstasy; it is as simple as hunger.
There is really nothing to be said about it. It is like the perfume
of a rose: you can smell it and that is all.
—*W. Somerset Maugham*

When we were teenagers, many of us started to dabble in make-up. The smart ones among us went to a professional make-up artist or two for some lessons, so we could learn how to work with our features. And didn't we look fabulous!

In our youth, we could pile on contrasting pinks, blues, and golds all at once from lid to brow (okay, I'm talking about myself here!) and look absolutely adorable. We could use a thick eyeliner, glob on the mascara, and line our lips with a precision that could have cut glass. Ah, the good old days.

But now the story takes a ghastly turn. Many of us are still using the same colors and techniques that made us look delightful in our teens when our skin was plump, dewy, and wrinkle-free. The problem is that our skin is no longer plump, dewy and wrinkle-free. Heavy eye make-up tugs at the corners of our eyes, and gravity does the same for our once pouty lips. Crèmes, powders, and colors cake in lines and wrinkles, making us look older by the hour. Yet despite the evidence in the mirror, many of us persist in our teenage ways. Now I'm not suggesting that you give up your love affair with make-up after you turn 21. I'm suggesting that, in order to look your best, you need to tweak your technique as you age. As much as make-up is about self-expression, a rainbow of color or extra-thick liner on your lids stops working for you shortly after you graduate from high school. As we mature, we realize that the goal is to have people notice *us*, not our make-up. For daytime, it's best to look healthy, natural, and glowing.

So it's probably time for you to visit a make-up artist again, but be sure to choose wisely: find someone who's about your age and who wears tasteful make-up herself. (It's more difficult to determine the style a male artist would use unless you know his work.) Be cautious of department store make-up artists who are tied to a product line and are therefore motivated to sell you as much of that line as possible, whether you need it or not. And don't just rely on the advice of your friends, who may be afraid to tell you the truth or who may not want you to change a thing, so they feel more comfortable changing nothing about their own make-up style!

As with every new direction you take in your life, changing your make-up style can be a bit frightening. If you're used to seeing yourself a certain way, it's not easy to get used to looking any different. And it's hard to acknowledge that these changes are necessary because we're no longer 16. But those old techniques may actually be making you look older than you are.

I'm not immune to this process either. I worked as a make-up artist years ago, and although I've since moved on to other things, I've held to my fascination with the fantasy. Over the years, I also tried to make changes to my make-up style to reflect the changes in my life, and I seriously cut down on the amount of eye shadow I wore. (You should have seen me in the 80s!) But even I had a thing or two to learn when I asked my friend Rose-Marie Swift for a critique. Now, I know I told you not to talk to your friends about this rather sensitive issue, but Rose-Marie is a celebrity make-up artist living and working in New York City. She has beautified the famous faces of Celine Dion, Isabella Rossellini, Kim Cattrall, Sheryl Crowe, Jessica Lange, Rebecca Romijn, Gisele Bündchen, and many others. Her work has appeared in *Harper's Bazaar*, *Vogue*, *Elle*, *Glamour*, and *Marie Claire*, and she's done make-up for several major fashion companies, including Victoria's Secret, Hugo Boss, The Gap, Banana Republic and more. (For a quick example of Rose-Marie's talent, please see my photo on the cover of this book.) When Rose-Marie talks about make-up, a wise woman listens.

Fortunately for me, I was in the right head space to listen to Rose-Marie's advice. I suspected I could do more to enhance my looks, and I learned rather quickly that "more" translated into still "less" than I was wearing! When Rose-Marie finished my "make-under," I was thrilled—so thrilled, in fact, that I asked her to contribute her ideas to this book. In the next several pages, you'll learn tips for creating a radiant daytime look from one of New York City's top make-up artists. Because Rose-Marie and I met through our mutual interest in the dangerous ingredients found in many cosmetic products, you'll notice several suggestions for healthy and natural alternatives to using chemical-laden items. Read with an open mind, ladies, and watch the transformation in the mirror!

Step One: The Eyebrows

The fastest, easiest, cheapest, and most natural way to change your appearance is to shape your eyebrow. A properly shaped brow frames the face, lifts the eyes, and softens your appearance. And after a good brow job, you might need less make-up to look your best! If you've abused your brow-line in the past, the first step in your facial re-creation will be to let your brows grow in. This might be an uncomfortable time for you, but the results will be well worth it. Once you have eyebrows to work with, and it's in your budget, schedule an appointment with a professional to tweeze you into shape. Tweezing is much more accurate than waxing—which can leave you with bald patches—and, unlike threading, you can do it yourself at home afterwards.

After your tweezing, follow the line made by the pro and pluck only the little hairs that come in. To decide whether or not to pluck a hair, use the tweezers to move it out of the way first. If losing the hair will leave you with a "hole" in your brow, it's better to leave it where it is. Always pluck hairs in the direction that they grow. Tugging from every angle can move the root bulb, causing the hair to grow in the wrong direction. In fact, you can correct the growing pattern of an out-of-control hair by consistently plucking it in the direction you'd like it to grow. To correct bald spots or to fill in a brow that's been over-plucked, use a matte eye-shadow powder that matches your brow color (but not black!). You can also try to draw in brow hair with a pencil, but you might find that the waxes in the pencil will ball up on your skin. At night, treat your eyebrows to a nourishing crème.

> **The fastest, easiest, cheapest, and most natural way to change your appearance is to shape your eyebrow. A properly shaped brow frames the face, lifts the eyes, and softens your appearance. And after a good brow job, you might need less make-up to look your best!**

If you don't have the time, inclination, or luxury of having a professional pluck, these simple guidelines should help you with your brow overhaul. Take cues from your natural brow line as to the right shape for your brow.

Beautiful Brows

1. Facing the mirror, lay a pencil so that it runs vertically alongside your nose, crossing over the inside corner of your eye. Your brow should start where the pencil reaches the brow-line. (If it's easier for you, use a make-up pencil to mark the spot where the pencil reaches the brow.)

2. Shift the pencil so it creates a line from the tip of your nose to the outside corner of your eye. Your brow should end where the pencil reaches the brow-line. Mark the finish line if you like.

Classic Arch

3. For a classic arch, the arch of the brow should appear directly above the outside corner of your iris (the colored part of your eye.) Don't put the arch at the inside corner of your iris or you'll create a brow that looks like a tadpole or a comma. Mark the arch point with your make-up pencil.

4. Leave your brow thicker at the start (between the eyes), and gradually taper it toward the end. Draw in a line if that makes the plucking easier for you.

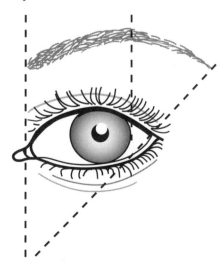

5. On the underside of the brow, pluck in a straight line from the beginning of the brow to the arch. Don't round the bottom of your brow or the tadpole will soon appear.

6. Make sure the outside of your brow is clean and free of strays, especially if your eyes appear to droop at the outside.

Other Brow Shapes

The Classic Arch doesn't work for everybody. Look to your brow-line for guidance. If it works for your face, for instance, a straight brow can be quite stunning. Sometimes a longer brow will work, and some people have beautiful semi-circle or half-moon brows that perfectly suit their face shape. Just be sure to keep the brow-line clean and remove any strays.

As a style tip, thin brows are out of fashion, so if you have that version, try to grow them in. If you're young and just starting to pluck your brows, don't overdo it. Eventually, over-plucked brows will no longer grow in.

Foundation: No Longer the Best Make-up Base

Most women overuse foundation and walk around with a mask of color blocking the visibility of their skin. Gone are the days when foundation covered everything, creating a palette on which to paint a new face. Instead, foundation should be used only where you need it to even out skin tone and cover imperfections. Most people require only a touch of foundation around the nose and chin. There's no need to put foundation on your eyelids or your mouth. And you should keep it far away from any crow's feet near your eyes.

It's important to remember that the more make-up you put on your face, the more it will get into your lines and wrinkles, calling attention to them. Too much foundation can also make your skin look dry and matte, rather than moist and dewy. In short, it will make you look older. That stops being a goal for most women somewhere around their 21st birthday!

Apply foundation with either a dampened sea sponge or slightly moist fingertips. The water will allow a smoother application and leave your skin more clean looking. Don't use foam sponges: they absorb more of the foundation than they apply and you'll just end up wasting a lot of make-up. Keep sea sponges clean by regularly boiling them for a few minutes. As your skin condition improves because of your new health habits and clean skin products, you'll need less coverage from a foundation. Try a tinted moisturizer, which will allow your skin to look more real. After all, this is the effect that we're trying to achieve. Without the heavy pigments, it's also possible that tinted moisturizers contain fewer toxic chemicals than foundations.

> ## Foundation Beauty Tip
> Foundation should match your skin tone exactly, but the lights in cosmetics stores can play tricks on your eyes. If you think you've found a good match, put some on your jaw-line and take a walk outside. A quick glance in your compact mirror will tell you whether you've found your color.

Concealer

When choosing a camouflage cream, look for a product with a slightly yellow tint that's still close to your skin color. Yellow helps counteract the gray of undereye circles. If your cover-up is too white, it will accentuate the gray underneath your eyes. The first mistake that most people make with concealers is that they put them on before they apply their foundation. If you use cover-up first, then rub foundation on top of it, you'll quickly undo all your concealing work.

• **Rule One:** Concealer goes on *after* foundation.
Most people also apply concealer incorrectly when trying to camouflage undereye circles. The crème should not go underneath the entire eye, for the same reason that you want to be sparse with your foundation: too much make-up will quickly find your creases and draw attention to them. Instead of looking refreshed, you'll look older! To camouflage undereye circles, tip your head down slightly as you look in the mirror. You'll see a darkened hollow near your nose and the inside corner of your eye. With your fingertips, apply your concealer only to that hollow area. If the area is very small, use a tiny brush to paint in the concealer. Remember that you're trying to create the illusion of a smooth surface, and focus on your school art-class lessons.

• **Rule Two:** Dark recedes and light brings forward.
Putting your light crème in the darker hollow will help create the illusion
that the hollow does not exist. But putting the light crème on the ridge of
skin underneath the hollow as well will make that
area come out too, effectively rendering your
concealer useless. Put the crème only in the hollow. Likewise, putting a light concealer on a puffy
eye "bag" will accentuate the bag even more, so
make sure you avoid any puffy areas. Stay completely away from the tiny lines and crow's feet—
unless, of course, you want people to see them.

> ### Concealer Beauty Tip
> To cover an inflamed red blem-
> ish, use a concealer that is tint-
> ed green. Green counteracts the
> redness of the pimple. Cover
> with tinted moisturizer.

When using cover-up to camouflage a pimple, a pointed brush will help
you apply a dot of crème on the blemish only. Avoid getting crème on the
area around the pimple, or you'll make the blemish appear larger.

Powder

As you try to create a healthy beauty look, it's important to avoid the
overprocessed, overpowdered face. The matte face is not only painfully
out of style; it also looks dry. Remember that healthy skin looks moist
and dewy. Use powder only on the nose and chin so these areas do not
look shiny. You can also use a bit of powder to set the undereye camouflage crème or concealer that you've used on a blemish.

Rather than using a talc powder that's often too grainy (and maybe
contaminated with asbestos), opt for a rice or corn powder. These fine
powders give a much smoother finish than talc. To apply, press your
powder-puff into the powder and shake off the excess. With light pressure, touch the puff on the undereye camouflage crème or concealer.
Unless you have a very light hand, using a brush to apply your powder
can actually remove the crème. You might also find that putting some
powder on blackheads will help camouflage them until your dietary
changes and use of healthy cosmetic products combine to help you
banish them from your skin.

Eye Shadow

Because eye-shadow powders can fall during application, it's wise to
put on your eye make-up *before* perfecting your foundation and cover

up. If you're planning to wear very little eye make-up, however, you can apply it last. If you aren't a professional, use sponge-tip applicators for your eye shadow. The sponges hold make-up better than a brush, so less powder is likely to fall onto your cheeks. Sponge applicators are also easier for most people to use, and they're excellent for blending. Shadows should always be blended, by the way, so you can't see where they start and stop. When applicators become dirty, simply clean them with organic shampoo. Don't use dish detergent or any other cleanser that might damage your eyes.

There are as many eye shapes as there are people on the planet, and we all have our own unique concerns. You'll have to do a little experimenting to find the right look for your face, and you should remember the rule about dark colors giving the illusion of receding and light colors bringing things forward. Apart from these general pointers, here are a few specific eye issues that many people have.

- **Close-Set Eyes.** To create a sense of more space between your eyes, concentrate darker colors on the outside corners of your eyes.

- **Wide-Set Eyes.** To create a sense that eyes are set closer together, concentrate darker colors on the inside corners of your eyes.

- **Low Eyebrow.** Lift a low brow by tweezing to a classic arch and adding highlight (a light color) just under the brow bone.

- **Heavy Lid.** Use a bit of a darker color along the lid to downplay the heaviness.

- **Sunken Eyes.** Use light colors to bring out a deep-set eye.

The best way to make your lids look beautiful is to attract light with a luminous shadow or, for a healthier approach, put a dab of light-reflecting organic oil on your lid. You can also use a moist, light-colored, natural lip balm for a dash of sparkle. Forget the idea that you need separate products for your lips, cheeks, and eyes. Many cosmetic companies package these products separately to part you from your hard-earned money. And, fortunately, many natural lip products work very well—in addition to being good for you! Just be sure that they don't contain ingredients that could damage your eye.

Lining Eyes

Many women struggle with getting their eyeliner just right, ending up with gaps between the rim of the eye and the liner or a wobbly line that draws attention to the make-up, rather than the eye. But eyeliner doesn't have to be difficult to apply.

> **Beauty Tip: Take It Back!**
>
> You can always return a cosmetic product to the store if you have a reaction to the product or if it doesn't work out for you as you'd planned. Don't be stuck with a product you can't use!

First of all, don't even think about using liquid liner unless you have wrinkle-free, 16-year-old skin and the steady hands of a surgeon. Pencils will work, as long as you choose ones that won't ball up on your lid. If you'd like a professional look, however, you'll need a thin eyeliner brush and a dark brown or black eye shadow, depending on the intensity of your eye. Using an almost microscopic drop of water, wet your brush and then mix it in a small amount of the eye shadow. With color on your brush, trace the line of your upper lashes. You actually want to rest the brush on the base of your lashes and follow the natural line of your eye. This way, you'll see the color fill in the area around your lashes. Keep the line as thin as possible at the inner corners of your eyes, gradually making it thicker as you head toward the end. Experiment to find the best finishing point for your liner. Stopping at the end of the eye will give you a round eye suitable for daytime; elongating the line past the end of the eye will create drama; and slanting the liner upward at the end will create an almond-eye effect.

Most people should omit a harsh line on the bottom of the eye, as this will harden the look of the area and accentuate lines. If you like some definition on the bottom, use well-blended eye shadow or smudge the liner after you apply it. Remember to keep the look soft. Be sure to discard unused eye shadow after three months to limit your exposure to bacteria. Never share your eye make-up or eye brushes— even with your teenaged daughter!

Lovely Lashes

Curling your eyelashes is one of the easiest ways to make your eyes look pretty, but the trick is to keep them looking natural. After getting all your lashes into the curler, move the curler as close to your lid as

Beauty Tip for Mascara and Curly Lashes

If you've taken the time to curl your lashes, make sure you use only waterproof mascara. Regular formulations contain too much water, which will cause your freshly curled lashes to lose shape.

possible. Gently press the curler closed. This is not the time to test your hand strength! Move the curler out slightly and gently press again. Continue the process, moving gradually out to the tips to create a beautiful curve. Turn your head sideways and check in the mirror to make sure you've created a curve, rather than a reverse "L" shape. If you don't like the shape you've created, simply wet your lashes with water to release the curl, wait until your lashes dry, and start again. Curlers come in various sizes, so you can curl a few or all of your lashes. Don't try to curl the bottom lashes.

Mascara

Mascara really helps to open up the eyes. If you use lots of it, applied well, you might find that you don't need eye shadow! The trick to putting on mascara without getting it all over your lids is to tilt your head back and look upwards into the mirror when coating the top lashes. Place the wand at the root of your lashes, wiggle it slightly, and comb out to the ends. And let your top lashes dry before starting to coat your bottom lashes.

Mascara Removal Beauty Tip

Let's face it: mascara isn't good for your lashes! So if you don't pamper them, they'll start to look like tree branches or they'll simply fall out altogether. Remove mascara with a nourishing organic oil to make amends for the damaging affects of the chemicals. And don't be afraid to put that moisturizing oil on your lashes even on days when you aren't wearing mascara!

When working on your bottom lashes, don't try to use the full length of the wand if doing so leaves more mascara on your skin than on your lashes! Tilt the wand so that only a few bristles make contact with your lashes at any time. Then use an eyelash brush or comb to remove clumps from lashes. Discard mascara three months after opening the tube, whether or not you've used it regularly. Mascara can be a breeding ground for germs!

You're Making Me Blush!

Not so long ago—it was in the 80s, as a matter of fact—we were taught to follow the line of the cheekbone to apply our blush. It was a two-in-

one contour and blush procedure. The problem now is that the con-
toured look ages you (unless you're the same age now as you were in
the 80s!) It's time to remember why we call it
"blush." We want to look healthy, vibrant, and
full of energy. We want our make-up to give us a
little lift while still looking natural. So let's put
the blush where our "blush" really is! All you
have to do is smile at yourself in the mirror and
put your blush on the plump "apple" of your
cheek. Dip your brush into the powder and
remove any excess. Make sure you don't paint in
a little circle. Instead, blend your blush out to
nothing. And don't be afraid to take the blush

> **Beauty Tip: Choosing Your Blush Color**
>
> Whether you opt for powder or crème, choose your blush based on your skin tone. Coral-pinks work on most skin colors, and they are also very modern looking. Finding the perfect color might take a little experimenting.

upward, toward your eye. Blending so that the outer edge disappers is
the secret to avoiding big clown circles on your face.

Lip Service

When it comes to lips and style, there are a few things you need to
know:

1. Using a lip-liner darker than your lip is "out"

2. Using a lip-liner to match your lipstick is "out"

3. Using a lip-liner that matches your natural lip color is fresh
   and modern, and keeps you looking younger!

If you look at your naked lip in the mirror, I'm quite sure you won't
find a dark line around your mouth. That only happens in coloring
books. And if you add a dark line, you might have to worry about people noticing it after you eat, drink, or talk. So use a liner that matches
your natural lip color. That will allow you to make minor corrections to
your lip-line without drawing people's attention for the wrong reasons!

Minor Corrections

As we age, the tug of gravity pulls our upper lips downward, making
them seem thinner. Gravity can also cause the corners of our mouths to
fall, making us look less happy than we might feel. Fortunately, a few
tricks can be used to restore a youthful pucker.

Thin Lips

To thicken your lips, line each lip just outside the natural lip-line, slightly rounding the lip-line from the bow (the indent at the center of the upper lip) to the corner of the lip.

Droopy Corners

To lift a mouth that has started to droop at the corners, round the upper lip-line from the peaks of the bow to the corners. A curved line fills out the upper lip and detracts attention from the nasolabial fold. (The nasolabial fold is the line in your skin that stretches from the side of your nose to the corner of your mouth on both sides. It tends to become accentuated with age.) Rounding the top lip will also give the illusion of softening a pointed nose.

Working the Bow

To keep your mouth looking youthful, don't accentuate the bow by sharpening its peaks. A sharp-looking mouth can be frightening! Keep peaks rounded and move the center of the valley slightly upwards. This will create the appearance of a fuller upper lip.

Organic Lipstick Beauty Tip

Want some value for your money? Use organic lipstick on your lips, apply it with your fingers to your cheeks as a blush, and if it's a light enough color, put some on your eyelid. You'll look fresh, and you'll also have the comfort of knowing that you haven't slathered chemicals on your face! Be sure that products do not contain ingredients that are harmful to your eyes.

To Prevent Lipstick Bleeding

Before applying your lipstick, use a ricepaper blotter so you can start with a matte mouth. The fine rice powder in these papers won't pile up in the tiny lines around your mouth. Use a lip brush to apply your color. This way, you can accurately follow the lip-line you've created, and you'll be almost guaranteed not to use too much lipstick. If you've never used a lip-brush before, you might be surprised to learn how much longer a tube of lipstick will last when you start using a brush! Blot again after applying the lipstick. Add a touch of gloss only to the center of your top and bottom lips. Glossing all over is for teenagers, and it will encourage color bleeding.

If your lipstick bleeds a lot, change the brand. Some products contain too much moisture or too many synthetic oils that don't absorb into the skin, so they slide around and bleed into the tiny lines around your mouth. Look for a lipstick or lip stain that contains more natural ingredients.

Coming Clean

As you change your whole body health routine, you'll want to encourage your new glow with the right skin care regime. Choose your skin products with care, being aware of ingredients that can dehydrate or irritate skin. Two essential steps need to be take for good skin care: cleansing and moisturizing. (While you'll certainly benefit from treatments that exfoliate and masks that purify or nourish, these products also generally fall into the categories of "cleanse" or "moisturize.") The most important thing to remember before you ever touch your face is to wash your hands. There's no sense in adding extra germs to the mix.

Removing Eye Make-Up

When working around this delicate area, remember that the skin here is neither as thick nor as resilient as the skin on other parts of your body (and it's not nearly as tough as the skin on your fingers and feet). So the key to protecting your eyes is to be very gentle.

> ### Label Lesson
>
> Beware of the word "organic" in the name of a beauty product. There are no laws governing the use of this word, and it is used with abandon to name everything from shampoo to lipstick. To determine whether a product is truly organic, look at the list of ingredients on the label: the word "organic" will appear in front of each ingredient in the formulation that is actually organic. Any ingredient that isn't described as organic is not organic.

If you wear eye make-up, it's important to remove it thoroughly at the end of the day. Depending on its formulation, your facial cleanser might be adequate for removing most eye products. This is often true of the milky cleansers. Of course, you must always remember to keep your eyes closed as you clean them! If you wear waterproof mascara, however, you'll need an oil-based product such as organic jojoba oil or olive oil to clean your lashes. First of all, run some warm water into your sink and make sure your facial cleanser and face cloth are nearby. (You don't want to open your eyes to search around for your cleanser and cloth halfway through this process!) Simply add a few drops of the oil to your fingertips or to an unbleached cotton ball, close your eyes, and gently massage the oil into your lashes to break up the mascara. You should be able to feel when the lashes are no longer coated.

Either use another cotton ball to remove the smudge from your face or use the face cloth when you cleanse. When you've finished removing the mascara, proceed with your normal cleansing. Your facial product should be able to remove traces of dirt and oil on your face.

Cleansing

If you wear make-up, cook supper, have young kids, or ever leave your house, it's very important that you clean your skin at the end of the day. Dirt, oil, and germs coat your skin, and if they're not removed, they'll block pores, leading to blemishes. Reduced cell turnover from lack of contact with a soft cloth will lead to a dull, lifeless complexion, and germs will have more time to find a suitable entry point into your body. But cleansing involves walking the fine line between being clean and stripping our skin of important defense mechanisms. So when it comes to cleansing your skin, it's important to remember that a certain amount of naturally present oil is necessary to protect you from bacteria. That's why you should use a very gentle product.

Myriad formulations for cleansers are available on the market, but look for the simplest one you can find, made with natural ingredients and minimal or no synthetic preservatives and other additives.

If you have normal to dry skin, on a day that you've spent lazing around the house without sunscreen or make-up, a quick splash of warm water and a gentle massage with a cotton face cloth should provide you with adequate cleansing. But on a make-up or sunscreen day—or if you have naturally oily skin—you're going to need a little help. Oil, along with some make-up and sunscreen products, is not water soluble.

Myriad formulations for cleansers are available on the market, but look for the simplest one you can find, made with natural ingredients and minimal or no synthetic preservatives and other additives. Avoid disposable cleansing wipes that are soaked in synthetic preservatives—for three reasons: they might have long-term implications for your health, they're a burden on the environment; and they don't give you the same gentle exfoliation that you get from your cotton face cloth.

Soaps and cleansers help remove grime because they're made of molecules that have an affinity for both oil and water. The oil-loving end

of these molecules attaches to the oils and disperses them into the surrounding water, leaving your skin clean. The foaming action results
because soaps and cleansers are surface-acting agents, or surfactants,
that can decrease the surface tension of water. Some surfactants, like
soapwort, are found in nature and have been used for centuries. Many
modern versions, like sodium laurel sulfate, have led to skin irritation,
redness, blisters, and eczema. (See Chapter 13.)

When choosing your cleanser, opt for a product containing natural
saponins like soapwort. Castile soap is also a natural product made
from olive oil and salt. If your skin demonstrates an allergic reaction like
redness or stinging after using *any* product, discontinue using it and
return it to the place of purchase with your receipt.

Always wash with warm water, never hot. Hot water can melt the
lipids in your skin, and you need those to keep your skin soft and supple. With clean hands, pour some cleanser into your palm, then apply a
small amount to each cheek and to your forehead and your chin.
Massage the cleanser into your hairline to remove traces of any hair
product you use.

Use a cotton face cloth for gentle exfoliation, and never tug on your
skin. Cleanse in an upward circular motion so you don't encourage the
effects of gravity. This gentle massage also increases circulation to the
area and makes your face feel great!

Exfoliation

With exfoliation, dead cells are removed from the surface of the skin
and healthy new skin is exposed. The cell-replacement process occurs
naturally every 28 days, but the cycle is influenced by age, sun damage,
poor diet, and insufficient exercise. The process is not purely cosmetic:
skin works to purge toxins from the body, and if the pores are clogged
with dirt and debris, impurities will be trapped. This forces the other
eliminative organs, the kidneys and liver, to work harder, and eventually they become exhausted. There are two basic methods of exfoliation.
Mechanical exfoliation refers to using something rough like an abrasive
sponge to slough off dead cells. With chemical exfoliation, on the other
hand, a chemical product is used to remove the cells.

Although the name sounds frightening, chemical exfoliations often use vitamins to achieve their effect. Vitamin C, for example, allows cell generation, which in turn, helps remove old cells. Vitamin B3, or niacinamide, helps to speed up epidermal turnover, while vitamin A (retinol) is useful as an antioxidant. Alpha Hydroxy Acids (AHA) are naturally occurring acids found in fruits and vegetables and milk. Most commercial AHA products are derived from milk, citrus fruits, apples, grapes, or sugar cane. They work to normalize cell renewal and encourage the formation of healthy skin by peeling away the dead cells. AHA products may also reduce the appearance of fine lines and wrinkles. For an at-home spa treatment, cover your face for 5–10 minutes with a cold, milk-soaked face cloth after cleansing, then rinse.

If you have sensitive skin, you might find AHA products too irritating for you, as they can cause blisters, dry patches, and redness. So you might want to try Beta Hydroxy Acids (BHA) instead. Derived from wintergreen leaves, willowtree bark, berries, papaya, or pineapple, BHA works by digesting the bonds that attach dead skin cells to live ones. Since they don't penetrate as deeply as AHAs, they may be better for people with sensitivities. BHA clears away dirt and oils that can clog pores, and it helps prevent acne eruptions. It also seems to work better than AHAs at smoothing skin. Chemical products may be irritating, and they should be used less often if your skin is sensitive. Whether you try AHA or BHA, do not combine them with a mechanical exfoliation like a loofah, a scrub, or a peel. If you do, you will likely damage your skin.

If you have mature or oily skin, you might prefer to use a more familiar product—the abrasive "scrub." Look for one containing crushed walnut, almond, or oatmeal. Try to find products that contain beneficial essential oils. Passion flower and black currant, for example, help to firm skin and reduce lines.

Always use a gentle, circular motion, and stay away from the area around your eyes. If you want to make your own scrub, combine one tablespoon of cornmeal and one tablespoon of mashed pineapple with one teaspoon of water (for oily skin). If you have dry skin, replace the water with one teaspoon of olive oil. Over a sink, apply the scrub to your face using a circular motion. Remove with a warm, wet face cloth. If you prefer, add one tablespoon of raw oatmeal to your regular moisturizer and massage into your face using a circular motion. Rinse with cool water after 5 minutes. You should always follow your shower with a moisturizing cream, but also consider using an AHA or BHA product for added effect—or try rubbing your elbows and knees with the inside of a fresh avocado peel. Its grainy texture will help remove alligator skin, and it's full of skin-nourishing vitamins A, D, and E. (Read Chapter 8 for more healthy-skin tips.)

> You should always follow your shower with a moisturizing cream, but also consider using an AHA or BHA product for added effect—or try rubbing your elbows and knees with the inside of a fresh avocado peel. Its grainy texture will help remove alligator skin, and it's full of skin-nourishing vitamins A, D, and E.

Unfortunately, you can't peel back the years through exfoliation, so don't overdo it! Exfoliate once a week for dry and sensitive skin and up to three times a week for oily skin. If you have acne, more is not necessarily better, as overscrubbing can stimulate oil production and irritate the skin. You will need to exfoliate less in the dry-aired winter than in summer, when you're likely to produce more bacteria-friendly oil and sweat. Whatever method you choose, it shouldn't hurt, sting, burn, or make your skin feel raw afterwards. And don't forget to protect your new skin—especially when you go outdoors.

What Is Toning Anyway?

The purpose of a toner is to return your skin to its natural pH of 5.5. You see, washing off oils leaves your skin too alkaline, and the toner makes it more acidic again, in order to protect it from invading bacteria. Toning is not a step that helps to remove traces of make-up that you missed—that's what cleansing properly is supposed to do. There are misconceptions about astringents, as well. Some people, for instance, believe that they sop up excess oil. Technically, astringents cause tissues to draw together and shrink by reducing their ability to absorb water. In doing so, they also help reduce tissue secretions. So applying astringent with a cotton ball doesn't soak up oil, but rather reduces the oils that get to the surface of the skin. If not properly formulated or if misused, however, astringents can lead to skin dehydration (even if your skin is oily!), since they reduce the skin's ability to absorb water. When choosing an astringent, find one that does not contain synthetic alcohols, which only serve to dehydrate the surface of the skin. Or you could try this simple and natural toner. Prepare a sinkful of warm water, add a bit of apple-cider vinegar, and splash it on your face!

Moisturizing

We've talked about the importance of nourishing your skin from the inside, but now it's time to take a different perspective. Some skin nutrients work best when they're applied directly to the skin. Moisturizers are designed to keep your skin hydrated, and this is accomplished either by adding water or by trapping water that's already there (occlusive moisturizers.) Occlusive moisturizers are particularly important if you live in an area that has harsh weather. There's nothing like a strong wind or a dry winter to sap the water from your skin.

Using a barrier cream like shea butter or cocoa butter, particularly when you are outside, helps you hold onto the moisture you have! But do be aware that occlusive moisturizers can clog pores. Other moisturizers work by different means. Hyaluronic acid (HA), for example, is a conditionally essential nutrient: our bodies produce plenty of it when we're young, but supply can't keep up with demand as we age. Think of a baby's soft, plump skin to see the benefits of a plentiful supply of HA. As we age, our ability to produce this compound weakens until, by the age of 50, we're producing less than half the HA we created in our diaper days. Loss of HA leads to loss of moisture, and this leads, in turn, to dehydration, wrinkles, and loss of skin tone and elasticity. Great.

The role of HA is to hold cells together to provide structural support to the skin, while at the same time retaining precious moisture. HA is a "humectant," which means that it draws water from the bloodstream into the skin. And as a humectant, HA is the master. It can hold up to 1,000 times its weight in water! It's no wonder, then, that skin starts to plump, fine lines flatten, and deeper wrinkles become less noticeable when you use HA. Because no food sources have been proven to increase levels of HA in skin cells, it must be applied topically. When encapsulated in liposomes (tiny hollow spheres similar to a human cell membrane in structure), HA can penetrate skin layers to prevent and diminish wrinkles while improving tone and elasticity. It has also proven to aid wound repair and has been used to heal surgical incisions, first- and second-degree burns, and various other skin lesions. Use an encapsulated HA product that contains no animal source of HA, so you can avoid possible contamination with allergy-causing protein derivatives and heavy metal toxins.

Remember that HA draws moisture into the skin, but it can't walk to the cooler to get a refill. Be sure to drink eight to ten glasses of pure, filtered water every day to make the most of your HA!

Certain skin conditioners and lubricants called "emollients" work by remaining on the skin's surface or by penetrating only to the top-most layers. Natural emollients include almond oils and other oils (such as castor oil). Protein has emollient properties, as does the beneficial Omega-6 Essential Fatty Acid gamma linolenic acid (GLA) in borage oil when applied topically. Try using an organic jojoba oil or almond oil on your skin. These oils do not clog pores, and they give your skin a beautiful, healthy sheen.

Whatever moisturizer you choose, make sure that you apply it morning and night for best results.

CHAPTER FIFTEEN

Living Beauty

To see our bodies as beautiful is not vanity. To learn to cherish that which not only houses the soul, but enables the soul access to the planet on which we live, is a joyful thing.

—*Rosemary Altea,* You Own the Power

In the early stages of writing this book, a friend recommended that I be sure to include my own story. My immediate reaction to his comment was shock and disbelief, because I thought my story really wasn't that interesting. I am not a reformed drug addict. I never weighed seven hundred pounds and had to lose bucketsful of weight through diet and lifestyle changes. What about my life could possibly be interesting and inspiring to others?

On the surface, in fact, my life may be very much like yours. I have two beautiful, amazing, exhausting, intelligent, clueless, loving, generous, and selfish children, who at times, need my guidance but very often prove to be my most valuable teachers. From them I have learned patience, tolerance, creativity, and negotiating skills, and I've experienced the joy of unconditional love. If anyone out there needs inspiration in their life, I'm telling you there's nothing that "inspires" you out of your chair faster than the sound of a loud crash followed by an ear-splitting "Mooooooomm!" We live in a single-parent household, which means I'm on double-duty and "doing it all" is my only option. And yet I wouldn't change a thing in my life. I have failed in love, and yet, perhaps more often I have been lifted by love. I have made horrible errors in judgment that, in hindsight, proved to be important turning points in my life. I've grown. I've changed over the years. Just like you. Although I am still very young, I feel as if it has been a long journey to the writing of this book. And the story starts in high school, where I loved writing. Not fiction or poetry, really, but more contemplative editorial stuff. I told people I would be a writer, and everyone encouraged me—everyone except a a certain high school teacher who told me I couldn't write an essay to save my life.

As I reflect on that now, I realize how much power we give the one dissenting voice in our lives (or in our heads), even when we are getting regular positive reinforcement everywhere else. I think we sometimes latch onto the dissenting voice because it has given form to our unspoken fears, and somehow the speaking of our fears gives them more clout. The criticism from that teacher stayed with me a long time, and I allowed it to keep me from my passion about writing. It's not that person's fault; it's mine. I gave those dissenting words the power to control my life.

I survived high school and graduated at the age of 17. I promptly turned down an offer of admission to a local journalism college. I don't remember why. But by the age of 21, I'd had enough of jobs that required long hours for little pay and decided it was time for higher education.

In university, I studied English literature. I remember tentatively approaching my first-year professor when the deadline for my initial essay assignment was drawing near—ever mindful of the negative remarks of my high school teacher I asked the prof if she would mind reading my work early and offer criticism so I could fix it before the due date. Anxiously, I watched her scroll through the handwritten sheets and held my breath as she passed the papers back to me. "Looks great," she said. "Make sure you type it before you hand it in." I got an A on that paper and every subsequent English paper that I wrote before graduating with a Bachelor of Arts. During my last year at university, I met one of my professors for coffee, and the topic of conversation rolled around to my future. This prof told me that I was really talented, and that I should consider pursuing my Master's degree. Knowing that academia was not my calling, I promised that I would continue writing. "I'm going to write a novel someday," I told her, "but not yet. What does a 24-year-old have to say that anyone would care about? I'll wait until I have more life experience."

In hindsight, I realize that you should be careful what you wish for! I then turned down another offer of admission, this time to a prominent school of journalism in Toronto. Why? My boyfriend at the time wondered why I wanted to incur more student debt. (The power of one dissenting voice.) Instead, I started a career path in finance that I stayed on for nearly a decade, a path I did not really enjoy. But as life progressed, and bills collected, I was trapped in the security of the regular paycheck.

Finally, after years of excuses and ignoring opportunities that would have allowed me to live my passion, I was put in a situation in which I had no choice—or perhaps I was finally free to make a choice. Drowning in debt, I decided late one night that I had to sell my house in order to retain my sanity. The next day, I lost my job. A week later, my marriage ended. Other than my children (whom I credit for keeping me out of the self-pity pool), I finally had nothing to lose by taking a chance on my dream. People say that money buys you freedom, but I'm telling you, so does a complete lack of it! With no job and no debt, I was finally free to live my life fully. I now look at that week of losses as a positive turning point in my life. The more I thought about my friend's comment, the more I began to value my story. I realized that my goal in sharing it is not to inspire you to make changes in your life, but rather to encourage you to find your own inspiration. And you'll probably find it in your own story. I'm not referring to the details of your life (spouse, parent, home owner, athlete) as much as how you are living your life.

> One day, in retrospect, the years of struggle will strike you as the most beautiful.
>
> —*Sigmund Freud*

Are you doing what you were put on the planet to do? Are you struggling with that question? The answer is simpler than you realize, and you probably already know but are afraid, for some reason, to pursue it. You knew when you were a kid, before the details of life started to confuse you. A looming mortgage can keep you in a meaningless job way past the stale date. Think about how you used to answer the question, "What are you going to do when you grow up?" Chances are that, as a child, your answer was based on the things that you loved doing and were good at. Very often, they *are* the same thing. Very often, that "thing" makes your heart sing. Are you still feeling the music?

Find the courage to live your passion. Ignore the dissenting voices. Don't give them any power. You're going to hear a lot of them as you work to make changes in your life. People are afraid of change, and the people who love you are afraid of how your changes will affect them. You will be mocked on occasion, as you politely decline an offer of a second helping of dessert or choose salad over pizza. People will say that they're "only kidding," but in reality, they're scared. They know that if it's possible for you to change the way you live, it's also possible that they can change the way that they live. And they may not be ready to do that. To them, it's much easier to try to keep you as you are.

Understanding the fear of change gives you the power to continue on your own path. The dissenting voices have held you back long enough—especially your own.

Do a life inventory to determine what gives you joy and what takes it away, and then make some changes. If you feel overwhelmed by financial circumstances that keep you bound to a job that drains your energy and leaves you feeling miserable, consider selling the house, the cottage, the extra car. Often, we hold onto the obligations in our lives as a means of avoiding our passion because we are afraid to live it. So you want to quit your fancy-schmancy job to paint watercolor pictures? Find a way to make that happen. It doesn't matter what anyone else thinks of your decision.

Your respect for and appreciation of your body will escalate, and this respect will eventually extend beyond your physical body to touch the world that surrounds you.

Don't scoff and mentally chide me because I "can't possibly know about your problems and how difficult it would be for you." You're right. I don't know your problems, but I do know how difficult it can be to walk through the fear and live the life you were put on this earth to live. Two marriages, two babies, several financial start-overs, four houses, a sprinkling of hard life lessons, and a smorgasbord of jobs later, I have exactly what I asked for as a naïve university student: life experience. Lots and lots of life experience. And, of course, you may remember from the beginning of the book that I became seriously interested in health when my son was diagnosed with a heart defect. So here I am, finally writing because I have something to say. And I've never been happier. My heart sings.

Following the instructions in this book will be an excellent first step in your journey to remembering your own passion. And once you've taken steps to live a more healthy lifestyle—even if you do that simply so your skin clears up or your nails stop splitting—you will, as a side effect, start to feel better. Having more energy, fewer distracting aches and pains, and the seemingly miraculous disappearance of problems that may have annoyed you for years might encourage you to increase your knowledge so you can make even more healthy changes. When you do so, you'll notice not only that your body is improving, but also that your mind is starting to clear. You may be able to remember things better and focus longer on tasks, and your head may no longer feel as if it's stuffed with cotton.

In a gradual and natural evolution, this new mental clarity will help you reconnect with the world around you. I'm not referring to the friends and family that you spend your time with (although they will surely notice a difference too). I'm talking more about how you will start to experience life in a more deliberate way. You'll start to feel the need to live to your full potential. Your respect for and appreciation of your body will escalate, and this respect will eventually extend beyond your physical body to touch the world that surrounds you. From a starting place of wanting to improve your own personal beauty, you will come to appreciate, again, all the beauty that surrounds you. You'll notice birds again, and you'll stop to admire the blooms in spring. Mothers holding babies, lovers holding hands, children squealing with delight on the playground. And along with an appreciation for this amazing, beautiful life, as you live in a healthy way, you'll start to feel your personal power build.

You'll start to feel fearless again, as if you're just starting out in life. With maturity, you've learned that you have nothing to prove, but you have much to do. You may be reading this book because you want to look your very best. We are surrounded by beauty in this world, and you are no exception. But when you're looking fabulous and feeling even better, I want you to use some of your newfound extra energy to live your life. I have faith that you'll know what that is. Use your talents; share your gifts. I can't imagine anything more beautiful.

Candida-Free
Menu Plan and Recipes

Five-Day *Candida*-Free Menu Plan

Day	Breakfast	Lunch	Supper
1	**Egg and Vegetable Scramble** *Vegetables will keep you feeling full.*	**Lettuce Sandwich** *Convenience of a sandwich without adding bread.*	**Poached fish with steamed vegetables** *Eat fish at least twice per week as a good source of FFAs.*
2	**Flax 'n' Oatmeal** *Excellent way to add more EFAs to your diet.*	**Cleansing Soup with Rice Crackers** *Will help clean out digestive tract.*	**Falafel, hummus, and green salad. Try it in a wrap!** *Chick peas (garbanzo beans) and grains combine to create an excellent source of protein.*
3	**Lentil Soup (with Home-made Tortilla if desired)** *Shake it up a bit! A hearty soup is a nutritious and delicious start to the day.*	**Easy Spinach Salad with slice of Rye or Spelt Bread** *Grains, spinach is a good source of protein.*	**Broiled Chicken with with grilled vegetables** *A simple dinner that is also easy to to digest.*
4	**Baked Millet** *Millet is high in the essential amino acid lysine, making it a good protein source.*	**Curried Garlic and Broccoli-Stuffed Potatoes with Grilled Vegetables** *Eating a good assortment of vegetables will help you feel satisfied and not deprived.*	**Ratatouille on a bed of brown rice** *The key to enjoying vegetables daily is to vary the preparation.*
5	**Puffed Kamut Cereal with Rice Milk and Ground Flaxseed** *Try any puffed grain cereal (except wheat) Kamut is a good source of protein.*	**Rice with Lentils Garden Salad** *Combining legumes with grains creates a complete protein and fiber, and easy to digest.*	**Vegetarian chili with toasted spelt bread** *Many of the spices we use in meal preparation have nutritional and healing benefits.*

Candida-Free Recipes

BAKED MILLET

Use a slow cooker overnight to have breakfast ready when you wake up!

1 cup millet, washed
3 cups pure water

Place in a casserole dish with a cover. Bake at 200°F for about 4 hours, or cook in a slow cooker overnight. You can add any of the following: nuts, cinnamon, nutmeg, sesame seeds, flaxseeds, butter, sea salt, rice or nut milks that you can purchase at the store or make yourself at home, or unsweetened soy milk. When you reach the point in your diet where you wish to start eating fruit again, try adding raw diced apples.

CLEANSING SOUP

When preparing this soup, leave the vegetables slightly crispy. This will help to clear out your system.

Half a shallot
1 bunch of scallions
1 leek
2 cloves garlic or 1 tsp liquid
  Aged Garlic Extract
Half a zucchini
Half a cucumber
Broccoli florets

1/2–1 cup green cabbage
1/2–1 cup Chinese cabbage
1 tomato
Half a red pepper

1 fresh chili pepper
2 stalks celery
Vegetable broth to cover

Cut all veggies and throw into your pot. Cover with the broth and bring to a boil. Let simmer for about 8–10 minutes. If you want the soup to be "cleansing," leave vegetables slightly crispy. Add salt, pepper, fresh cilantro/coriander, or other fresh herbs.

CURRIED GARLIC AND BROCCOLI-STUFFED POTATOES

1 large potato or 2 small potatoes
1 cup broccoli florets
2 cloves garlic (crushed)
1 tsp curry powder (no sugar added)
1 tbsp olive oil
Sea salt and fresh ground pepper to taste

Bake potatoes. Crush garlic and sautée over low heat with curry powder and oil for about 2–3 minutes. Steam broccoli to desired tenderness. Cut open baked potato(es). Fill with broccoli and pour garlic-curry oil over it. If you wish, add sea salt and fresh ground pepper to taste. Avoid eating potato skin in the first stage of the diet.

EASY SPINACH SALAD

Put washed baby leaf spinach in a bowl. Add chopped cauliflower pieces, chopped red bell pepper, shredded carrots, and sliced almonds, and top with a dash of ground flaxseed. For dressing, combine light olive oil and squeezed lemon juice and a dash of salt or garlic.

EGG AND VEGETABLE SCRAMBLE

Stir-fry your favorite vegetables in a bit of olive oil: combine broccoli, asparagus, any color of pepper, onion—whatever inspires you. Turn down heat, and add one or two beaten eggs. Cook through.

FALAFEL

Baked, rather than fried, these falafels are lower in fat than traditional falafel. Leftovers can be frozen. To make a sandwich, roll the falafel in a homemade tortilla (see the recipe for Homemade Tortillas) with fresh vegetables. For topping, use hummus, tahini, or tzatiki sauce.

3 cups cooked organic garbanzo beans (chick peas)
1 small onion, finely chopped
1 garlic clove, finely chopped (I use more)
1/4 cup minced fresh parsley

3 tbsps fresh ground flaxseeds
1 tsp paprika
1 tsp Braggs Liquid Amino sauce
2 tbsp wheat germ (if avoiding wheat, you can use oat bran instead)
1/4 cup whole grain flour of your choice (try spelt)

Preheat oven to 350°F. Combine all of the ingredients in a food processor, or mash in a bowl and mix well. With wet hands, form the mixture into 1-inch balls. Bake on a lightly oiled cookie sheet for 10 minutes on one side, then roll over and bake 10 minutes on the other side.

Gas Relief

If eating beans gives you gas, try soaking dried beans overnight before using them. (Discard the soakwater.) Soaking starts the process of sprouting, which not only improves the enzyme-providing potential of your meal, but also cuts down on gas production.

FLAX'N' OATMEAL

Cook 1/4 cup oatmeal in 1/2 cup water with a little sea salt and a sprinkle of cinnamon. Remove from heat. Add 2 tbsp ground flaxseed. Let cool slightly. Add 1 tbsp flax oil.

GARDEN SALAD

Let your imagination run wild, but remember our guidelines about food combining for this cleanse: avoid including protein sources such as egg, meat, or cheese with your greens. Toss some fresh, organic lettuce or spinach into a bowl, along with a serving of tomatoes, cucumber, celery, carrots, sliced cabbage and other vegetable favorites. Experiment by adding chick peas, almonds, or pinenuts for some variety. Mix up your choice of greens by alternating Romaine lettuce, Boston lettuce, or mesclun. Salad does not have to be predictable!

GRILLED VEGETABLES

1 tbsp olive oil
1 clove garlic, minced
2 tsp snipped fresh rosemary or 2 tbsp snipped fresh basil
  or 1/2 tsp dried rosemary or 1 tsp dried basil, crushed
1/4 teaspoon salt
4 cups mixed vegetables (such as eggplant; summer squash or
zucchini; green beans; red onion; and red, green, or
yellow sweet pepper)

In a medium-sized mixing bowl, combine the olive oil, garlic, rosemary or basil, and the salt. Add the vegetables to this oil mixture, tossing to coat. Spoon vegetable-and-oil mixture into a grilling basket. Grill vegetables on a grill rack directly over medium-hot coals about 20 minutes or until the veggies are tender. Turn often, to be sure they don't burn. (Or bake vegetables in a 350°F oven about 25 minutes or until tender.) Season vegetables to taste with pepper.

HOMEMADE TORTILLAS

1 1/2 cup spelt flour (or whole wheat)
1 tsp baking powder
1 tsp sea salt
1/4 cup olive oil
1/2 cup warm water

Mix dry ingredients. Add oil until mixture is crumbly. Then add the water. The mixture will form a slightly sticky ball (if not sticky, just add more water).

   Knead the dough a little. Divide it into fist-sized balls (or smaller) and roll each ball out onto a floured surface. In a large skillet, heat 3 tbsp of oil (I prefer olive oil) on medium-high heat. Place rolled dough in pan and let it fry for 2 minutes. When you see it forming bubbles, turn it over for 30 seconds to 1 minute. Cool and eat. Use as a crust for pizza with pesto, onions and peppers!

HUMMUS

Hummus can be used as a dip for raw vegetables, or it can be spread on rice or dipped up with pieces of tortilla.

1 16-oz. can organic garbanzo beans (chick peas)
1/3 cup tahini
juice of 1 small lemon
2 cloves garlic (or more if you like), crushed in blender
1/2 tsp salt
pinch of little white pepper
2 tbsp toasted sesame seeds (optional)

Drain the beans well, and in a blender or food processor, combine all ingredients (except the sesame seeds) and purée until smooth. You may have to turn off the blender or food processor frequently to scrape the sides. If using sesame seeds, toast them in a bit of olive oil in a hot heavy skillet until they begin to pop. Then stir them into the puréed hummus with a spoon. Store in a tightly covered glass container. You can also use dried chick peas. Just soak and cook as you would for any dried bean. Then use in the recipe. Makes approximately 2 1/2 cups.

Lentil Soup

3 cups dry lentils	*10 cups water*
2 tsp salt	*7 crushed garlic cloves*
2 cups chopped onion	*2 medium carrots, diced*
2–3 medium-ripe, peeled tomatoes	*1 large potato (optional)*
1 tsp basil	*1/2 tsp thyme*
1/2 tsp oregano	*freshly ground black pepper*

Bring to boil lentils, water, and salt in a large pot. Lower heat and bring to the lowest possible simmer, partially covered, for 20–30 minutes. Add garlic, basil, thyme, and oregano. Then add onions, carrots, and potato. Partially cover, and let simmer another 20–30 minutes, stirring occasionally. Squeeze seeds out of tomatoes, chop, and add to soup. Cook for 5 more minutes.

Lettuce Sandwiches

Chop chicken into bite-sized pieces or strips and stir-fry in olive oil. Add chopped zucchini, red pepper, and shredded carrots. When cooked to taste, wrap in a lettuce leaf. For added crunch, add raw almonds if you are not allergic to these nuts. Try wrapping tuna, salmon, and boiled or scrambled egg in a lettuce leaf!

Pesto

In a blender, blend:

2 cloves garlic	*Handful of toasted pine nuts*
1 bunch fresh (washed)	*Sea salt*
basil leaves	*Flax oil or hazelnut oil to*
	make a paste

Toss with rice or spelt pasta, or spread on tortillas with onions and peppers to make a pizza.

Ratatouille

3 tbsp olive oil	*1 1/2 tsp salt*
4 medium cloves garlic (chopped)	*1 1/2 tsp basil*
2 cups onion (chopped)	*1 tsp marjoram or oregano*
1 medium eggplant (cubed)	*1/2 tsp rosemary*
1 medium zucchini	*1/2 tsp thyme*
2 medium bell peppers	*freshly minced parsley (optional)*
2 cups tomatoes (chopped)	*olives (chopped) (optional)*
1 bay leaf	*ground black pepper*

Sautée garlic, onion, and bay leaf in oil in a Dutch oven for about 5 minutes. Add eggplant, salt and herbs, and stir. Cover and cook over medium heat, stirring occasionally for about 15–20 minutes or until eggplant is soft. Add zucchini, bell peppers, ground black pepper, and tomatoes. Cover and simmer for 10 more minutes or until zucchini and bell peppers are tender. Serve hot, warm, or at room temperature. Garnish with chopped olives or parsley if desired.

Rice with Lentils

1 cup lentils (any color)	*Olive oil*
1–2 onions (diced)	*2 tsp cumin*
2 cups brown or wild rice	*1 tsp salt, pepper*
5 1/2 cups boiling water	*1–2 garlic cloves (crushed)*

First soak lentils in plenty of water for at least 1 hour. Stir-fry diced onions and crushed garlic in olive oil until brown. Add rice and stir-fry for a few more minutes. Add boiling water, lentils, and cumin. Cover and cook over medium heat until all the water is absorbed. Enjoy!

Taco Salad

Mix up a salad with lettuce, onions, tomato, and peeled cucumber. Put salad either in a deep bowl or on a dinner plate and pour a serving of Vegetarian Chili on top. Serve with corn chips.

VEGETARIAN CHILI

3 garlic cloves (finely chopped)
3 tbsp olive oil
1 large Spanish onion
  (coarsely chopped)
3 celery stalks with leaves
3 carrots
2 green peppers
3 cups frozen corn

4 cups cooked kidney beans
4 cups cooked pinto beans
3 1/2 cups chopped tomato
2 tbsp chili powder
1 tbsp paprika
1 1/2 tsp salt
pepper to taste

(This recipe is also delicious with some cooked ground chicken. Of course, then it would no longer be a vegetarian dish!)

Add olive oil to large pot over medium heat. Add finely chopped garlic and coarsely chopped onion, stirring occasionally until onions soften. Cut celery, carrots, and green peppers into 1/2-inch pieces and add to pot. Cut tomatoes into 1-inch pieces and stir into mixture.

Add chili powder, paprika, salt, and pepper. Then add kidney and pinto beans and bring to a low boil. Simmer for 1 hour. Add frozen corn and cook on low for 15 minutes.

Eat as is or use in a Taco Salad.

Dictionary of Ingredients

All substances are poisons; there is none which is not a poison. The right dose differentiates a poison and a remedy.

—*Paracelsus, 1493–1541*

A s you read through and reference this dictionary, it is important that you keep several things in mind. As I have already mentioned, I am not a chemist. Instead, I am a researcher who spent many hours in the local library, on the Internet, and rifling through books, sorting through thousands of pages of information in an attempt to create a dictionary that includes chemicals frequently used in personal-care products. Although I made every attempt to create accurate definitions, I invite you to bring errors to my attention.

It's also important to remember that a "chemical" is not necessarily a bad thing. Every single person, plant, animal, or mineral—anything on this planet—is an amalgam of chemicals. Water is nothing more than two parts hydrogen and one part oxygen, or H_2O. And it is possible to have too much of any one thing—even a good thing like water or oxygen. Your task is to decide how much of any particular chemical you are willing to expose yourself to.

Next, as I read through various sources, I realized that dictionaries are not entirely objective. The definitions that they provide are sometimes flavored by the bias of the writer. A definition created by a present-day chemist, for instance, might not include the traditional use of a chemical. ("Traditional" refers to how our ancestors would have used a plant, for example.) A dictionary written by a person with a product line to support will focus on the benefits of the ingredients in their formulations, possibly glossing over some of the more unpleasant aspects of a chemical. Telling you that a chemical in a product might not be good for you is bad for business. So I caution you to use judgment in reading dictionaries written by people selling a product.

Finally, I have to admit to my own bias. My intention in creating this dictionary is to motivate you to think about the dangers that might lurk in products you use on a regular basis. I'm also of the mind that our bodies are better equipped to process ingredients that grew from the ground than those that came from a test tube. My goal is to inspire you to opt for safer choices as often as possible. I have included information from scientific journals and herbal resource guides to give you input on both natural and synthetic ingredients. Some ingredients are scientifically proven to do what they are used for, while others have been used for centuries for a certain purpose and have undergone no clinical testing.

I encourage you to challenge my bias. I would be thrilled if you took it upon yourself to do your own research and create your own informed opinion about the use of chemicals not only in our personal-care products but also in every aspect of our lives. A selection of the resources I used are listed at the back of this book, and these will offer you an excellent starting point for your research. A more complete list of publications I consulted is posted on my website, (www.iamlivingbeauty.com).

I should add an important caution: as you compare the definitions in this dictionary with the products you are using, note that any time a label states "from," as in "from coconut," the ingredient has been altered in some way and may no longer be natural. It may therefore now be considered synthetic. Also be watchful of the word "organic" in product listings: only those ingredients listed on product labels that are directly preceded by the word "organic" (or denoted with a symbol such as an *) are, in fact, organic. You can assume that other ingredients lacking the "organic" description are *not* organic.

In addition, many ingredients, such as essential oils, can be either natural or synthetic. If your goal is to avoid synthetic ingredients, I recommend that you contact the manufacturer of a product to determine the origin of chemicals listed on the product label.

Finally, I want to remind you that there are no perfect products on the market. There will be someone, somewhere who is allergic or sensitive to a particular chemical, whether it comes from a natural source or a factory. Your task is to determine what products will work for you in the short term, without potentially making you very sick in the long term. By all means, report any adverse reaction you experience after using a beauty product to the manufacturer: they can't fix a problem that they don't know exists. I also encourage you to report adverse reactions to the FDA, Health Canada, or the governing body in your country so that trends can be recorded. And be sure to see your health-care provider for advice and treatment.

A

Acacia Senegal Usually used as a thickening agent, this herb also has anti-inflammatory properties.

acetic acid Acid found in milk, apples, grapes and other fruits, vinegar, and human sweat; can also be synthetic. Used as a solvent, astringent, acidifier, and disinfectant. It can be a skin irritant.

acetone This strong solvent can be synthetic or natural and is used to remove nail polish. Toxic by inhalation and ingestion; irritant to nose, throat, eyes; can elicit confusion, nausea, and vomiting.

acetylated castor oil Used as an emollient and to thicken cosmetic formulations. *See also* castor oil.

acetylated hydrogenated cottonseed glyceride Used as an emollient and to thicken cosmetic formulations.

acetylated lanolin Emollient derived from lanolin. *See also* lanolin.

acetylated palm kernel glycerides Used as an emollient and to thicken cosmetic formulations.

Achillea millefolium *See* yarrow extract.

Aesculus hippocastanum *See* horse chestnut extract.

agar This colloid extract from red marine algae is strongly hydrophilic and can hold 20 times its weight in water; occasionally causes allergic reaction.

AHA (Alpha Hydroxy Acid). In low concentrations, AHAs are used as moisturizers due to their water-binding ability. AHAs can also increase the skin content of hyaluronic acid. (*See* hyaluronic acid.) As concentrations increase, AHAs are used to exfoliate skin cells by dissolving the material that binds cells together.

If you are looking for an exfoliating product, be sure that the concentration of AHA is 4% in a formulation with a pH of 4. The most common natural AHAs are glycolic acid (found in sugarcane) and lactic acid (found in milk). Malic acid (found in apples) and citric acid (found in citrus fruits) are also used. AHAs should be used with caution, as they can increase photosensitivity and may lead to skin irritation.

Ahnfeltia concinna extract A form of algae. *See* algae.

ahnfeltia extract A form of algae. *See* algae.

Alaria esculenta Extract A form of algae. *See* algae.

albumen Derived from egg or bovine sources, this group of water-soluble simple proteins act as emulsifiers, film-forming agents, and astringents. Often used in masks.
   May cause an allergic reaction.

alfalfa extract Mild, natural cleanser and exfoliant containing saponins. Also used in face
   masks. *See also* saponins.

algae These simple life forms provide an excellent source of amino acids, chlorophyll,
   lipids, minerals, proteins, and vitamins and are useful in cosmetics, as well as in the
   diet. May cause skin irritation.

algin Water-soluble polysaccharide found in brown algae and used for thickening.
   (Polysaccharides are formed from many sugar units.)

alginic acid Emulsifier and thickening gel produced by acidifying seaweed; soothes and
   protects skin. Derived from algae. *See also* algae.

alkyloamides Synthetic alcohols used as thickeners, emulsifiers, emollients, lubricants,
   foam boosters. Used in bubble baths, shampoos, liquid soaps, etc. Can combine
   with other ingredients to form carcinogenic nitrosamines.

allantoin Although the version derived from comfrey root is superior, most allantoin
   used in cosmetics now results from oxidizing uric acid; anti-irritant, anti-inflammatory; used to clean wounds of skin debris; healing, moisturizing; non-toxic. *See also*
   comfrey extract.

almond butter Emollient and skin conditioner made from sweet almond oil.

almond meal Used as an exfoliant in scrubs; made by grinding the kernel of sweet
   almond. Is absorbent.

almond oil Emollient oil extracted from the seeds of almonds. May cause allergic reactions. *See also* bitter almond oil; sweet almond oil.

Aloe barbadenis (aloe extract, aloe juice, aloe vera) Can reduce inflammation of wounds
   with concentrations of bradykinase, salicylic acid, and magnesium lactate. Also
   known to relieve pain and itching and prevent wound infection. Gel taken directly
   from the leaf may be useful as a remedy for psoriasis.

alpha bisabolol *See* bisabolol.

alpha lipoic acid A potent antioxidant known to boost the effectiveness of other antioxidants when taken internally.

alpha-tocopherol (or dl-alpha-tocopheral) Synthetic vitamin E.

althea extract Used as a demulcent; for bee stings, wound healing.

alum Astringent used in anti-perspirant products; may cause lung irritation if inhaled.
   Always contains aluminum. *See also* aluminum.

alumina (also known as aluminum oxide) Used as an abrasive, absorbent, and thickening agent.

aluminum Some studies suggest a link between aluminum and Alzheimer's disease, since those with the disease seem to have more aluminum in their brain tissue. It is unclear whether the disease causes aluminum retention or if the aluminum is a causative factor in the disease. It is probably best to avoid exposure to aluminum.

aluminum chlorohydrate This common antiperspirant ingredient can be extremely irritating to broken or irritated skin.

amino acid Amino acids are the building blocks of protein, and they are essential to every cell in our bodies. Because our hair consists of 18 amino acids, plant or animal amino acids are often included in hair-care formulations. Amino acids also support proteins in the skin, help to bind water, and provide antioxidant protection.

aminomethyl propanol Synthetic, mildly alkaline ingredient used to adjust pH in cosmetics.

ammonia Although the word ammonia might not appear on the product label, it is commonly used in the creation of formulations that include nitrates, sulfates, and sulfites; common skin irritant.

ammonium chloride Synthetic or mineral alkaline salt used as a pH balancer in cosmetics. Also used to thicken cleansers and shampoos.

ammonium laureth sulfate While product labels may state "from coconut," this surfactant is synthetic. Used largely as a detergent.

ammonium lauryl sulfate While product labels may state "from coconut," this surfactant is synthetic. Also manufactured from other sources. Used largely as a detergent or cleansing agent. Highly irritating; should not remain on skin. Rinse off immediately.

anisaldehyde Synthetic fragrance. *See also* fragrance.

annatto extract A deep yellow-orange to red natural colorant. Derived from a South American shrub. Color is known to fade over time. No known toxicity.

apple cider vinegar This mildly acidic astringent ingredient lowers the pH of a formulation; helps to slow over-productive oil glands. Often recommended for an at-home facial toner.

apple oil *(Pyrus malus)* Extract from the peel of apples used as an antioxidant, pH adjuster, and exfoliant; fragrance.

apricot kernel Provides a natural exfoliant when finely ground; used in scrubs.

apricot kernel oil Light, absorbent non-fragrant plant oil; useful as a skin softener, emollient, and lubricant.

arachidonic acid Taken from peanut oil, this non-irritating oil is a source of fatty acids. Used as an emollient, lubricant, and thickening agent. No known toxicity; may cause allergic reaction.

arbutin Found in the leaves of the bearberry shrub, and in cranberry, blueberry, and most types of pears. Used for its hydroquinone content. (Hydroquinone inhibits melanin production, thereby lightening skin.) Used as antioxidant and skin conditioner in cosmetic formulations. Can also be synthetic.

argan oil Emollient oil obtained from the nuts of the argania tree.

arnica extract (*Arnica montana*) (Wolf's Bane) Traditionally used to treat bruises or aches. Anti-irritant, anti-inflammatory, antiseptic, stimulates blood circulation. Rich in fatty acids, as well as vitamins A, B, C, and D. Do not use on broken skin; contains sesquiterpene lactones. Toxic if ingested. *See also* sesquiterpene lactones.

ascorbic acid Form of vitamin C that may be a skin irritant. It is difficult to formulate and stabilize, and oxidizes rapidly when exposed to air. Often combined with ascorbyl palmitate. *See also* ascorbyl palmitate.

ascorbyl palmitate A more stable, non-acidic form of vitamin C (salt of ascorbic acid). More effective than BHA or BHT in inhibiting rancidity of vegetable oils. Non-toxic. *See also* BHA; BHT.

Avena sativa *See* oatmeal.

avobenzone (butyl methoxydibenzoylmethane) Synthetic sunscreen ingredient commonly known as Parsol 1789. Protects against UVA rays; also prevents sun degradation of product. Should not be used in a formulation with PABA and PABA esters.

avocado oil Light-feeling, edible, emollient oil pressed from avocados and similar to other non-fragrant plant oils. Offers some UV protection and is high in vitamins A and E, as well as EFAs. No known toxicity.

awapuhi (also known as wild ginger) *See* ginger.

Azadirachta indica *See* neem extract or oil.

azelaic acid Dicarbonic acid made from a fatty acid in castor oil. Used as an acne treatment, as well as for skin discolorations, in place of hydroquinone. *See also* hydroquinone.

Azo colors The largest group of coal tar colors. *See also* coal tar colors.

azuki beans These legumes are used in ground form as abrasives in scrub products.

azulene From German chamomile, this extract is used primarily as a natural blue-to-green coloring agent in cosmetics; anti-inflammatory, anti-irritant, antioxidant. *See also* chamomile.

B

babassu oil An edible plant oil that is used as an emollient, lubricant, and moisturizer.

baking soda *See* sodium bicarbonate.

balm mint extract Extract from this fragrant plant was traditionally used in Palestine as a soothing medication. May cause skin irritation.

banana extract Used for antioxidant properties; also used for dry skin.

barberry (*Berberis vulgaris*) This plant contains the alkaloid berberine, which is known to have antibacterial and anti-inflammatory properties; can kill staphylococcus and streptococcus on external wounds and may help with eruptions of psoriasis. Used for gargle for mouth and throat irritations and to strengthen gums. May cause skin irritation.

barium Flammable and toxic Earth element.

barium sulfate This Earth mineral is used as a whitening agent but can be a skin irritant. Also used as a base for lake colors. *See also* lake colors.

barium sulfide Used in depilatories and to relax hair, this ingredient is considered a toxic skin irritant. Do not apply to broken skin. Fatal if swallowed.

bay leaf oil Antioxidant. May irritate skin.

bearberry extract (*Uva ursi*) Contains arbutin. (*See also* arbutin.) Bearberry is well known for contributing antibiotic activity in urinary tract.

beeswax *(cera alba)* Created by bees to build the honeycomb. Used as an emollient, softening agent, thickener, and emulsifier. Found in hair-removal products and various baby and beauty products. May cause pollen-allergic reactions. Look for organic beeswax, as some waxes could contain harmful pesticide or fungicide residues.

behenic acid This natural fatty acid is a mild solid alcohol used as an emulsifier, emollient, surfactant, and thickener. No known toxicity.

bentonite Colloidal clay used as an absorbent or thickening agent or to stabilize cosmetics. Used for acne treatments or to clean pores. Often found in facial masks. Can be drying for skin.

benzalkonium chloride Highly toxic antimicrobial agent used as a preservative in skincare products. Effective against staphylococcus. Avoid eye area.

benzene Carcinogen used in nail polish remover and as a solvent for oils, resins, and waxes. This highly absorbable chemical is flammable, poisonous, and irritating to mucous membranes and is known to cause photosensitivity. Toxic by inhalation; causes chronic damage to bone marrow.

benzocaine A topical anesthetic that can cause contact dermatitis.

benzoic acid Natural astringent, antioxidant, antifungal agent, and preservative that can be made from an organic acid found in berries, herbs, and roots. However, synthetic varieties are often used in cosmetics. Check with the manufacturer. Toxic if ingested; may cause allergic reactions.

benzoin extract Balsam resin that has some antioxidant, disinfecting, preservative, and fragrant properties; may also be a skin irritant. Found in benzoin gum.

benzophenones These chemicals are used in sunscreen, as well as to protect a product from UVB degradation. Toxic if ingested; allergic reactions include hives and photoallergic sun reactions.

benzoyl peroxide This chemical is a potent antibacterial, but it is highly irritating. Toxic by inhalation; can also be a skin allergen.

benzyl alcohol Made with essential oils from balsam, jasmine, ylang-ylang. Used as a solvent and antibacterial; useful for relief of insect bites. Can be irritating and corrosive to skin and mucous membranes.

berberine A potent antibacterial derived from various plants.

bergamot oil *(Citrus bergamia)* Cold-pressed or steam-distilled from the peels of the fruit of this tree. Used as antibacterial, astringent, and anti-perspirant; normalizes oil production; used as treatment for acne, dandruff, eczema, and oily skin; fragrance. May be photosensitizer; may cause contact dermatitis.

beta carotene Precursor to vitamin A that is converted in the body to the vitamin. This oil-soluble carotenoid is responsible for coloring red and orange vegetables. Derived from algae, vegetables, and palm fruit. In sufficient quantity, beta carotene will turn a formulation yellow. When used topically, it improves the effectiveness of sunscreens while providing antioxidant protection. Can also be synthetic.

Beta Hydroxy Acid (BHA) *See* also salicylic acid.

beta-glucan A polysaccharide that can be derived from yeast; antioxidant, anti-inflammatory, anti-irritant. May help stimulate collagen and elastin production in skin. Used for wound healing. Offers some UV protection.

Betula alba *See* birch bark extract.

BHA Butylated hydroxyanisole; a synthetic chemical used as an antioxidant. According to the National Toxicology Program, this chemical preservative is reasonably anticipated to be a carcinogen.

BHA (Beta Hydroxy Acid) *See* salicylic acid.

BHT Butylated hydroxytoluene; a synthetic antioxidant used to prevent oxidation of oils. Can cause allergic reactions and contact dermatitis; also has carcinogenic properties. No longer permitted for use as a food additive in England.

bilberry extract Mild antiseptic, astringent. May be of use in the treatment of varicose veins when taken internally.

bioflavonoids Components of fruits and vegetables (e.g., berries, gingko biloba, citrus fruits, and green tea) that are responsible for imparting color; antioxidant, beneficial against cancer. May help to stimulate collagen production.

biotin Water-soluble vitamin; part of the B complex group of vitamins. Necessary for the metabolism of amino acids, carbohydrates, and fats. Used in hair products to add body and shine. Non-toxic.

birch bark extract (extract of *Betula alba* bark) Traditional astringent with a high methyl salicylate content; antiseptic, anti-inflammatory, antimicrobial. Used in creams and shampoos.

bisabolol Can be extracted from chamomile or created synthetically. It is an anti-irritant; for wound healing.

bismuth Naturally occurring metallic element; found in the earth's crust. Used to impart a reddish tinge to eye shadows and lipstick. May contain impurities such as lead, iron, and copper. Flammable in powder form. Can cause allergic reactions when used on skin; may be associated with memory loss, confusion, and trembling.

bitter almond oil This essential oil has a mild scent and is used as a skin softener.

black alder *(Alnus glutinonsa)* An external wash for lice and scabies; also used as an astringent.

blackberry Potent antioxidant. Astringent. Also helps to constrict blood vessels and stop minor bleeding; used for wound healing.

black currant oil Natural fruit acid used in face masks and lotions for exfoliation. Excellent emollient and source of EFAs.

black elderberry Potent antioxidant.

black raspberry Potent antioxidant when applied topically.

bladderwrack extract *(Fucus vesiculous)* Seaweed extract rich in alginic acid. (*See also* alginic acid.) Essential oil is a tonic and stimulant; good for massage lotions, hair and scalp products. Also soothing in foam baths and gels. No known toxicity.

bluet extract *See* cornflower.

blueberry leaf tea Non-drying skin tonic.

blue cypress oil Essential oil with a woody fragrance; used as a natural disinfectant.

blue-green algae The earliest form of life on earth, this form of algae is a good source of antioxidant enzymes and minerals. Readily absorbed into skin. Used in hair products for protein content; conditions damaged hair.

blush A cheek colorant that can be either crème, liquid, or powder. May contain: alcohol, brilliant red lake, carnauba wax, carmine, cellulose, cetyl alcohol, coloring, glycerin, isopropyl palmitate, kaolin, lanolin, liquid tragacanth, mineral oil, mucilage, ozokerite, perfume, petrolatum, polyvinyl pyrrolidone, potassium hydroxide, propylene glycol, propyl paraben, sorbitol, talc, titanium dioxide, and/or zinc oxide.

borage seed oil *(Borago officinalis)* Contains gamma linolenic acid (GLA); may contain allantoin. Anti-irritant, anti-inflammatory; may repair cell membranes. Excellent topical treatment for dry skin and eczema.

borates Used primarily as pH adjusters or as antimicrobial agents. Highly toxic by ingestion and absorption; affect central nervous system, gastro-intestinal tract, kidneys, liver, and skin. Can be significant skin irritants.

borax Also known as sodium borate decahydrate, this mineral found in salt lakes and alkaline soils is composed of sodium, boron, oxygen, and water. It has properties of an insecticide, disinfectant, fungicide, herbicide, and preservative; often used with beeswax. Has bleaching properties, as it can convert water molecules to hydrogen peroxide; this also generates free radical damage in the skin. Toxic; significant skin irritant.

boric acid This mineral acid is used primarily as an antimicrobial and preservative in cosmetics; also pH adjuster. Toxic if ingested; irritant to skin; should not be used in baby products or on broken skin.

boron This compound occurs in nature. May cause skin irritation, and high-level exposure can harm stomach. Long-term effect is unknown. Lethal at one ounce for adults.

boron nitride A synthetic, inorganic powder used as an absorbent similar to talc.

Boswellia carterii *See* frankincense extract.

boysenberry Potent antioxidant.

Brassica campestris Polymer made from canola oil and chinawood; used as moisturizer and film-former to increase shine and water resistance.

bromelain This enzyme found in pineapple helps to break down the bonds that hold skin cells together, thereby promoting exfoliation; used for light skin peels. May cause irritation.

bronopol This formaldehyde-releasing preservative may also contain nitrosamines. Toxic; causes skin irritation. Used in face creams, mascara, bath oils. *See also* formaldehyde.

burdock root *(Articum lappa)* Anti-inflammatory, antioxidant, antiseptic, antibacterial, anti-fungal due to polyacetylenes. Used to smooth and neutralize hair and promote hair growth; also found in anti-itch products and products for treating oily skin, healing acne and eczema, and restore skin smoothness.

butcher's broom extract Astringent, anti-inflammatory, and diuretic. Used in anticellulite preparations and to treat sensitive skin.

butyl acetate Solvent used in nail polish and many other products. Toxic by inhalation; narcotic, depresses central nervous system.

butyl alcohol Used as a solvent, this chemical is known to cause skin and eye inflammation; may cause contact dermatitis. Toxic by inhalation.

butylene glycol Synthetic solvent. Often used in place of propylene glycol. *See also* propylene glycol.

Butyl ester of PVP/MA Copolymer Synthetic polymer used to cover hair and hold it in position.

butyl methoxydibenzoylmethane *See* avobenzone.

butylparaben *See* parabens.

Butyrospermum parkii *See* shea butter.

Buxus chinensis *See* jojoba oil.

C

C18-36 Acid Triglyceride Emollient, emulsifier, moisturizer, stabilizer, and thickener derived from plants. Provides rigidity in stick products.

cade wood oil Analgesic essential oil traditionally used in Europe as a scalp cleanser and toner; to clear up flakes and treat hair loss. Also used for eczema, wounds.

calaguala extract To condition skin and clean and tone scalp.

calamine Blend of zinc oxide and ferric oxide; used to reduce itching and rash. May contain substantial phenol; could lead to phenol poisoning with repeated use.

calcium ascorbate Non-acidic, stable form of vitamin C used as a food preservative. Could be plant-derived or synthetic.

calcium carbonate Chalk; mineral source. Used as white coloring, as abrasive in toothpaste, and absorbent in cosmetics. Also used as filler and to reduce acidity. No known toxicity.

calcium pantothenate *See* pantothenic acid.

calendula extract *(Calendula officinalis)* This extract from the common marigold is used as an antibacterial, antioxidant, anti-inflammatory, and antiseptic for rashes, burns, wounds, bruises, boils, and warts. Also used in sensitive-skin lotions, baby lotions, sun products, and face powders. The marigold also contains saponins and is sometimes used to provide natural yellow color.

Camellia sinensis *See* green tea.

camphor *(Cinnamomum camphora)* Aromatic substance from trees more than 50 years old found in China, Japan, Brazil, and Taiwan. Can be synthetic. Known for its pungent odor, this chemical is antiseptic, astringent, and anti-inflammatory. Used in after-shave; skin tonics. Can cause contact dermatitis.

Canadian willowherb extract Containing proanthocyanidins and salicylic acid, this extract has anti-inflammatory, anti-irritant, anti-itch, and antioxidant properties. Used for wound healing. (Proanthocyanidins are compounds involved in the production of the most vibrant colors found in fruits and flowers.)

candelilla wax Natural wax from candelilla plants; used as a thickening agent and emollient; gives lipsticks and stick products rigidity and gloss. Also a substitute for rubber; hardens other waxes. No known toxicity.

Cannabis sativa oil *See* hempseed oil.

canola oil Rapeseed oil; used as lubricant in beauty products.

caprylic/capric triglyceride Derived from coconut oil; used as moisturizer, emollient, solubilizer, lubricant, and thickener. Non-greasy.

capsaicin Component of dried, ripe fruit of capsicum, or African chili plant. Blocks pain and stimulates circulation. Also a topical irritant that can trigger allergic reactions; do not apply to broken skin. Often used to create heat in sore-muscle-and-joint preparations.

caramel Natural coloring agent created by concentrating sugar or corn syrup through the use of heat. Also found in soothing skin lotions.

carbomers Synthetic thickening agents used primarily to create gel-like formulations. Avoid products with high benzene levels; contact manufacturer for details.

carbon tetrachloride A type of chlorinated hydrocarbon. *See* chlorinated hydrocarbons.

cardamom Essential oil of a plant from the ginger family; used as fragrance in cosmetics. Can be a skin irritant and sensitizer due to its terpene content.

carmine Natural red color that comes from the dried bodies of Latin American female cochineal beetles; traditionally used for dyes and inks. Sometimes used to color lip gloss, lipsticks, and other cosmetics.

carnauba wax Vegetable wax from buds and leaves of the carnauba palm; used in cosmetics as thickening agent; used in lipsticks, mascara, deodorant. Can also be formed into spheres for use as an exfoliating agent in mechanical scrubs. Rarely causes allergic reactions.

carrageenan (also known as Irish moss) Used for hundreds of years in India, this seaweed gum and mucilage comes from red algae. Readily absorbs water; binding agent; natural thickener. Also suspends or stabilizes ingredients; emulsifier and emollient.

carrot oil This emollient plant essential oil is rich in vitamin A and beta carotene. Excellent for cell regeneration and production of sebum; found in sunscreen formulations Also used as a natural coloring agent. No known toxicity. *See also* beta carotene; vitamin A.

cassia oil Chinese cinnamon oil; contains cinnamic aldehyde. Used for flavoring, perfumes. *See also* cinnamon.

Castile soap Mild soap made from olive oil and sodium hydroxide (table salt); named for the Spanish region where it originated. May be drying, depending on skin type.

castor oil High-viscosity vegetable oil derived from the castor bean; used to suspend pigments; often used in lipstick. Contains linoleic, oleic, and stearic fatty acids; used in hair products and ointments. Soothing to skin; irritation not common.

cellulose gum Cellulose is part of the cell wall of plants, making this sugar-based ingredient the most abundant natural polymer. Used as setting agent in hair sprays, gels, mousse; also binder and thickener in cosmetic products. Absorbent.

centaury Strong antiseptic useful for cuts and scratches.

cera alba *See* beeswax.

cera microcristallina *See* petrolatum.

ceramides These lipids (fats) occur naturally in skin and are major components of the skin's structure. They are responsible for cell regulation and water retention. Cosmetic formulations could contain ceramides derived from plant or animal sources, to mimic our own lipids. Can also be synthetic.

ceresin Waxy ingredient created through purifying ozokerite; used interchangeably with beeswax and paraffin. Petroleum product. Used as a thickening agent or to increase rigidity in stick products. May cause allergic reactions

ceteareth-5 Derived from cetyl alcohol and ethylene oxide. *See* ethylene oxide.

ceteareth-20 Derived from polyethylene glycol ether and cetearyl alcohol. *See* polyethylene glycol.

cetearyl alcohol Mixture of fatty alcohols; used as an emollient, emulsifier, thickener, and carrying agent for other ingredients. Can be natural coconut fatty alcohol or synthetic.

cetyl alcohol This reduction of palmitic acid is used as an emollient, emulsifier, thickener, and carrying agent for other ingredients. Solid alcohol; can be natural coconut fatty alcohol, or synthetic. May cause allergic reaction; hives.

chamomile *(Matricaria chamomilla)* This herb contains azulene, giving it antioxidant, anti-irritant, anti-inflammatory, antibacterial, astringent, and soothing properties. Kills both *Candida albicans* and *staphylococcus* bacteria. Used to soften and hydrate dry skin; also a treatment for eczema and inflammatory skin conditions and burns. Used as fragrance and to accentuate natural highlight for blondes. May cause pollen allergic reactions. Contains sesquiterpene lactones. May cause contact dermatitis.

chapparal extract *(Larrea mexicana)* From the Dwarf evergreen chapparal tree; antibiotic, antiseptic, antibacterial, antiviral; may help inhibit cavities and gum disease. Previously used as preservative in lard and shortening, but since replaced. Potentially a liver toxin.

chaulmoogra oil This antimicrobial oil was once used around the world to treat leprosy. Used for infective skin disease. Possible skin irritant.

chicory extract *(Cichorium intybus)* Has antioxidant properties and may also have anti-inflammatory properties. Chicory plant is related to dandelion. Traditionally used as a narcotic.

China clay. *See* kaolin.

chitin This glucosamine polysaccharide is structurally similar to cellulose and is the main component of shells of crabs, beetles, and lobsters. Also found in some algae, fungi, and yeasts. *See also* chitosan.

chitosan Derived from chitin, this polysaccharide has antibacterial and anti-inflammatory properties that make it useful for wound healing. Also used as a film-former and to retain water; used in deodorant and sunscreen to improve water resistance. Absorbs heavy metals from water; dyeing assistant. *See also* chitin.

chlorella These inexpensive green algae contain all the essential amino acids. Also high in vitamin A and chlorophyll. Used as a skin hydrator.

chlorinated hydrocarbons Carcinogenic in animals and humans; accumulate in the tissues of humans and human fetuses.

chlorine This extremely strong oxidizing agent is used as a disinfectant. A military poison. Chlorine has been linked to skin irritation, eczema, asthma, and cancer.

cholesterol A natural steroid alcohol fat used in cosmetics as a lubricant, stabilizer, emulsifier, emollient, and water-binding agent. Used to keep skin more supple. Found in crèmes, lotions, and ointments. Sourced from animal fats, oils, and egg yolk.

chrysanthemum *(Chrysanthemum sinense)* This natural astringent and skin neutralizer also has anti-inflammatory properties.

cinnamon With antimicrobial and antiseptic properties, this spice can kill bacteria, fungi, and viruses. Also used as a natural colorant, fragrance, and flavoring. Can be a skin irritant; can cause mouth inflammation when used in toothpaste.

citric acid Obtained from citrus plants or through fermentation of crude sugars or molasses by yeasts; found in living cells. Mainly used to adjust the pH of products; also an astringent, detergent builder, dispersing agent, foam inhibitor, preservative, and sequestering agent.

Citrus medica limonium *See* lemon.

clary oil Cultivated in England and Europe and used as fixative for perfumes. Can be a skin irritant or sensitizer.

clay *See* bentonite; kaolin.

clematis extract *(Clematis vitalba)* This extract from the leaves of the biting clematis was traditionally used for its anti-inflammatory properties. May also have anti-fungal benefits. Possible skin sensitizer.

clove oil This spicy oil was traditionally used for the health of teeth and gums. It is an oral disinfectant and anesthetic that provides temporary relief of toothache pain. Used in perfumes. Skin irritant; repeated use may cause inflammation.

coal tar This semi-solid tar obtained from bituminous coal contains many components known to be carcinogenic, including benzene, creosol, and phenol. Used to make colors for cosmetics, including hair dyes. Frequent source of skin irritation.

coal tar colors Although now made from petrochemicals, these synthetic colors were initially made from coal tar. Individual batches of these colors must be sent to the FDA for testing. Historically, many of these colors have proven to be carcinogenic and some have subsequently been banned.

cocamide DEA and MEA Amides are used to increase foam or to thicken or solubilize other ingredients. They can combine with free diethanolamine (DEA) to form cancer-causing nitrosamines—even when found in health products store brands that are labeled "derived from coconut." *See also* alkyloamides; DEA (diethanolamine).

cocamidopropyl betaine Surfactant. Often combined with other surfactants such as sodium laurel sulfate; may combine with other ingredients to form cancer-causing nitrosamines.

cochineal A red dye derived from the dried bodies of Latin American female cochineal beetles. *See also* carmine.

cocoa butter Also known as theobroma oil, this non-fragrant plant oil is extracted from roasted cocoa beans and used as an emollient. As an occlusive moisturizer, it melts at body temperature. Cocoa butter is a rich emollient, used in crèmes, lipsticks, and moisturizers. May clog pores. *See also* theobroma oil.

coconut oil *(Cocos nuciferal)* This plant-kernel oil is solid at room temperature and is a highly saturated fat. It lathers easily and has de-greasing properties; usually blended with other fats. Although it resists oxidative rancidity, it is vulnerable to micro-organisms and molds. Emollient, moisturizer, base for many products. May cause allergic reactions.

collagen A major factor in the structure of skin; weakens with age and sun exposure. Collagen from plants and animals is used in cosmetics as a water-binding agent; moisturizing. Can cause allergic reactions. There is as yet no evidence that topical application of collagen improves skin structure.

colloid A suspension; containing particles too small to settle.

coloring Also listed as colorant, color. Refers to pigment; could be synthetic or natural.

comfrey extract *(Symphytum officinale)* Traditionally used for bruises, this extract contains allantoin to provide skin protection and promote the growth of new cells. Used as an anti-inflammatory, astringent, demulcent, and emollient, and to soothe skin. Contains pyrrolizidine alkaloids, which cause liver damage when ingested in large amounts. Use as topical treatment only. *See also* allantoin.

Commiphora myrrha extract *See* myrrh.

coneflower *See* echinacea.

Corallina officinalis extract *See* algae.

coriander The volatile oil of this herb is used as a fragrance. It is also used externally for rheumatic joints and muscles. Can cause skin allergic reactions.

corn glycerides Used as an emollient and thickening agent in cosmetics.

corn oil This fatty oil is used as an emollient and thickener; can promote acne and allergic reactions.

cornflower *(Centaurea cyanus)* (also known as blue bottle) Astringent, anti-flammatory, moisturizing, soothing. Used for wound healing; also eye wash, eye drops, eye compresses. Natural blue colorant. May cause photosensitivity.

cornmint (also known as wild mint) Can cause skin irritation.

cornsilk Used in face powders.

cornstarch This natural starch from corn is absorbent and often appears in non-talcum baby powders. Also used as a thickening agent or to coat containers to prevent sticking of product. Can cause skin irritation and trigger asthma.

corticosteroids *See* hydrocortisone.

cortisone *See* hydrocortisone.

costus root The dried root of this herb is used as a fixative in perfumes. No known toxicity; may inhibit immune response.

cottonseed oil High in linoleic acid (LA), palmitic acid, and oleic fatty acids, this oil is used as an emollient.

cucumber extract *(Cucumis sativus)* Traditionally used as an astringent for oily skin, this extract is soothing, cooling, and anti-inflammatory. Used as a skin softener, to treat burns and skin problems, and to promote healthy skin. Found in facial creams, lotions, and cleansers.

cyclamen aldehyde (methyl-*p*-isopropylphenylpropyl aldehyde) Synthetic fragrant constituent that can be a skin irritant.

cyclohexasiloxane *See* silicone.

cyclomethicone *See* silicone.

cysteine This sulfur-rich amino acid is beneficial to skin and hair. Antioxidant.

D

D&C A coloring agent considered by the FDA to be safe for use in drugs and cosmetics that can be ingested or have direct contact with mucous membranes. Not approved for food. Usually synthetic coal tar colors. *See also* coal tar; coal tar colors.

d-alpha-tocopherol Natural form of the antioxidant vitamin E.

DEA (diethanolamine) Used to alkalize formulas. DEA is often a suffix or prefix attached to another ingredient, such as DEA methoxycinnamate. DEA can react with other ingredients to form cancer-causing nitrosamines.

DEA methoxycinnamate Often used in sunscreen preparations, this ingredient ironically can trigger formation of cancer-causing nitrosamines when exposed to sunlight.

Dead Sea minerals Studies show that Dead Sea minerals may be useful in treating psoriasis.

deionized/demineralized water All water used in cosmetics is filtered to remove calcium, magnesium, nitrates, and heavy metals.

diazolidinyl urea This formaldehyde-releasing preservative is a cumulative skin irritant that can cause contact dermatitis. *See also* formaldehyde.

dibutyl phthalate Used as a solvent, fixative, and anti-foaming agent, and in the creation of synthetic fragrance, this commonly used colorless, oily ester is also employed as a plasticizer. Found in insect repellants, perfumes, and nail polish. The vapor is known to irritate eyes. As a xenoestrogen, this chemical caused testicular atrophy in animals in some studies.

diethanolamine *See* DEA.

diethylene glycol Derived from ethylene oxide, this synthetic glycerin is used as a surfactant and humectant. Also used in anti-freeze. Possibly toxic if absorbed into skin; can be toxic if ingested. *See also* ethylene oxide.

diethyl phthalate (DEP) Used to improve feel of a product, DEP is toxic by ingestion and inhalation; also a strong irritant to mucous membranes and eyes. Can cause depression of central nervous system when absorbed into skin. Xenoestrogenic.

Digenea simplex extract *See* algae.

dimethylaminoethanol (DMAE) Known as 2-dimethyl-amino-ethanol, this naturally occurring chemical stimulates production of the neurotransmitter acetylcholine. This means that it helps us with brain function. Recent studies are trying to determine its effect on aging skin.

dimethyl phthalate Xenoestrogenic preservative also known to irritate eyes and mucous membranes.

dimethyl sulfate According to the National Toxicology Program, this chemical is reasonably anticipated to be a human carcinogen. Used in the manufacture of perfumes and in the creation of methyl derivatives of amines, phenols, and thiols.

dimethyl sulfoxide (DMSO) Because this ingredient easily penetrates skin and other tissues, its use must comply with strict FDA regulations. Consider the toxicity of other ingredients found in a formulation that also includes this ingredient, as you can be assured that the product will be well absorbed.

dioxin One of the more than 70 chlorinated dioxins that are carcinogenic, teratogenic, and mutagenic. Dioxin is considered by some scientists to be the most toxic substance known to humans, possibly equal to plutonium. It is formulated as a byproduct of pulp-and-paper bleaching. Use only unbleached paper products on your body.

disodium EDTA *See* EDTA.

Di (2-ethylhexyl) phthalate (DEHP) This plasticizer is reasonably anticipated to be a human carcinogen. Also xenoestrogenic.

dl-alpha-tocopherol (or alpha-tocopherol) Synthetic version of vitamin E used in vitamin supplements and cosmetic products. Often used as a preservative.

DMDM hydantoin (1,3-Dimethylolo-5-5-dimethylhydantoin) This formaldehyde-releasing preservative is also known to cause dermatitis. *See also* formaldehyde.

dogwood Used as an anti-inflammatory and antioxidant.

dulcamara extract (also known as extract of bittersweet nightshade) Used by herbalists as a treatment for skin cancer. Anti-inflammatory; preservative.

dulse *See* algae.

Durvillaea antarctica extract *See* algae.

E

earth smoke This traditional Chinese herbal is used as a tonic and purifier; also mild bleaching and skin brightening.

earth wax General name for natural ceresin, montan, and ozocerite waxes. *See also* ceresin; ozocerite (also spelled ozokerite.)

echinacea (coneflower) This natural antibiotic contains antimicrobial echinacosides; also antibacterial, anti-fungal, antiviral. Echinacein neutralizes a germ's ability to dissolve tissue; also mends skin. Used in crèmes and lotions for wound healing, acne, eczema, and other skin problems; texturizer, firming agent.

EDTA (ethylene diamine tetra acetic acid) Synthetic chelating agent made through the addition of sodium cyanide and formaldehyde to ethylene diamine; also a preservative. Can combine with nitrogen compounds to form carcinogenic nitrosamines. *See also* formaldehyde and ethylene diamine.

elastin This major dermal protein gives skin its elasticity; weakens with age and sun exposure. Elastin attracts and retains moisture. In cosmetics, it is animal-derived. Unfortunately, any potential benefits of topical elastin might be destroyed by the chemical preservatives used in the formulation.

elderberry Potent antioxidant; skin softener. Also stimulates circulation.

elecampane Antiseptic, astringent, diuretic, and tonic; natural blue dye extracted from root. May irritate skin and trigger allergic reactions.

emollient An agent that helps keep skin soft and supple; emollients remain on the surface of the skin or within the topmost layers.

emu oil Oil from a large, flightless bird native to Australia. Anti-inflammatory, emollient; skin-penetrating properties. Not as likely to clog pores as mineral oil. *See also* mineral oil.

emulsifier You can't mix oil and water unless you are creating an emulsion. The emulsifier is the compound that allows oil and water to mix on a molecular level.

emulsion A stable blend of oil and water, including all crèmes and lotions.

Epsom salts *See* magnesium sulfate.

erythritol Natural sugar found in plants and animals; has water-binding properties.

essential fatty acids (EFAs) Fatty acids required for optimal health that must be obtained from the diet because the body cannot manufacture them. Also known as vitamin F. EFAs have also been found to be beneficial when used topically.

essential oil Volatile plant oil that contains the fragrance or flavor of the plant. Synthetic essential oils are increasingly used.

Ester-C Containing mainly calcium ascorbate, this form of vitamin C has been trademarked.

ethanol *See* ethyl alcohol.

ethanolamines Created through a reaction of ethylene oxide and ammonia. Can combine with other ingredients to form cancer-causing nitrosamines. *See also* ethylene oxide; ammonia.

ethyl acetate Volatile solvent made from acetic acid and ethyl alcohol in the presence of sulfuric acid. Used in nail polish and nail-polish removers. May cause irritation; toxic to skin through absorption. *See also* acetic acid; ethyl alcohol.

ethyl alcohol (also known as ethanol) Because this chemical removes protective lipids from the skin's surface, it can dehydrate or irritate skin; should not be used in products that remain on the skin.

ethylene A highly flammable, asphyxiant gas used to accelerate the ripening of fruits. Also used in the production of other chemicals.

ethylene diamine This ingredient is a strong irritant to skin and eyes. It is also toxic by inhalation and absorption.

ethylene glycol This chemical is toxic by ingestion and inhalation and demonstrates some possible toxic effects through skin absorption; causes contact dermatitis and contact eczema. Known to affect body chemistry by increasing acidity, which leads to metabolic problems. Some byproducts of this chemical have proven to cause reproductive and developmental damage when taken orally.

ethylene oxide Used as a surfactant and in the formation of other chemicals, including ethylene glycol and ethanolamines. Known to be a human carcinogen; irritant to skin and eyes. Highly flammable.

ethylparaben High risk of skin irritation and allergic reactions from this paraben. *See also* parabens.

eucalyptus extract *(Eucalpytus globulus)* This essential oil has antibacterial, anti-fungal, antiseptic, and antiviral properties; used to prevent the infection of burns, skin ulcers, and wounds. Used as fragrance in soaps, crèmes, lotions, and perfumes. May irritate broken skin; may cause allergic reactions.

evening primrose oil *(Oen othera biennis)* High in gamma linolenic acid (GLA). Used to repair the moisture barrier of skin; astringent, anti-inflammatory, emollient. Useful for inflammatory skin conditions such as rashes and eczema. Edible and safe for babies. Found in crèmes for dry skin and shampoos for dry hair.

eyebright *(Euphrasy)* Used medicinally since the 1300s, eyebright has traditionally been used as anti-inflammatory and to reduce redness and irritation. Has also been used as an eyewash.

eyeliner Liquid or pencil used to outline eyes. May contain: an alkylanolamine, antioxidants, fatty alcohol, cellulose ether, methylparaben, perfumes, polyvinyl pyrrolidone, titanium dioxide, etc.

eye shadow Crème or powder used to add color to the eye area. Can contain aluminum, beeswax, calcium carbonate, ceresin, lanolin, mineral oil, petrolatum, propyl paraben, talc, titanium dioxide, and/or other ingredients.

F

farnesol A molecule found in nature in essential oils of cassia, neroli, rose, and other plants. Used in perfumery.

fatty acid A natural component of skin that helps keep the cells strong and hydrated. Some fatty acids are essential to the diet, meaning that we need to eat them in order to be healthy because our bodies do not produce them. Fatty acids are used as thickening agents, soaps and detergents, and emollients. No known toxicity.

fatty alcohols Made from fatty acids and used as emollients and thickening agents; found in hair conditioners and crèmes. Cetyl and stearyl alcohol are fatty alcohols that form an occlusive, thereby creating a moisture barrier. *See also* fatty acid.

FD&C A type of coloring agent approved by the FDA as suitable for coloring food, drugs, and cosmetics.

fennel extract Derived from the fennel plant, this extract has anti-irritant, anti- inflammatory, astringent, moisturizing, tightening, cleansing, and detoxifying properties. The essential oil from the fennel plant is rich in EFAs. Also used for fragrance. May be a skin irritant; may cause allergic reactions.

feverfew extract This extract was traditionally used for its cooling and analgesic properties. Also anti-inflammatory; relieves pain and swelling of insect bites and skin irritations. May cause allergic reactions.

fibronectin A protein found in the skin which is similar to collagen and elastin; weakens with age and sun exposure. Although topical application will not rebuild your fibronectin, it is used in cosmetics as a skin conditioner and defense mechanism. Animal sourced.

film-forming agent Any ingredient that is applied wet but dries to a continuous film, such as in nail polish and hair products.

figwort *(Scrophularia nodosa)* This perennial plant is used to treat bruises, eczema, rashes, scabies, skin tumors, and wounds; also used to remove freckles.

fir needle oil This fragrant essential oil created through the steam distillation of twigs and needles of coniferous trees is antibacterial, antimicrobial, and soothing. Used for respiratory weakness, fragrance, and flavoring. Can cause skin irritation.

formaldehyde A colorless gas created through the oxidation of methyl alcohol; used as an inexpensive preservative and disinfectant in cosmetics. Also found in food. Can be created within the body as other chemicals are metabolized. Causes DNA damage, produces mutagenic and carcinogenic effects; highly sensitizing and known to cause dermatitis; toxic by inhalation; extremely irritating to mucous membranes. Can be fatal if swallowed.

foundation Used for coverage and to even out skin tone. Can be cake, crème, or liquid and may contain: beeswax, borax, cetyl alcohol, glycerin, gums, iron oxides, isopropyl myristate, kaolin, lanolin, mucilage, quince seed, silicone, sorbitol, spermaceti, stearic acid, propylene glycol, talc, triethanolamine (TEA), titanium dioxide, water, zinc, and/or other ingredients not listed here.

fragrance One of either volatile and/or fragrant plant oils or synthetically derived oils (or a blend of these) that imparts aroma to products; sometimes as many as 200 ingredients are used in a single fragrance. Fragrances are often skin irritants; frequently contain phthalates, which are known xenoestrogens. *See also* phthalates.

frankincense extract (extract of *Boswellia carterii*) Fragrant essential oil used as anti-wrinkle, astringent, and anti-inflammatory. Promotes new cell growth and soothes rough skin. Fragrance used in cosmetic products. Can be a skin irritant.

fructose Often called fruit sugar; the sweetest of all common sugars. Found in fruits and honey. Used as a water-binding agent and preservative.

fuller's earth Colloidal aluminum silicate, a naturally occurring mineral substance that is similar to kaolin clay. Used as absorbent in conditioning masks; also thickening agent.

fumaric acid This trans-isomer of maleic acid is used as a pH adjuster in cosmetics.

G

gardenia oil Essential oil of tropical gardenia flowers; used for fragrance and in aromatherapy. No known toxicity.

gelatin Edible protein from plants or animals used in cosmetics as a thickening agent. Strongly hydrophilic, absorbing up to 10 times its weight in water. Used for hair and skin conditioning. No known toxicity.

gentian violet extract Antibacterial properties; soothing to skin.

geranium oil Fragrant essential oil with antimicrobial, antibacterial, anti-inflammatory, anti-fungal, antiseptic, and astringent properties; excellent for oily skin, acne, and dermatitis. Promotes new cell growth. Fragrance in soaps and crèmes. May irritate skin.

ginger (also known as Hawaiian ginger, white ginger) This plant was traditionally used in China to treat baldness. Astringent, anti-irritant, and hair lubricant. Used as fragrance in cosmetics, male products, and bath oils. May cause skin irritation.

Gingko biloba This sacred Chinese herb is known for its properties as an antioxidant and vasodilator. (A vasodilator relaxes smooth muscles in the blood vessel wall, causing the blood vessels to widen, resulting in a drop in blood pressure.) Used to treat cellulite and varicose veins. Flavonoids may also help in the production of collagen and elastin. Used in perfumes, insecticides. No known toxicity.

ginseng Traditionally used to increase cell proliferation and prolongs the lifespan of cells. Used as demulcent in cosmetics. Hair tonic and stimulant; excellent in shampoos. No known toxicity.

glycereth Synthetic form of glycerin created with polyethylene glycol. See also polyethylene glycol.

glycerin Also called glycerol and created as a byproduct of soap manufacture. Naturally derived from vegetable oils for use in cosmetics, glycerol is present in all natural fats. It can be synthetically created by the hydrolysis of fats and the fermentation of sugars; also manufactured using propylene glycol and chlorine or through the use of propylene oxide. Check with manufacturer for source (natural or synthetic). See also propylene glycol; chlorine; propylene oxide.

glyceryl ester A group of chemicals that includes fats and oils. Used as emollients, lubricants, and thickening agents. Can cause contact dermatitis.

glycogen Liver starch that is converted into protein; can be derived from oyster shells. Water-binding properties for skin and conditioning for hair.

glycolic acid Component of sugarcane juice that can help to control the pH of a product. Used as an exfoliant. May irritate skin and cause photosensitivity.

glycolipid A crucial part of cell membranes that forms a barrier to keep water in place.

glycyrrhetic acid (also known as glycyrrhizin) The active component of the licorice root. Has anti-inflammatory properties. See also licorice extract.

goa This herb has astringent properties. Helps with acne, eczema, and other skin conditions. Calms itching, irritated skin.

goldenseal (Hydrastis canadensis) Traditionally used by Native Americans to treat sore eyes, this plant has antibacterial, antiviral, antiseptic, and antibiotic properties; contains berberine. Used for skin diseases, sores, ringworm, and dandruff. Can be a skin irritant. See also berberine.

gotu kola Herb used as a homeopathic remedy for psoriasis and other skin conditions. Anti-inflammatory; treatment for acne, skin soother, burn healing, for infection and dermatitis.

grapefruit seed extract Anti-inflammatory, antioxidant, astringent, bactericide, preservative. Fragrance in lotions, perfumes, and soaps. Non-toxic.

grapeseed extract Potent antioxidant, particularly for diminishing the damaging effect of the sun and reducing free radical damage.

grapeseed oil Antioxidant, emollient oil containing linoleic acid (LA). No known toxicity.

green tea *(Camellia sinensis)* Used as antioxidant, anti-inflammatory, astringent. Also has photoprotective abilities and is beneficial in a sunscreen formulation. Found in skin-care products, lotions, shampoos, and conditioners.

guanine Pearlizing agent from fish scales; used in powders.

guar gum *(Cyanmopsis tetragonoloba)* The ground seed of a plant found in India and used as a thickening agent and stabilizer; has a greater thickening ability than does starch.

gum Derived from acacia, guar, guaiac, karaya, locust bean, tragacanth, and other plants and trees. Obtained when bark is injured. Used for thickening and binding agents, as film-forming agents and for viscosity. Natural gums are hydrophilic. No known toxicity; may cause allergic reactions. *See also* hydrophilic; film-forming agent.

H

hazelnut oil Oil extracted from the hazelnut; used as an emollient.

hematite Mineral used to color face powders, make-up, and rouge throughout the ages. Hematite mining has been linked to lung cancer. www.ehp.niehs.nih.gov.

hempseed oil *(Cannabis sativa)* Not to be confused with marijuana, a plant of the same genus. Hemp contains almost none of the active ingredient (THC) found in marijuana. Emollient; excellent in lipsticks.

henna *(Hawsonia alba)* Coloring agent found only in the plant's leaves; anti-fungal, anti-bacterial. Traditionally used as a dye for hair, nails, fabric, and skin; works best at bringing out reds. Used in hair-care products; may cause allergic reaction.

hexylene glycol Widely used synthetic solvent. Toxic by ingestion and inhalation; irritant to eyes, skin, and mucous membranes.

honey Astringent, antiseptic, antibacterial, antimicrobial, emollient, and humectant. Helpful for oily skin and large pores. Used as thickening agent for crèmes, lotions, and masks. May cause pollen allergic reaction.

honeysuckle extract. Fragrant plant used in perfumes. May be a skin irritant. No known toxicity.

hops *(Humulus lupulus)* From the flowers of the plant; used for skin softening; also antimicrobial.

horse chestnut extract *(Aesculus hippocastanum)* Traditionally used to help stop wound bleeding and for circulatory and vein problems. Antioxidant, astringent, anti-inflammatory. Source of silica. Used for tonics and sensitive-skin lotions.

horsetail extract Traditionally used to help stop wound bleeding and for circulatory and vein problems. Modern herbalists use it to treat varicose veins. Also used for dandruff, eczema, to reduce swollen eyelids, and for wound healing. High in silica. No known toxicity.

humectant Attracts and holds water. Humectants are also used to prevent moisture loss from the product itself.

hyaluronic acid Natural skin component that exists in the spaces between the cells. An excellent water-binding agent that helps maintain smooth, elastic skin. Used in eye surgery to help keep eye moist. No known toxicity.

hydrocortisone (also known as ascortisone and corticosteroids) Natural adrenal hormone that can also be created synthetically. While a potent anti-inflammatory, repeated use can damage collagen, and this leads to fragile skin. Calcium loss and weakened immunity also result from prolonged use. Do not apply near eyes or mucous membranes. Do not use if you are experiencing a systemic fungal infection like *Candida albicans*.

hydrogen peroxide A powerful oxidizing agent made from barium peroxide and diluted phosphoric acid, hydrogen peroxide generates a tremendous amount of free radical damage, leading to impaired healing processes and cellular damage. Used as a permanent-wave neutralizer and bleaching agent. Concentrated solution is highly irritating and toxic to skin.

hydrophilic Any compound that has a strong tendency to bind or absorb water, which results in swelling and the formation of reversible gels. Examples include algin, gums, and pectin. The word literally means "water-loving."

hydroquinone Used as a skin bleach, it can lead to increased sun sensitivity over the long term. Can be fatally toxic by ingestion; toxic by inhalation. Must be used only with rinse-off products; may cause irritation and allergic reaction.

hyssop *(Hyssop officinalis)* Traditionally used for the pain of bruises, this fragrant plant extract has antibacterial, anti-inflammatory, and astringent properties. Used as a wash for burns, skin irritations, and infections. The essential oil helps to treat eczema, inflammation, and wounds. Fragrance. No known toxicity; may irritate skin.

I

imidazolidinyl urea This water-soluble, formaldehyde-releasing preservative ranks as the second-most-common cause of contact dermatitis. *See also* formaldehyde.

indigo *(Indigofera tinctoria)* Ancient dark blue natural dye from an herb native to Bengal, Guatemala, and Java. Not known to cause skin reaction, but prolonged use can dry out hair.

inorganic colors Colors from inorganic non-petroleum sources, including iron oxides, bronze powder, titanium dioxide, and zinc oxide.

iodine Naturally found in Earth's crust. Used as antiseptic and germicide in cosmetics.

Irish moss *See* carrageenan.

iron oxides Natural or synthetic oxides of iron, forming various shades used to color cosmetics.

isopropyl alcohol Synthetic alcohol made from propylene glycol with sulfuric acid. Toxic by inhalation; fatally toxic if ingested. *See also* propylene glycol.

isopropyl myristate This partially synthetic chemical causes blackheads, and allergic reactions are common. May increase absorption of carcinogenic NDELA by up to 230 times. *See also* NDELA.

isopropyl palmitate Double-distilled from coconut oil and used as a thickening agent and emollient. Can clog pores and promote acne.

J

jasmine oil Traditionally used for skin problems, this fragrant oil is anti-inflammatory and antibacterial. Soothing to skin and scalp. Fragrance used in perfumes. May cause allergic reactions, including skin irritation. Can also be synthetic.

jewelweed Anti-fungal properties; used to reduce inflammation.

jojoba oil *(Buxux chinensis)* Non-fragrant emollient oil from the seeds of the desert shrub. Resists rancidity better than vegetable oils, making it an ideal lubricant and non-comedogenic moisturizer. (A comedogenic substance is likely to promote acne or blackheads.) Used for dandruff prevention, damaged hair, and dry skin. May cause allergic reactions.

jojoba wax Semi-solid portion of jojoba oil used for lipsticks, lip balms, and occlusive moisturizers. *See also* jojoba oil.

juniper berry Traditionally used as an antiseptic, this berry also has anti-inflammatory and detoxifying properties for skin; high in vitamin C. The essential oil is used as a toner and acne treatment, as well as for its fragrance; also used for eczema, psoriasis, dermatitis. Ethanol content may cause skin irritation with repeated use.

K

kaolin Natural silicate of aluminum found in Mount Kaolin, China. Used for astringent and absorbent properties in facial masks; sometimes as a thickener or drying agent. Used in face powders, blush, and baby powders. No known toxicity for skin.

kava-kava extract *(Piper methysticum)* This extract has analgesic, antiseptic, and anti-inflammatory properties when applied topically; may cause skin irritation.

kelpadelie extract *See* algae.

kelp extract Rich in iodine, this extract remineralizes, stimulates circulation, and moisturizes. Used in anti-cellulite formulations, soothing bath products, crèmes, and gels. No known toxicity.

kiwi fruit extract Antioxidant, tonic, flavoring, and emollient; may cause skin irritation.

kojic acid A byproduct of manufacturing Japanese sake, this acid is an antibiotic and antioxidant; used as a bleaching agent to reduce pigment. Can be synthetic. Unstable in formulation; may turn brown and lose effectiveness upon exposure to air.

kola nut Anti-irritant used to reduce the probability of a formulation causing irritation. Also contains caffeine. Contains primary amines, which can combine with other ingredients to form carcinogenic nitrosamines. May cause irritation.

kukui nut oil Traditionally used for thousands of years in Hawaii to treat acne, dry skin, and psoriasis, this non-volatile nut oil is high in linoleic acid (LA) and alpha linolenic acid (ALA); excellent natural emollient and moisturizer. Often blended with other oils.

L

Labdanum oil (also known as rockrose oil) Results from the steam distillation of gums from various rockrose shrubs. Used as an anti-fungal, antibacterial, and fragrance. This fragrant resin hardens to create a solid film; used as fixative.

lactic acid An Alpha Hydroxy Acid (AHA) obtained from milk, beans, and sauerkraut; may also be produced synthetically. Exfoliates surface cells by dissolving the material that binds cells together. May irritate mucous membranes and skin.

lake colors Water-soluble colors created by precipitating dye into an absorbent material.

Laminaria digitata A form of algae. *See* algae.

lanolin (also known as wool fat or wool wax) Bears closer resemblance to human sebum than does any other natural raw material. Results from purification of a grease called degras that is obtained by solvent treatment of wool. May contain chlorfenvinphos, a toxin that affects the nervous system; may also contain insecticides used on livestock. Common sensitizer; may cause acne, skin reactions.

lanolin alcohol An emollient derived from lanolin. *See also* lanolin.

L-ascorbic acid A common form of vitamin C; antioxidant, anti-inflammatory. Stable only in a formulation with a low pH; may cause skin irritation.

lauramide DEA (or MEA) Used as surfactants or foam builders, these skin-irritating chemicals can combine with nitrates to form cancer-causing nitrosamines.

lavender extract and oil Traditionally used to disinfect wounds and acne; antiseptic, analgesic, antibacterial, anti-fungal, anti-inflammatory, and fragrance. Used for acne, eczema, oily skin, and sunburn and to promote new cell growth; also used as insect repellant and to prevent hair loss. May cause skin irritation and photosensitivity.

lead This poison is cumulative and overdose causes serious toxic effects, including risk of coma and death.

lecithin Naturally occurring mixture of compounds found in egg yolks, corn, soybeans, and the membranes of plant and animal cells. Antioxidant, emollient, emulsifier, moisturizer, water-binding agent; used to create liposomes. Also used as surfactant. Non-toxic.

lemon *(Citrus medica limonium)* From the fruit; antibacterial. May cause skin irritation and trigger allergic reactions.

lemon extract From the fruit; astringent, antiseptic. Often used for enlarged pores and oily skin.

lemongrass extract Antibacterial; may cause skin irritation.

lemongrass oil From distillation of the grass; anti-fungal, astringent, fragrance. Citronella content makes it a good insect repellant.

lemon oil From peel of lemon; antioxidant, antibacterial, astringent, anti-inflammatory. Used as skin freshener and to revitalize skin; promotes new cell growth. Also used to treat dandruff and as fragrance. May cause skin irritation, especially on broken skin; may cause allergic reactions.

lettuce extract Antioxidant, anti-inflammatory, and soothing.

licorice extract Traditionally used to control oil production of the scalp. Active component is glycyrrhizin; anti-irritant, anti-inflammatory. Prevents wound infections; no known skin toxicity. *See also* glycyrrhetic acid.

lime (oil or extract) From the fruit. Astringent, antioxidant; high vitamin C content. May cause skin irritation and photosensitivity.

linden extract Extract of flowers of the lime tree; emollient and soothing for skin.

linseed oil High in linoleic acid (LA). May clog pores.

liposome Microscopic cell-like structures made of fat that work as delivery agents to carry other ingredients directly to the cell level. They are non-toxic, but because of their efficiency, it is important that whatever they are delivering is also non-toxic.

lipstick Used to color lips; available in tube, liquid, or pot. May contain: bismuth compound, beeswax, candelilla wax, carnauba wax, castor oil, cocoa butter, color, guanine, hydrogenated vegetable oils, lanolin, lecithin, mineral oil, paraffin wax, petrolatum, polyethylene glycol, olive oil, ozokerite, and sesame oil, etc.

locust bean gum Anti-irritant, film-former, thickener; protects skin. No known toxicity for skin. *See also* gum.

Luffa cylindrica Exfoliant; used in body scrubs. Do not use near eye area. When the fruit from the luffa plant is dried, it is used as an abrasive sponge. Be sure to thoroughly clean and dry the sponge after use, as skin flakes left on sponge would be excellent fodder for bacteria.

lye (also known as sodium hydroxide and potassium hydroxide) This highly alkaline ingredient is used in small amounts to regulate the pH of a cosmetic product. In higher concentrations, it is a significant skin irritant. It is also a cleansing agent in some cleansers and is used in drain cleaners. Irritant to eyes, skin, mucous membranes; can cause blindness. *See also* sodium hydroxide; potassium hydroxide.

M

macadamia nut oil From the nut of a small evergreen tree; emollient. Excellent penetration of top layers of skin; may be too heavy for use on the face. Contains magnesium (mineral) and thiamine (vitamin).

Macrocystis pyrifera A form of algae. *See* algae.

magnesium Earth mineral that has strong absorbent properties and some disinfecting properties. Along with calcium, magnesium is essential for the maintenance of our bones.

magnesium aluminum silicate (also known as smectite clay) White solid used as thickening agent and powder in cosmetics; anti-caking agent, filler, stabilizer. Known to have caused kidney damage in dogs who ate it. Contains aluminum. *See also* aluminum.

magnesium ascorbyl phosphate This ingredient includes magnesium plus ascorbic acid as a stable form of vitamin C; antioxidant. Also whitens skin by inhibiting melanin production; allows skin penetration of ascorbic acid through natural phosphatase enzymes.

magnesium sulfate Better known as Epsom salts; mined in an extreme level of purity. Soothes aches and pains; detoxifies in bath. No known toxicity when used externally.

malic acid An organic acid found in herbs, apples, and other fruits; also made synthetically. Used as antioxidant and exfoliant.

mallow *(Althea officinalis)* (also known as marshmallow) Traditionally used for bruises, burns, inflammation, and wounds and as a wash for dry eyes; anti-inflammatory, emollient, soothing. Used for oily skin, acne, and as a thickening agent.

mango butter Butter of mango fruit; excellent moisturizer.

manuka oil Derived from the New Zealand tea tree and similar to tea tree oil. Analgesic, anti-fungal, antibacterial. *See also* tea tree oil.

marigold *See* calendula extract.

mascara Cosmetic used to coat eyelashes. May contain: beeswax, carbon black, carmine, carnauba wax, cetyl alcohol, chromium oxide, gum, insoluble pigments, iron oxides, isopropyl myristate, lanolin, mineral oil, paraffin wax, propylene glycol, spermaceti and triethanolamine stearate, nylon, and rayon, among other ingredients.

MEA (monothanolamine or monoethanolamide) Used as humectant and emulsifier. Can combine with other ingredients to form carcinogenic nitrosamines. *See also* ethanolamines.

Melaleuca alternifolia *See* tea tree oil.

melamine Derived from urea; used as a film-forming agent. Toxic by ingestion; skin and eye irritant.

Melia azadiracht *See* neem extract or oil.

menthol Derived from peppermint; cooling, soothing in small amounts. May cause skin irritation.

mercury This toxic metal arrives in the body via our food, water, and the environment and through mercury-release from dental work. Causes skin rashes, eye irritation, irritability, memory problems, and tremors and is a challenge to the liver.

methylparaben Preservative that should be used only in rinse-off products because it can be too irritating when left on skin. Also xenoestrogenic. *See also* parabens.

methylsilanol mannuronate A source of silicon that can be plant or mineral but also synthetic. Used as an anti-irritant or moisturizer.

mica Earth mineral used to give products sparkle and shine; can also be "grown" synthetically. Used for filler and for absorbing oil. Mineral irritant by inhalation; may damage lungs. Non-toxic to skin.

microcrystalline wax Derived from petroleum. *See also* petrolatum.

mimosa oil or extract Used as a fragrance; may cause allergic reactions.

mineral oil *(Paraffinum liquidum)* Petroleum product known to cause cancer in humans; contains carcinogenic polycyclic aromatic hydrocarbons. Allergenic; photo toxic (becomes toxic in sunlight); causes skin discoloration; can promote acne. Used because it is inexpensive and plentiful.

mink oil Similar to human sebum; emollient. No known toxicity.

monoethanolamine *See* MEA.

mint This natural antiseptic, anesthetic, stimulant, and freshener is used as fragrance for lip products, men's shaving products, soaps, and toothpaste. May irritate skin.

montan A plant- or mineral-based thickener.

montmorillonite One of the major constituents of fuller's earth and bentonite; natural clay used for stabilizing, suspending, or thickening. Used in masks. *See also* bentonite; fuller's earth.

mulberry extract Used as purplish-black dye. This extract may help to prevent melanin production due to its arbutin content. *See also* arbutin.

mucilage A sticky, semi-fluid substance obtained from the seeds of plants.

myristic acid Created through the distillation of coconut acid, nutmeg, and most animal and vegetable fats, this solid organic acid is used as a detergent and foam builder. Can be drying.

myrrh *(Commiphora myrrha)* Fragrant gum resin; antibacterial, antiseptic, anti-fungal, anti-inflammatory, antimicrobial, and astringent. Used in toiletries, mouthwashes, gargles; for wound healing; to fight bacteria that causes cavities; for dermatitis, dry skin, and eczema.

N

natural colors Colors derived from non-petroleum organic sources, including annatto, beet powder, caramel, carotene, chlorophyll, grapeskin extract, saffron, and turmeric.

natural ingredients "Natural" should mean "not synthetic," but no rules govern the use of this word. The word "natural" means very little when applied to the label of a cosmetic. Your best defense is to have a good understanding of what ingredients are in the products that you choose.

NDELA (n-nitrosodiethanolamine) This chemical is cancer-causing for animals and reasonably anticipated to be a human carcinogen. According to the National Toxicology Program, NDELA is a known contaminant of cosmetics, lotions, and shampoos.

neem extract or oil (extract of *Melia azadiracht*) From leaves of the neem tree. Antibacterial, antimicrobial, antiviral; used in ointments for eczema and ringworm.

neptune kelp extract *See* algae.

neroli oil Fragrant plant oil; anti-inflammatory; promotes new cell growth; used for dry and sensitive skin. May cause skin irritation.

nettle extract Traditionally used to stimulate hair growth when applied to scalp; analgesic, anti-inflammatory. Used topically for skin problems and for stimulating hair growth.

niacinamide (also known as niacin, nicotinic acid, and vitamin B3) Stimulant; used in cellulite and scalp treatments to increase circulation. No known skin toxicity.

niaouli oil This extract comes from a plant similar to the tea tree. Antibacterial; healing; promotes new cell growth; used to treat acne and burns. *See also* tea tree oil.

nitrogen Used as a propellant or preservative, this chemical generates free radical damage.

nitrosamines Some chemicals, such as DEA methoxycinnamate, can combine with amines in a formulation to create carcinogenic nitrosamines.

O

oatmeal *(Avena sativa)* Traditionally used as a facial mask; anti-irritant, anti-inflammatory. Used for cleansing, dry skin, flaky skin, frostbite, and wounds.

octocrylene Synthetic petrochemical used as sunscreen.

octyl dimethyl PABA Also called padimate-o. The irritation potential of this ester of PABA increases along with the Sun Protection Factor (SPF) of the product.

octyl methoxycinnamate Sunscreen agent used to protect against UVB rays. Xenoestrogenic; linked to breast cancer.

octyl palmitate Used in cosmetics as a thickening agent and emollient; can promote acne.

octyl stearate Used in cosmetics as a thickening agent and emollient; can promote acne.

oleic acid This essential dietary monounsaturated fatty acid is a mild surfactant used in cosmetics, ointments, and soaps. In higher concentrations can promote acne.

oleth-2, -3, etc. Polyethylene glycol esters of oleyl alcohol; used as surfactants. More likely to cause skin irritation as number increases.

olibanum extract *See* frankincense extract.

olive oil High in EFAs; demulcent, emollient, lubricant. Also healing and soothing. Used in soap and surfactants; for treatment of bruises, burns, insect bites. A frequent foundation for linaments and ointments; excellent for dry hair and scalp. Superior absorption; offers some UVB protection. May cause allergic reaction. *See also* Castile soap.

orris root Has a scent similar to a violet's; used mainly as a fragrance; may cause skin sensitivity or trigger allergic reactions.

oryzanol From rice hulls or rice bran oil. Has some antioxidant and sunscreen properties. Also used as flavoring and fragrance.

Oryza sativa oil *See* rice bran oil.

oxalic acid Occurs naturally in plants and molds; used in skin-bleaching products. Caustic and corrosive to skin; toxic to kidney and intestines.

oxybenzone (also known as benzophenone-3) Protects against UVB and some UVA radiation. Sensitivity to this sunscreen agent is increasing.

ozokerite Mineral wax for thickening; found in lipsticks and stick foundations. Also synthetic from petroleum waxes.

P

PABA *See* para-aminobenzoic acid.

Palma Christi oil *See* castor oil.

palm glyceride Used as an emollient and thickening agent in cosmetics.

palmitates This salt of palmitic acid is used as a thickening agent and emollient. May clog pores. *See also* palmitic acid.

palmitic acid Obtained from palm oil, but when used in cosmetics, it often contains petrochemicals such as propylene glycol. *See also* propylene glycol.

palm oil Similar to coconut oil; has emollient and antioxidant properties for skin. Used to make soap.

pantothenic acid Also called vitamin B5. Used for scalp diseases, to condition hair, and to make hair look fuller. Hygroscopic; skin hydrator; wound healing. Non-toxic. *See also* hygroscopic.

papain Traditionally used to remove freckles and to soften skin, this protein-digesting enzyme is extracted from papaya. Used as an exfoliant in light peels to dissolve dead skin cells. Hygroscopic; skin softener. No known toxicity. *See also* hygroscopic.

para-aminobenzoic acid (PABA) Should not be confused with the water-soluble B vitamin of the same name known for its sun-protective qualities when included in the diet. When used in sunscreen products, ironically, can lead to photosensitivity; causes contact dermatitis and allergic eczema.

parabens Group of preservatives, including butylparaben, propylparaben, methylparaben, and ethylparaben. Most frequently used preservatives in cosmetics; only water is used more often in formulations. Not effective with products that contain proteins. Toxic and allergenic; have an additive xenoestrogenic effect.

paraffin or paraffin wax Waxy, petroleum-based substance used as a stabilizer and thickener for cosmetics. May contain recognized carcinogens benzo-a-pyrene and benzo-b-fluroanthene. May cause eczema and irritations.

Paraffinum liquidum *See* mineral oil.

Parsol 1789 *See* avobenzone.

partially hydrogenated vegetable oils (also known as "trans-fats") Oils treated with hydrogen to alter their molecular structure. Trans-fats interfere with the body's normal metabolism of fats, promoting inflammation and chronic conditions such as diabetes and heart disease. No better on your skin than in your diet.

peanut oil (*Arachis* oil) Emollient plant oil similar to all non-fragrant plant oils; used in the manufacture of soap. May cause skin irritation or cause allergic response.

pecan oil Emollient plant oil.

pecan shell powder Edible colorant.

pectin Natural edible substance from apples, citrus peel, and the cell walls of other plants; emulsifier, thickener, film-forming agent.

PEG compound Synthetic glycol compound. Used as emollient, binding agent, stabilizer, and surfactant. May contain potent toxin dioxane as a byproduct of manufacturing. May combine with other ingredients to form carcinogenic nitrosamines; may cause hives and eczema. *See also* polyethylene glycol.

PEG -4, -6, -8, -10, -12, -14, -16, -18, -32, -40, -150, -200, -350 Polymers of ethylene oxide. *See* ethylene oxide.

Pelargonium graveolens oil *See* geranium oil.

pentasodium penetrate Used as a chelating (binding and removal) agent and dispersing ingredient. Used in cleansing creams and lotions. Ingesting can lead to violent vomiting; may be irritating to skin and mucous membranes.

peony root extract Traditionally used as antibacterial, anti-fungal, and anti- inflammatory.

peppermint Cooling, antiseptic, anti-inflammatory. Used in shampoos for toning scalp; externally for itching and skin inflammation. Also for acne, blackheads, dandruff, dermatitis, pimples, and itchy skin.

perfluorononyl dimethicone Fluorine-modified silicone. *See also* silicone.

perfume Also listed on labels as fragrance. May contain up to 200 ingredients to create one fragrance; manufacturers are not required to list each ingredient individually. Some natural essential oils are used, but most often synthetic ingredients are used in non-organic cosmetic products. Some perfumes can cause breathing difficulties, dizziness, headache, skin irritation, nausea, and vomiting. Some chemicals used to create perfumes are also xenoestrogenic.

petrolatum *(Cera microcristallina)* (also known as petroleum jelly, paraffin jelly) Semi-solid hydrocarbons from petroleum; used as occlusive (barrier cream to prevent water loss). May contain recognized carcinogens benzo-a-pyrene and benzo-b-fluroanthene. May cause eczema and irritations; can cause skin discoloration.

phenol First isolated in coal tar, phenols occur widely in nature from amino acids in proteins to blistering agents in poison ivy; also synthetic as a caustic poisonous crystalline compound derived from benzene. Toxic by absorption, ingestion, and inhalation; strong skin irritant.

phenoxyethanol This common preservative does not release formaldehyde; usually synthetic by treating phenol with ethylene oxide. Topical antiseptic, fixative, insect repellant. Strong eye irritant when not diluted. *See also* phenol; ethylene oxide.

phosphatidylcholine Naturally occurring phosphatidylcholine exists in cell membranes; active ingredient in lecithin. Water-binding agent; improves penetration of other ingredients into the skin. *See also* lecithin.

phospholipid Lipid essential to the structure of cell membranes; well-known examples include cholesterol and lecithin. Water-binding agent. Cosmetic formulations typically obtained from lecithin, egg yolks, and soy. *See also* lecithin.

phosphoric acid Used to adjust the pH of formulations; also sequestering agent. Toxic by ingestion and inhalation; irritant to skin and eyes.

phthalates Used as plasticizers and fragrance, these chemicals are mutagenic, carcinogenic, and xenoestrogenic. Worldwide manufacture of these chemicals is estimated to be many millions of tons annually.

phthalic acid Created by oxidizing benzene derivatives. Irritating to skin and mucous membranes. *See also* benzene.

phytonadione Synthetic vitamin K; antibacterial. Used to stimulate circulation in foot and leg products. May redden skin if used on face. Degrades in sunlight.

pilewort extract See *Ranunculus ficaria* extract.

pineapple extract Contains the enzyme bromelain; anti-inflammatory. Exfoliant; dissolves bonds between skin cells. No known toxicity. *See also* bromelain.

pine cone extract *(Pinus sylvestris)* Contains gamma linolenic acid (GLA) and linoleic acid (LA); antioxidant, antibacterial.

pine needle extract/pine oil Antibacterial, anti-inflammatory, antimicrobial, antioxidant, antiseptic, antiviral; solvent, disinfectant. Used in deodorant. Pine tar is used in hair tonics. Potent irritant; do not use on broken skin.

pistachio nut oil (from *Pistaclum* tree) A readily absorbed emollient plant oil from the pistachio nut; high in the emollient EFA linoleic acid (LA).

placenta extract Extracted from the mother's placental lining, expelled after birth. While a source of proteins and amino acids, there is no proof that this ingredient prevents wrinkles. Typically bovine sourced; mad cow disease is a concern.

plantain Traditionally used for skin ailments; astringent, antiseptic. Used for wound healing and to soothe irritated skin, treat blemishes.

polyethylene glycol Often shown as "PEG" on product labels. This product of petroleum gas is created through the condensation of ethylene glycol or ethylene oxide and water. Ingestion can cause kidney and liver damage. *See also* ethylene glycol; ethylene oxide; petrolatum.

polypropylene glycol Often shown as "PPG" on product labels. This petroleum product is highly absorbable and can cause irritation and dermatitis. Used as a wetting ingredient in liquid make-up, but also used in hydraulic fluids and paint formulations. Used widely because it is inexpensive. *See also* petrolatum.

polyquaterniums *See* quaternary ammonium compounds.

polysorbates Prepared from sorbitol (a sugar); emollient, thickening agent. Used to reduce irritation potential of the product formula.

polyvinyl alcohol The vinyl monomer content of this synthetic plasticizing agent and lipstick resin is potentially carcinogenic.

polyvinyl pyrrolidone Also shown as "PVP" or "PVP copolymer" on product labels; synthetic. Petroleum-derived chemical used in hairstyling products to hold hairstyles. Inhalant toxicant; may cause the formation of foreign particles in the lungs. May cause lung or kidney damage. *See also* petrolatum.

potassium chloride Mined salt; used interchangeably with sodium chloride in cosmetic formulations. Used as an abrasive in scrub products. Toxic if ingested; large amounts can cause gastrointestinal irritation, vomiting, and weakness.

potassium cocoate Cleanser made from potassium chloride and coconut oil fatty acids; leaves residue in hard water. May cause skin irritation.

potassium hydroxide (also known as lye) An alkaline ingredient used to alter the pH of a product. Cleansing agent. Toxic by inhalation and ingestion; ingestion can cause pain, bleeding, and death. Corrosive.

potassium myristate Potassium salt of myristic acid; detergent. Can be dehydrating and irritating to skin. *See also* myristic acid.

PPG *See* polypropylene glycol.

propolis Brownish, resinous material used to construct a beehive; antibacterial, anti-inflammatory.

propylene carbonate Synthetic, petroleum-derived solvent and plasticizer; used in nail-polish removers, lipsticks, deodorants, and mascara. *See also* petrolatum.

propylene glycol Petroleum product derived from ethylene oxide or propylene oxide; used as a humectant, preservative, and film-former. After water, the most widely used vehicle to transport moisture. Increases body acidity levels, leading to metabolic problems. Can increase the absorption of other irritating ingredients in a formulation. Allergic and toxic reactions. *See also* ethylene oxide; petrolatum; propylene oxide.

propylene oxide Clear, colorless, flammable liquid used in the production of propylene glycol and glycol ethers; solvent, emollient, plasticizer. A known carcinogen for animals and reasonably anticipated to be a human carcinogen according to the National Toxicology Program.

propylparaben Preservative that can cause allergic reactions and dermatitis; xenoestrogen. *See also* parabens.

proteases Enzymes like papain from papaya that help to decompose amino acids and proteins; skin softener, exfoliant.

PVP *See* polyvinyl pyrrolidone.

PVP copolymer *See* polyvinyl pyrrolidone.

pycnogenol From the French maritime pine tree; also found in apples, grapeseeds, and red wine; powerful antioxidant. Excellent free radical scavenger.

Pyrus cydonia *See* quince seed.

Pyrus malu The pectin from this apple is used to thicken cosmetics.

Q

quaternary ammonium compounds (also known as polyquaterniums) These chemicals can cause the death of mucous membranes, yet are present in mouthwashes. Also used in after-shave and hair products as film-formers. May cause skin irritation.

quaternium-15 Synthetic formaldehyde-releasing preservative; might contain dangerous cancer-causing nitrosamines. Causes birth defects in animals (teratogen). May
be linked to birth defects when absorbed through skin. May cause skin irritation.

quaternium-90 bentonite Synthetic or mineral- or animal-sourced; used to allow sunscreens to spread more easily; skin barriers. Known to cause irritation.

quillaja (or quillaya) extract (also known as soap bark) Natural saponins in this extract
have excellent foaming properties; used for shampoo and to control dandruff and
scalp problems. Relieves itchiness of psoriasis; used for douches; also for athlete's
foot. No known toxicity. *See also* saponins.

quince seed (seed of *Pyrus cydonia*) This expensive ingredient is used to thicken and
emulsify cosmetics. May cause allergic reactions.

R

Ranunculus ficaria extract (pilewort extract) Antibacterial, anti-fungal; traditionally
used to treat tuberculosis. For treatment of hemorrhoids; may cause skin irritation
and dermatitis. No known toxicity.

rapeseed oil (canola oil) This non-fragrant, edible oil is high in unsaturated fats, including oleic and linoleic acid; emollient, antioxidant, lubricant. Removed by solvent or
extraction. Can cause skin eruptions.

red raspberry extract Fruit extract; anti-irritant, anti-inflammatory, antioxidant, astringent, and flavoring. Soothing to skin; can also cause irritation due to its tannin content. No known toxicity.

retinol Unstable form of vitamin A; can be absorbed into the skin. Promotes healthy
skin; useful for acne treatments and wound healing and to improve elasticity. This
form of vitamin A is more likely to irritate than other forms.

retinyl palmitate Form of vitamin A; combination of retinol (pure vitamin A) and
palmitic acid; antioxidant. Derived from plants and animals; can also be synthetic.
Healing for skin; also used for acne treatments.

rice bran oil (also known as *Oryza sativa* oil) Emollient oil rich in vitamin E; has sunscreen
properties.

rice bran wax An edible wax made from the oil of rice bran.

rice powder Non-toxic starch powder; used in face powder and as a drying ingredient.

rice starch Absorbent, demulcent, emollient; used to replace talc. May block pores or
support bacterial growth; may cause allergic reaction.

rosehip oil Natural flavoring, antioxidant, emollient; rich in EFAs. Used for skin burns,
scars; soothes and hydrates. Avoid use on oily skin. No known toxicity.

Rosmarinus officinalis extract *See* rosemary extract.

rosemary extract (*Rosmarinus officinalis* extract) This extract was traditionally used as a
preservative and to promote healthy skin; analgesic, antibacterial, antimicrobial,
astringent, antioxidant, purifier, and toner. Good rinse for auburn hair or to darken
graying hair. Used to stimulate hair follicles and encourage scalp circulation when

massaged into scalp; regulates oil balance; for acne, dermatitis, dandruff, dry skin, eczema, and hair. Non-irritating. No known toxicity when used externally; ingesting the oil can cause illness or death

rose oil This fragrant essential oil was traditionally used for wound healing; anti-inflammatory, astringent, fragrant, healing. Used as moisturizer; promotes new cell growth for aged skin. Used for eczema, broken capillaries. Good for sensitive and dry skin. Non-toxic. May cause skin irritation in high concentrations; may cause allergic reaction.

rosewood *(Aniba rosaeodora)* Essential oil used for fragrance; mild analgesic, stimulant.

royal jelly Milky white, nutritive secretion fed to bee larvae; may have some immune-modulating benefits. Concentrations used in cosmetics are not likely to improve skin quality. No known toxicity.

S

saccharin Artificial sweetener used in dental products and mouthwash; carcinogen in animals and potential human carcinogen. May be mutagenic; may also affect reproduction.

St. John's Wort Traditionally used for wound healing, this herb is used to treat scratches, swelling, and burns. Soothing anti-inflammatory. Non-toxic.

safflower oil Emollient, non-fragrant plant oil; antioxidant. Used to soften skin and condition hair.

sage oil Traditionally used as an antiseptic and astringent; antibacterial, antiperspirant, stimulant, purifier, tonic; used in antiperspirant and insect repellant. Good for scalp or hair loss or to cover gray hair. Skin purifier and tonic; also used for wound healing. Regulates oil production for acne. No known toxicity.

salicin *See* white willow bark extract.

salicylic acid Can be derived from wintergreen oil, but also produced synthetically by heating phenol with carbon dioxide. Salicylic acid is used to manufacture aspirin. Also referred to as Beta Hydroxy Acid (BHA), salicylic acid dissolves the material that binds dead cells to the skin's surface; can penetrate the pore, offering more complete exfoliation than Alpha Hydroxy Acids (AHAs). Is also a preservative. Look for natural wintergreen oil.

sandalwood oil *(Santalum album)* Fragrant oil; antibacterial, anti-inflammatory, astringent. Healing, moisturizing, soothing; promotes new cell growth. For acne, dry skin, itch; also for dark-hair care. May cause skin irritation or trigger allergic reactions.

Santalum album *See* sandalwood oil.

saponin Natural compounds obtained from sugars and used for their ability to foam in water. Used in cleaners and detergents and as an emulsifier. No known toxicity; may be synthetic.

Saponaria officinalis extract. *See* soapwort.

sea salt Salts from evaporated seawater, mostly sodium chloride. Sometimes used as a mechanical scrub; if left on skin, can lead to increased photosensitivity to UVB radiation.

sebum Oily secretion made up of oils and waxes produced by the sebaceous glands in skin. Sebum works to protect and lubricate skin. Too much sebum may contribute to clogged pores, while not enough sebum is associated with dry skin.

sepia Natural red-brown tint obtained from cuttlefish.

sesame seed oil Edible, non-fragrant emollient oil extracted from the seed; high in linoleic and oleic fatty acids. Light, versatile oil often used as a carrying agent. For skin and hair care. May cause allergic reactions.

Sesamum indicum *See* sesame seed oil.

sesquiterpene lactones More than 50 of these naturally occurring compounds have been found in essential oils; in arnica, chamomile, yarrow, and other plants. Known to cause allergic contact dermatitis.

shea butter From the karite tree *(Butyrospermum parkii)*; also known as karite butter or African butter. Traditionally used for skin healing and as an occlusive-type emollient; anti-inflammatory. Rich in fatty acids; moisturizing. Good for sun care. Widely used; no known toxicity.

shellac *(Coccus lucca)* A natural resin obtained from insects and used as a fixative in hair-sprays, gels, lipsticks, and eyeliners. Flammable; may cause contact dermatitis.

silica This natural mineral is abundant in sandstone, clay, and granite; also found in plants and animals. Can increase collagen production when used internally. Used as absorbent; thickening agent; stabilizer. Increases effectiveness of sunscreen. Toxic by inhalation; powdered form should not inhaled.

silica gel Absorbs water readily, so it is used for dehydrating. Non-combustible; no known toxicity.

silicate Inorganic salt; absorbent, thickener.

silicone Obtained by heating silicon in methyl chloride (chloromethane); a chemical known to have toxic effects on the liver, kidney, and spleen of animals. It is also a narcotic. Human cancer data are limited. Used as water-binding agent and to improve feel of a product. Might be listed as cyclohexasiloxane or cyclomethicone.

silk protein Also listed on product labels as silk. From the silkworm *(Bombyx mori)*. Amino acids used in hair and skin conditioners, moisturizers, make-up powders. Improves the feel of formulas; anti-irritant. Can cause hives on contact.

silver Metal used as disinfectant; prolonged contact can lead to a blue-gray cast to skin. May irritate skin and mucous membranes.

soapwort *(Saponaria officinalis)* This perennial herb was traditionally used for skin com-plaints. Lathers well in water; has cleansing properties. Also used for dermatitis and skin itch. No known toxicity.

sodium bicarbonate Also listed on product labels as bicarbonate of soda, baking soda. Used to raise the pH of formula or as an abrasive. Also effervescent. Relieves the itch of insect bites; burn treatment; used in mouthwash. May irritate dry skin. May con-tain aluminum; look for aluminum-free variety for home cooking and use. *See also* aluminum.

sodium borate (borax) A natural hydrated sodium borate found in salt lakes and alkali soils; detergent, emulsifier, preservative. Used to neutralize beeswax. May cause hair to become dry. Do not use on babies or on broken skin; may cause irritation.

sodium chloride Table salt; astringent, antiseptic. Used as a binding agent or an abrasive in scrub products. Necessary to make soap. Found in mouthwash and dental products. May be drying to skin.

sodium hydroxide (also known as lye) An alkaline ingredient used to alter the pH of a product. Cleansing agent. Toxic by inhalation and ingestion; ingestion can cause pain, bleeding, and death. Corrosive to tissue when combined with water. Irritant to eyes and mucous membranes. Inhalation may cause lung damage.

sodium laureth sulfate Can be derived from coconut; used primarily as a detergent cleansing agent. May contain toxic ethylene oxide and/or dioxane as a manufacturing byproduct. Can combine with other ingredients to form carcinogenic nitrosamines. Can cause skin irritation, dermatitis. *See also* ethylene oxide.

sodium lauryl sulfate Can be derived from coconut; often synthetic. Used as wetting agent, detergent, emulsifier, and thickener. May contain formaldehyde as a preservative. Combines with other ingredients to form carcinogenic nitrosamines. Skin irritant; can cause severe inflammation, cracking, contact eczema. Eye irritant.

sodium metabisulfite Inorganic salt, bacterial inhibitor. Preservative; reducing agent. Alters the structure of hair; can be a skin irritant.

sodium PCA (also known as sodium pyrrolidone carboxylic acid) A natural component of skin that is also a very good water-binding agent. Synthetic versions can absorb water from skin, leading to dehydration.

sodium salicylate Salt form of salicylic acid; does not have exfoliating properties of salicylic acid. Antiseptic, analgesic, preservative. Used to filter sun radiation. May cause allergic reactions.

sodium sulfite Preservative; reducing agent to alter hair structure. Those with impaired kidney may not be able to break down sulfites in the body. May release sulfur dioxide; may cause skin irritation. May trigger asthma attack. May also destroy thiamine.

sorbitol A sugar alcohol used to flavor toothpaste, mouthwash. Also used as humectant.

soy extract Extract that is high in linoleic, oleic, and other fatty acids that are necessary for healthy skin; excellent emollient, antioxidant, anti-inflammatory. Used in bath oils, shampoos, soaps. May cause allergic reactions and skin eruptions.

soya sterol From soybeans; excellent emollient, anti-inflammatory.

spearmint oil Fragrant, volatile oil; cleanser, analgesic. Used to treat acne and dermatitis. May cause skin irritation and allergic reactions.

spermaceti (cetyl palmitate) Derived as wax from the head of the sperm whale. May cause irritations. Used as a thickener and emulsifier.

squalene A component of skin; occurs naturally in sebum and is a precursor of cholesterol. Also found in an oil derived from shark liver or from plants. Antioxidant, bactericide, emollient, lubricant. May stimulate immune system Used in crèmes, cleansers, hair products, and lipsticks.

stearalkonium chloride Originally created as a fabric softener, it is now used extensively in hair products because it is inexpensive and plentiful. Known to damage hair over the long term. Opt for a formulation using lecithin instead.

stearic acid This fatty acid from animals and plants is a wax-like solid used as an emollient and lubricant. Often neutralized with triethanolamine (TEA) or sodium hydroxide. Found in crèmes and lotions. May cause irritation. *See also* TEA (triethanolamine).

stearyl alcohol Fatty alcohol; emollient, emulsifier, and thickener. Used in perfumes and cosmetics. Usually produced by hydrogenating stearic acid. May cause dermatitis and allergies.

strawberry extract Astringent; excellent for oily skin.

sugarcane extract A natural source of glycolic acid. *See also* glycolic acid.

sulfur This non-metallic element is found in Alberta, Japan, Louisiana, Mexico, Sicily, and Texas. Sulfur-containing amino acids are essential to healthy hair and skin; antibacterial, anti-fungal. Herbal sulfur is used to reduce scalp problems and repair damaged hair. May cause skin irritation. Do not eat.

sunflower oil This non-volatile plant oil is an emollient; rich base for massage oils and lotions. High in vitamin E. No known toxicity

sweet almond oil This edible oil is high in Omega-6 EFAs; emollient. For dry skin; smoothing and moisturizing. Promotes spreading and feel of product; used in perfumes and soaps. No known skin toxicity.

T

talc (also known as soapstone, French chalk, hydrous magnesium silicate) Finely ground mineral used as absorbent; main ingredient in baby powders, eye shadows, face powders. Often contaminated with asbestos, a known lung irritant and carcinogen. Toxic by inhalation; do not use near babies. Do not use on open wounds; avoid talc in feminine pads.

tallow An animal fat used to make soap and candles and in the creation of stearic acid and oleic acid. Used as lubricant and emollient base, and in lipsticks, shampoos. May cause eczema and blackheads.

tangerine oil Fragrant oil from the peels of the ripe fruit; astringent, flavor, fragrance. May cause skin irritation.

tannic acid A natural substance found in tree barks, nutgalls, and plant parts, traditionally used as a burn treatment; antioxidant, astringent. May cause irritation; may increase pigmentation.

tannin A plant-derived phenolic compound found in many plants; astringent. Can be beneficial or toxic. Soothes skin and mucous membranes; used by herbalists to treat wounds and burns.

tartrazine FD&C Yellow#5. Bright yellow and orange colorant used in cosmetics and foods; known allergen and may be carcinogenic.

TEA (triethanolamine) Widely used amino alcohol synthesized from ammonia and ethylene oxide. Used to balance the pH of a formulation; surfactant, dispersing agent. May combine with other ingredients to form carcinogenic nitrosamines. May cause skin irritation; extreme sensitizer. Should be used only in rinse-off products, yet frequently found in make-up.

tea tree oil *(Melaleuca alternifolia)* Disinfectant, germicide, antibacterial, anti-fungal, antiseptic; used to kill bacteria that cause blemishes; also effective against *Escherichia coli (E. coli)*, *Staphylococcus*, *Candida albicans,* athlete's foot. Used for treatment of dandruff and nail infections and used in therapeutic masks. Penetrates skin quickly; accelerates skin healing. No known toxicity. Similar to niaouli oil.

theobroma oil Fat extracted from seeds of cocoa plant by expression, decoction, or extraction by a solvent. *See also* cocoa butter.

thimerserol Preservative derived from mercury; sometimes used in eye shadows. *See also* mercury.

thioglycolic acid Compounds that break the sulfide bonds in hair; used in permanent waves and depilatories. Toxic by ingestion and inhalation; strong skin irritant. May cause severe allergic reactions.

Thuja occidentalis extract An essential oil also known as extract of red or yellow cedar; antibacterial. Can help to treat warts. May cause skin irritation.

thyme extract/thyme oil (oil of *Thymus vulgaris)* An extract of the herb; antioxidant, astringent, antiseptic, anti-fungal, fragrance, preservative; topical treatment for skin rashes; used in bath water to relieve aching muscles; used for skin infections; also used in toothpaste. Promotes perspiration. May cause skin irritation and hay fever.

thymol From thyme oil; also synthetic. Antioxidant, anti-fungal, antiseptic, preservative; used in mouthwash, toothpaste. Helpful in treating warts; also to encourage blood flow to the skin surface. May cause allergic reactions.

titanium dioxide An inorganic salt used as whitener, opacifier, and for reflectivity in sunscreen and make-up. Also thickening, lubricating. Provides barrier protection from UVA and UVB radiation; great covering power. Generally inert; no known toxicity when used externally. Toxic by inhalation.

tocopherol Synthetic form of vitamin E.

toluene Petroleum-derived solvent used in nail polishes, dyes, pharmaceuticals. Flammable. Toxic by ingestion, inhalation, and absorption. Narcotic; may affect central nervous system, leading to dizziness, sleepiness, and unconsciousness. May cause liver damage.

tragacanth Natural gum found in Southwestern Europe, Greece, Iran, and Turkey. Used as a thickener, film-former, emulsifier, and binding agent in cosmetics. Also helps to increase viscosity.

trichloroethylene (TCE) A chlorinated hydrocarbon known to cause cancer in animals and reasonably anticipated to be carcinogenic for humans according to the National Toxicology Program. It concentrates in fatty tissue in the liver, brain, and fat stores, and is readily absorbed through the stomach and lung. This chemical has been used as a solvent for fats, dyeing, dry cleaning, and waxes, and is considered to be pervasive in the environment. The FDA regulates the presence of TCE as a residue in color additives and bottled water.

triclosan An antibacterial agent added to deodorant and antibacterial soaps. Believed to cause a bacterial imbalance on the surface of the skin. Studies show that exposure to sunlight causes triclosan to chemically convert into a dioxin. May also be contaminated with carcinogenic nitrosamines. *See also* dioxin.

triethanolamine *See* TEA.

2-Ethylhexylmethoxycinamate (Octyl methoxycinnamate) Sunscreen agent. The higher the SPF of the product, the more potentially irritating the formula.

U

urea A product of protein metabolism, urea is a natural component of urine; also synthetic, created with liquid ammonia and carbon dioxide. Can affect skin function and cause thinning of epidermis. Frequently used in deodorants, mouthwashes, hair colorings, shampoos, hand crème. *See also* ammonia.

V

valerian root extract *(Valeriana officinalis)* Traditionally, the distilled roots and rhizome of the plant were used for wound healing; antioxidant. Also used for fragrance and flavors.

Vanilla planifolia fruit extract Vanillin extracted from the vanilla bean. Used in perfumes and flavors. Synthetic forms are now often used in cosmetic formulations. May cause skin irritation or contact eczema.

vegetable glycerin Used as a humectant, emollient, and lubricant. Derived from vegetable oils.

vegetable protein Combines with fatty acids and amino acids to coat damaged hair in hair-care formulas. Applied topically, provides hydration for skin.

verbena extract *(Verbena officinalis)* Traditionally used as an acne treatment and for other skin problems. Also used for wound healing, eczema, and fragrance. May cause skin irritation.

vinegar *See* acetic acid.

violet Analgesic and soothing agent containing salicylic acid. Often used as fragrance; used in face powders; natural coloring. May cause allergic skin reaction.

vitamin A Considered a topical antioxidant in some of its various forms, particularly as retinol and retinyl palmitate. *See also* retinol.

vitamin B5 (also known as pantothenic acid) *See* pantothenic acid.

vitamin C Considered a potent antioxidant for skin; neutralizes free radical damage from sunlight. Stimulant; useful for wound healing.

vitamin E Fat-soluble antioxidant vitamin. Protects skin from free radical damage; wound healing.

W

walnut oil Emollient, non-fragrant, edible plant oil. Source of EFAs; moisturizing.

walnut-shell powder Abrasive used in scrub products; exfoliant.

water Solvent, suspending agent, cleanser, moisturizer. The most widely used cosmetic ingredient.

watercress extract *(Citrullus vulgaris)* Emollient; soothing, conditioning. Beneficial for oily skin. To strengthen and thicken hair.

wheat germ oil *(Triticum vulgare)* Non-fragrant emollient plant oil; natural source of vitamin E; high in gamma linoleic acid (GLA). Anti-inflammatory, preservative. Amino acid content is good for dry skin and hair. Low sensitivity.

white willow bark extract *(Salix alba)* Natural source of salicylates; also known as salicin. Analgesic, astringent, antiseptic. For wound healing and eczema. External wash for skin eruptions, sores, burns, and sweaty feet.

wild ginger *See* ginger.

wild strawberry *(Fragaria vesca)* Astringent; used for acne and eczema.

wintergreen oil Used as fragrance, flavor, astringent; source of methyl salicylate. Used in body rubs, bath oils, toothpaste, mouthwash. Absorbed rapidly; may irritate skin and mucous membranes.

witch hazel *(Hamamelis virginiana)* Herb used as an astringent, anesthetic, anti-inflammatory, and vasoconstrictor (causes narrowing (constriction) of the blood vessels). Used for skin irritations, bruises, insect stings and bites, burns, and poison ivy. Can also cause contact dermatitis, hemorrhoids. An extract from the bark and leaves is helpful for oily skin.

Y

yarrow extract (*Achillea millefolium*) Related to chamomile, this herb was traditionally used to stop bleeding and to promote wound healing; antiseptic, astringent, anti-inflammatory. Helps with blood coagulation. May cause photosensitivity. Contains sesquiterpene lactones; may cause skin irritation. *See also* sesquiterpene lactones.

yeast One-celled organisms that can be a source of vitamins, enzymes, and antioxidants. Can also cause infections such as *Cryptococcus* and *Candida albicans*. Used in skin conditioners; moisturizers. No known toxicity.

ylang-ylang *(Cananga odorata)* Fragrant essential oil that regulates oil production; also scalp stimulant for hair growth; good for oily skin. May cause skin irritation and allergic reactions.

yucca extract Plant extract with high saponin content; used as foaming agent. Also anti-inflammatory. Used in soaps, shampoos, and hair fixatives; also used to treat burns and scrapes.

Z

zinc oxide Made by oxidation of vaporized pure zinc or by heating zinc oxide ore (Franklinite) with coal and oxidizing in air; occlusive; lubricant. barrier sunscreen, whitening agent. Also astringent, antiseptic, and protective. Fumes are toxic by inhalation; may block pores. May not be suitable for dry skin.

zirconium chloride Active ingredient in antiperspirants; may be highly irritating. Also used to make other zirconium compounds.

Selected References

I researched hundreds of sources in the preparation of this book, but space limitations prohibit recording them all here. Please visit my website (www.iamlivingbeauty.com) to access the complete list.

General References

Balch, James F., and Phyllis A. Balch. *Prescription for Nutritional Healing*. New York: Avery Publishing, 2000.

Berkow, Robert et al., ed. *Merck Manual of Medical Information Home Edition*. New York: Pocket Books, 1997.

Castleman, M. *The New Healing Herbs*. Rodale Inc., 2001.

Hampton, A. *Organic Hair and Skin Care: Including A to Z Guide to Natural and Synthetic Chemicals in Cosmetics*. 1st ed. Tampa: Organika Press, 1987.

Lewis, R.J., Sr. *Hawley's Condensed Chemical Dictionary*. 13th ed. New York: John Wiley and Sons, Inc., 1997.

Lust, J. *The Herb Book*. New York: Bantam Books, 1974.

Marieb, E.N. *Essentials of Human Anatomy and Physiology*. 6th ed. San Francisco: Addison Wesley Longman Inc., 2000.

Matsen, J. *Eating Alive: Prevention thru Good Digestion*. Vancouver: Crompton Books, 1987.

Murray, M.T. *The Healing Power of Herbs: The Enlightened Person's Guide to the Wonders of Medicinal Plants*. 2nd ed. Rocklin, CA: Prima Publishing, 1995.

National Institute of Environmental Health Sciences (www.niehs.nih.gov)

Ody, Penelope. *The Holistic Herbal Directory*. East Sussex: The Ivy Press Limited, 2004.

Roberts, A.J., M.E. O'Brien, and G. Suback-Sharpe. *Nutraceuticals: The Complete Encyclopedia of Supplements, Herbs, Vitamins and Healing Foods*. New York: Perigree, 2001.

Rutledge, M. *Product of Misinformation: Demistifying Cosmetics and Personal Care Claims, Terms, and Ingredients*. Irving: Tapestry Press, 2001.

Smeh, N. *Health Risks in Today's Cosmetics*. Garrison: Alliance Publishing Company, 1994.

Watson, F. *Aromatherapy Blends and Remedies*. London: Thorsons, 1995.

Winter, R. *A Consumer's Dictionary of Cosmetic Ingredients*. New York: Three Rivers Press, 1999.

The following references are listed in order of their appearance in the text.

Pedersen, B.K. "Influence of Physical Activity on the Cellular Immune System: Mechanisms of Action." *Int J Sports Med* 12 Suppl 1 (June): S23–9.

Brenner, J. *Essential Fatty Acids and the Skin*. Saskatoon: Bioriginal Food and Science Corp., 2003.

Mindell, E., and V. Hopkins. *Prescription Alternatives.* 2nd ed. Lincolnwood: Keats Publishing, 1999.

Donaldson, M.S. "Nutrition and Cancer: A Review of the Evidence for an Anti-cancer Diet." *Nutr J* 3 (October 20, 2004): 19.

Van Loo, J.A. "Prebiotics Promote Good Health: The Basis, the Potential, and the Emerging Evidence." *J Clin Gastroenterol* 38 (6 Suppl) (Jul 2004): S70–5.

Pappas, P.G., J.H. Rex, J.D. Sobel, W.E. Filler, T.J. Dismukes, and J.E. Edwards. "Guidelines for Treatment of Candidiasis." *Clinical Infectious Diseases*   38 (2004): 161–89.

Gaby, Alan R. "Fungus Allergy as a Cause of Sinusitis." *Townsend Letter for Doctors and Patients* (August-September, 2002).

Savolainen, J., K. Lammintausta, K. Kalimo, and M. Viander. "*Candida albicans* and Atopic Dermatitis." *Clin Exp Allergy 23* (April 1993): 332–39.

Buslau, M., H. Hanel, and H. Holzmann. "The Significance of Yeasts in Seborrheic Eczema." *Hautarzt* 40 (October 1989): 611–13.

Dovzhanskii, S.I., V.F. Orkin, A.K. Myshkina, and L.B. Pavlenko. "Secondary Candidal Infection in Patients with Chronic Dermatoses." *Vestn Dermatol Venerol* 11 (1989): 41–45.

Shahidi Bonjar, G.H. "Inhibition of Clotrimazole-resistant *Candida albicans* by Plants Used in Iranian Folkloric Medicine." *Fitoterapia* 75 (January 2004): 74–76.

Appleton, N. *Lick the Sugar Habit*. New York: Avery Publishing Group, 1996.

Hirasawa, M., and K. Takada. "Multiple Effects of Green Tea Catechin on the Antifungal Activity of Antimycotics against *Candida albicans.*" *J Antimicrob Chemother* (December 19, 2003).

Tadi, P., et al. "Aged Garlic Extract Hastens Clearance of *Candida albicans*." *Int Clin Natr Rev* 10 (1990): 423–29.

Jabbour, S.A. "Cutaneous Manifestations of Endocrine Disorders: A Guide for Dermatologists." *Am J Clin Dermatol* 4 (2003): 315–31.

Van Thiel, D.H., and R. Lester. "Editorial: Sex and Alcohol: A Second Peek." *N Engl J Med* 295 (October 7, 1976): 835–36.

Gooren, L.J., and A.W. Toorians. "Significance of Oestrogens in Male (Patho)physiology."*Ann Endocrinol* (Paris) 64 (April 2003): 126–35.

Olivo, J., G.G. Gordon, F. Rafii, and A.L. Southren. "Estrogen Metabolism in Hyperthyroidism and in Cirrhosis of the Liver." *Steroids* 26 (July 1975): 47–56.

Facemire, C.F., T.S. Gross, and L.J. Guillette, Jr. "Reproductive Impairment in the Florida Panther: Nature or Nurture?" *Environ Health Perspect* 103 (Suppl 4) (May 1995): 79–86.

Eichler, O., H. Sies, and W. Stahl. "Divergent Optimum Levels of Lycopene, Beta-carotene and Lutein Protecting against UVB Irradiation in Human Fibroblasts." *Free Radic Biol Med* 32 (June 2002): 1293–303.

Wei, H., R. Saladi, L. Yuhun., Y. Yan Wang, S.R. Palep, J. Moore, R. Phelps, E. Shyong, and M.G. Lebwohl. "Isoflavone Genistein: Photoprotection and Clinical Implications in Dermatology." *J Nutr* 133 (2003): 3811S–3819S.

Tobi, S.E., M. Gilbert, N. Paul, and T.J. McMillan. "The Green Tea Polyphenol, Epigallocatechin-3-gallate, Protects against the Oxidative Cellular and

Genotoxic Damage of A-RAY Radiation." *Int J Cancer* 102 (December 2002): :439–44.

Cordain, L., S. Lindeberg, M. Hurtado, K. Hill, S.B. Eaton, and J. Brand-Miller. "Acne vulgaris: A Disease of Western Civilization." *Arch Dermatol* 138 (December 2002): 1584–90.

Lucky, A.W. "Endocrine Aspects of Acne." *Pediatr Clin North Am* 30 (June 1983): 495–99.

Isolauri, E., et al. "Probiotics in the Management of Atopic Eczema." *Clin Exp Allergy* 30 (2000): 1605–10.

Yasumoto, R., H. Fujita, and T. Yamamoto. "The Effectiveness, Safety and Usefulness of Borage Oil on Atopic Dermatitis." *Acta Dermatologica* 92 (1996): 249–51.

Vanderhaeghe, L.R., and K. Karst. *Healthy Fats for Life: Preventing and Treating Common Health Problems with Essential Fatty Acids.* 2nd ed. Toronto: John Wiley and Sons, 2004.

Bittiner, S., et al. "A Double-Blind, Randomized, Placebo-controlled Trial of Fish Oil in Psoriasis." *Lancet 1* (1988): 378–80.

Diaz, C., C.J. O'Callaghan, A. Khan, and A. Ilchyshyn. "Rosacea: A Cutaneous Marker of Helicobacter pylori Infection? Results of a Pilot Study." *Acta Derm Venereol* 83 (2003): 282–86.

Johnson-Henry, K.C., D.J. Mitchell, Y. Avitzur, E. Galindo-Mata, N.L. Jones, and P.M. Sherman. "Probiotics Reduce Bacterial Colonization and Gastric Inflammation in H. pylori-infected mice." *Dig Dis Sci* 49 (August 2004): 1095–102.

Tsukahara, K., Y. Nagashima, S. Moriwaki, T. Fujimura, M. Hattori, and Y. Takema. "Relationship between Physical Parameters and Blood Flow in Human Facial Skin." *J Cosmet Sci* 54 (September-October 2003): 499–511.

McGrath, K.G. "An Earlier Age of Breast Cancer Diagnosis Related to More Frequent Use of Antiperspirants/Deodorants and Underarm Shaving." *Eur J Cancer Prev* 12 (December 2003): 479–85.

Crawford, G.H., J.R. Sciacca, and W.D. James. "Tea Tree Oil: Cutaneous Effects of the Extracted Oil of *Melaleuca alternifolia*." *Dermatitis* 15 (June 2004): 59–66.

Boorman, G.A. "Drinking Water Disinfection Byproducts: Review and Approach to Toxicity Evaluation." *Environ Health Perspect* 107 (Suppl 1) (February 1999): 207–17.

King, W.D., and L.D. Marrett. "Case-control Study of Bladder Cancer and Chlorination By-products in Treated Water (Ontario, Canada)." *Cancer Causes Control* 7 (November 1996): 596–604.

United States Environmental Protection Agency (www.epa.gov)

Rosen, C.J., M.F. Holick, and P.S. Millard. "Premature Graying of Hair Is a Risk Marker for Osteopenia." *J Clin Endocrinol Metab* 79 (September 1994): 854-57.

Chen, W., C.C. Yang, G.Y. Chen, M.C. Wu, H.M. Sheu, and T.S. Tzai . "Patients with a Large Prostate Show a Higher Prevalence of Androgenetic Alopecia." *Arch Dermatol Res* (October 28, 2004).

Prager, N., K. Bickett, N. French, and G. Marcovici. "A Randomized, Double-blind, Placebo-controlled Trial to Determine the Effectiveness of Botanically

Derived Inhibitors of 5-alpha-reductase in the Treatment of Androgenetic Alopecia." *J Altern Complement Med* 8 (April 2002): 143-52.

Trueb, R.M. "Association between Smoking and Hair Loss: Another Opportunity for Health Education against Smoking?" *Dermatology* 206 (2003): 189-91.

Bengt, Ljung. "EU Reaches Agreement to Impose Ban on Use of Toxics in Cosmetic Products." *Chemical Regulation Reporter* (December 2, 2002).

Aligne, C.A., et al. "Passive Smoke Causes Dental Caries: Association of Pediatric Dental Caries with Passive Smoking." *JAMA* 289 (2003): 1258-64.

Merchant, A.T., W. Pitiphat, B. Ahmed, I. Kawachi, and K. Joshipura. "A Prospective Study of Social Support, Anger Expression and Risk of Periodontitis in Men." *Journal of the American Dental Association* 134 (December 2003): 1591.

Danscher, G., P. Horsted-Bindslev, and J. Rungby. "Traces of Mercury in Organs from Primates with Amalgam Fillings." *Exp Mol Pathol* 52 (June 1990): 291-99.

Hezberg, M.C., and M.W. Meyer. "Dental Plaque, Platelets and Cardiovascular Diseases." *Annals of Periodontology* 3 (1998): 151-60.

Hellwig, E., and A.M. Lennon. "Systemic versus Topical Fluoride." *Caries Res* 38 (May-June 2004): 258-62.

Marshall, T.A., S.M. Levy, J.J. Warren, B. Broffitt, J.M. Eichenberger-Gilmore , and P.J. Stumbo. "Associations between Intakes of Fluoride from Beverages during Infancy and Dental Fluorosis of Primary Teeth." *J Am Coll Nutr* 23 (April 2004):108-16.

United States Food and Drug Administration (www.fda.gov)

Environmental Health Perspectives (ehp.niehs.nih.gov)

Guidotti, S., W.E. Wright, and J.M. Peters. "Multiple Myeloma in Cosmetologists." *Am J Ind Med* 3 (1982): 169-71.

Koch, H.M., H. Drexler, and J. Angerer. "An Estimation of the Daily Intake of Di(2-ethyl-hexyl)phthalate (DEHP) and Other Phthalates in the General Population." *Int J Hyg Environ Health 206* (March 2003): 77-83.

Silva, M.J., D.B. Barr, J.A. Reidy, N.A. Malek, C.C. Hodge, S.P. Caudill, J.W. Brock, L.L. Needham, and A.M. Calafat. "Urinary Levels of Seven Phthalate Metabolites in the U.S. Population from the National Health and Nutrition Examination Survey (NHANES) 1999-2000." *Environ Health Perspect* 112 (March 2004): 331-38.

Seo, K.W., K.B. Kim, Y.J. Kim, J.Y. Choi, K.T. Lee, and K.S. Choi. "Comparison of Oxidative Stress and Changes of Xenobiotic Metabolizing Enzymes Induced by Phthalates in Rats." *Food Chem Toxico* 42 (January 2004): 107–14.

Vrijheid, M., B. Armstrong, H. Dolk, M. van Tongeren, and B. Botting. "Risk of Hypospadias in Relation to Maternal Occupational Exposure to Potential Endocrine Disrupting Chemicals. *Occup Environ Med* 60 (August 2003): 543–50.

Duty, S.M., N.P. Singh, M.J. Silva, D.B. Barr, J.W. Brock, L. Ryan, R.F. Herrick, D.C. Christiani, and R. Hauser. "The Relationship between Environmental Exposures to Phthalates and DNA Damage in Human Sperm Using the Neutral Comet Assay." *Environ Health Perspect 111* (July 2003): 1164–69.

Carlsen, E., A. Giwercman, N. Keiding, and N.E. Skakkebaek. "Evidence for Decreasing Quality of Semen during Past 50 Years." *Br Med J* 305 (1992): 609–13.

Davis, D., H. Bradlow, M. Wolff, T. Woodruff, D. Hoel, and H. Anton-Culver. "Medical Hypothesis: Xenoestrogens as Preventable Causes of Breast Cancer." *Environmental Health Perspectives* 101 (October 1993).

Oishi, S. "Effects of Butyl paraben on the Male Reproductive System in Mice." *Arch Toxicol* 76 (July 2002): 423–29.

Harvey, P.W. "Parabens, Oestrogenicity, Underarm Cosmetics and Breast Cancer: A Perspective on a Hypothesis." *J Appl Toxicol* 23 (September-October 2003): 285–88.

Oishi, S. "Effects of Propyl paraben on the Male Reproductive System." *Food Chem Toxicol* 40 (December 2002): 1807–13.

Occupational Safety and Health Association (www.osha.gov)

Agency for Toxic Substances and Disease Registry (www.atsdr.cdc.gov)

Vondracek, J., A. Kozubik, and M. Machala. "Modulation of Estrogen Receptor-dependent Reporter Construct Activation and Go/G1-S-phase Transition by Polycyclic Aromatic Hydrocarbons in Human Breast Carcinoma MCF-7 cells." *Toxicol Sci* 70 (December 2002): 193–201.

Rier, S., and W.G. Foster. "Environmental Dioxins and Endometriosis." *Semin Reprod Med* 21 (May 2003): 145–54.

Knowland, J., E.A. McKenzie, P.J. McHugh, and N.A. Cridland. "Sunlight-induced Mutagenicity of a Common Sunscreen Ingredient." *FEBS Lett* 324 (June 1993): 309–13.

Rajapakse, N., E. Silva, and A. Kortenkamp. "Combining Xenoestrogens at Levels below Individual No-observed-effect Concentrations Dramatically Enhances Steroid Hormone Action." *Environ Health Perspect* 110 (September 2002): 917–21.

Melnick, R.L., J. Mahler, J.R. Bucher, M. Hejtmancik, A. Singer, and R.L. Persing. "Toxicity of Diethanolamine. 2. Drinking Water and Topical Application Exposures in B6C3F1 Mice." *J Appl Toxicol* 14 (January-February 1994): 11–19.

Mindell, Earl. *Earl Mindell's Anti-Aging Bible.* New York: Simon and Schuster, 1996.

Cosmetic Ingredient Review (www.cir-safety.org)

Index

For an alphabetical listing of product ingredients, see Appendix II, pages 267–306

Biographies

Lisa Petty, B.A., R.H.N., R.N.C.P., is a registered holistic nutrition consultant, health advocate and writer specializing in anti-aging and family nutrition. She is a regular contributor to *Canada's Healthy Living Guide* and *alive* magazine. Visit www.iamlivingbeauty.com for more information.

CONTRIBUTOR

Rose-Marie Swift has been a make-up artist for over 20 years, and her work has been featured in *Vogue, Harper's Bazaar, I.D., Allure, Numero, Marie Claire, Glamour, 10* and *Elle*. Her make-up has appeared in ads for Calvin Klein, Hugo Boss, Max Mara, The Gap, Victoria's Secret and others. Her portfolio includes the famous faces of Celine Dion, Jessica Lang, Giselle Bundchen, L'il Kim and Sheryl Crow among many others. Rose-Marie has also developed a line of organic make-up called *beautytruth*™, because she believes that make-up shouldn't cause problems with our health. Visit www.beautytruth.net for more information.

FOREWORD

Angela Lindvall is one of the world's most recognized supermodels. She has graced the covers of countless fashion magazines, and has appeared in ad campaigns for Chanel, Prada and Gucci and many others. She is also a wife and concerned mother. Recently, Angela founded *Collage*, a public service organization that focuses on environmental concerns. *Collage* not only brings awareness to issues including animal extinction, water pollution and environmental sustainability, but also helps to connect people, organizations and resources so that individuals can take action. Visit www.collage foundation.org for more information.